SPRINGER SERIES IN NEUROPSYCHOLOGY

Harry A. Whitaker, Series Editor

Springer Series in Neuropsychology

Harry A. Whitaker, Series Editor

Yves Joanette   Hiram H. Brownell
Editors

Discourse Ability and Brain Damage

Theoretical and Empirical Perspectives

With 17 Illustrations

Springer-Verlag
New York Berlin Heidelberg
London Paris Tokyo Hong Kong

Yves Joanette, Ph.D.
Centre de Recherche
Centre hospitalier Côte-des-Neiges
Montréal, Québec H3W 1W5
Canada

Hiram Brownell, Ph.D.
Department of Psychology
Boston College
Chestnut Hill, Massachusetts 02167
USA

Library of Congress Cataloging-in-Publication Data
Discourse ability and brain damage : theoretical and empirical
  perspectives / Yves Joanette and Hiram H. Brownell, editors.
     p.   cm. — (Springer series in neuropsychology)
  Includes index.
  1. Aphasia. 2. Brain damage—Complications and sequelae.
3. Discourse analysis. I. Joanette, Yves II. Brownell, Hiram.
III. Series.
  [DNLM: 1. Brain Damage, Chronic—complications. 2. Brain
Injuries—complications. 3. Language Disorders.
4. Neuropsychology 5. Psycholinguistics. 6. Speech Disorders.
WL 340 D6045]
RC425.D57 1989
616.85′52—dc20
DNLM/DLC   89-11430

Printed on acid-free paper.

Typeset by Publishers Service, Bozeman, Montana.
Printed and bound by Edwards Brothers, Inc., Ann Arbor, Michigan.
Printed in the United States of America.

9 8 7 6 5 4 3 2 1

ISBN 0-387-97044-4 Springer-Verlag New York Berlin Heidelberg
ISBN 3-540-97044-4 Springer-Verlag Berlin Heidelberg New York

Foreword

Nonspecialists are often surprised by the issues studied and the perspectives assumed by basic scientific researchers. Nowhere has the surprise traditionally been greater than in the field of psychology. College students anticipate that their psychology courses will illuminate their personal problems and their friends' personalities; they are nonplussed to discover that the perception of geometric forms and the running of T-mazes dominates the textbooks. The situation is comparable in the domain of linguistics. Nonprofessional observers assume that linguists study exotic languages, that when they choose to focus on their own language, they will examine the meanings of utterances and the uses to which language is put. Such onlookers are taken aback to learn that the learning of remote languages is a marginal activity for most linguists; they are equally amazed to discover that the lion's share of work in the discipline focuses on issues of syntax and phonology, which are virtually invisible to the speaker of a language.

Science moves in its own, often mysterious ways, and there are perfectly good reasons why experimental psychologists prefer to look at mazes rather than at madness, and why linguists study syntax rather than Sanskrit. Nonetheless, it is a happy event for all concerned when the interests of professionals and nonspecialists begin to move toward one another and a field of study comes to address the "big questions" as well as the experimentally most tractable ones.

Discourse Ability and Brain Damage reflects this trend in scientific research. A decade or two ago, that odd breed of researchers called psycholinguists was devoting its efforts to those topics that, however fascinating to a professional researcher, would have seemed hopelessly arcane to the layperson. During the last several years, however, researchers in psychology and language have taken as their concern problems of language that adhere much more closely to a "common sense" understanding of this domain. And so, for the first time in the modern era, one encounters serious scientific workers who are concerned with stories, jokes, conversations, figurative language—more broadly, with the domain of discourse.

Analogous trends have touched the neurosciences as well. Although never quite so exclusively fixated on the colorless building blocks of language, neuropsychologists and neurolinguists had, in past decades, ignored most of the larger topics and problems of language. Yet in conjunction with—and in some cases even ahead of—their colleagues in cognate disciplines, neuropsychologists have begun to study the fate of discourse capacities under conditions of brain damage.

What a rich harvest they have reaped! Counter to what basic teachings implied, it is the right cerebral hemisphere that seems especially predisposed to deal with linguistic communication above the level of the sentence. Aphasic patients with left (or dominant)-hemisphere damage often show surprisingly preserved abilities to deal with specimens of discourse. In contrast, right-hemisphere-damaged patients exhibit significant, and often enduring, problems in apprehending texts and, more generally, in "getting the point" of a narrative.

Going beyond this striking dissociation among linguistic functions across the two cerebral hemispheres, the authors represented in this collection inform us in many ways. I doubt that many prospective readers can already distinguish between cohesion and coherence in a text, outline forms of the mutual knowledge that speakers and hearers must share; review various representations of discourse and the operations habitually performed on them; distinguish among the levels of hierarchy involved in different kinds of mnemonic and narrative representations; describe the connections, as well as the disjunctions, between production and perception of discourse; analyze the linguistic productions that distinguish aphasics, polylinguals, Alzheimer's patients, and patients who have sustained right hemisphere disease; and anticipate the kinds of differences in discourse that might characterize individuals of different social classes or gender. And yet, readers who carefully read this book will gradually attain an expert's level of understanding of the topics at hand.

What does one look for in a collection of articles in neuropsychology? At the very least, one hopes to receive a state-of-the-art report from some of the leaders in the respective fields. If one is more fortunate, these articles will be written in a clear voice, without jargon, and will make explicit the links to past work and to work in other laboratories and research traditions. And, if one is more fortunate still, the collection will strike a proper balance among theoretical work in the area, experimental studies, and clinical applications even as the innovative research will engage in a dialogue with the informing theory.

Readers of this volume can count themselves lucky. Dr. Joanette and Dr. Brownell have included in their survey the relevant populations, the most articulated theories, and the proper methods of investigation. They have assembled a provocative set of articles, each one interesting in itself; taken together, these essays describe—indeed, define—a new area of study. As happens in an effective specimen of discourse, the whole is indeed greater than the sum of the individual chapters.

I am confident that seasoned researchers will feel edified by this compendium and that newcomers to the field will be stimulated to carry out further studies that will, in rapid course, dictate a need for a second edition.

Boston Veterans Administration Medical Center   Howard Gardner
Boston University School of Medicine
Harvard Graduate School of Education

Contents

Contributors

LEE ALLARD   The State University of New Jersey Rutgers, Center for Molecular & Behavioral Neuroscience, Newark, New Jersey 07101, USA

ROBERT J. BRACEWELL   Laboratory of Applied Cognitive Science, and Department of Educational Psychology, McGill University, Montréal, Québec H3A 1Y2, Canada

ALAIN BREULEUX   Laboratory of Applied Cognitive Science, and Department of Educational Psychology, McGill University, Montréal, Québec H3A 1Y2, Canada

HIRAM H. BROWNELL*   Department of Psychology, Boston College, Chestnut Hill, Massachusetts 02167, USA; Boston V.A. Medical Center, Boston, Massachusetts 02130, USA; Aphasia Research Center, Department of Neurology, Boston University School of Medicine, Boston, Massachusetts 02115, USA

SANDRA BOND CHAPMAN   University of Texas at Dallas, Callier Center for Communication Disorders, Dallas, Texas 75235, USA

MAUREEN DENNIS   Psychology Department, The Hospital for Sick Children, Toronto, Ontario M5G 1X8, Canada

WOLFGANG U. DRESSLER   Department of Linguistics, University of Vienna, A-1090 Vienna, Austria

CARL FREDERIKSEN   Laboratory of Applied Cognitive Science, and Department of Educational Psychology, McGill University, Montréal, Québec H3A 1Y2, Canada

HOWARD GARDNER   Boston V.A. Medical Center, Boston, Massachusetts 02130, USA; Aphasia Research Center, Department of Neurology, Boston University School of Medicine, Boston, Massachusetts 02115, USA; Project Zero, Longfellow Hall, Harvard School of Education, Cambridge, Massachusetts 02138, USA

JOAN GOLDBERGER   The Parker Jewish Geriatric Institute, New Hyde Park, New York 11042, USA

---

*Editor.

PIERRE GOULET   Laboratoire Théophile-Alajouanine, Centre de Recherche du Centre hospitalier Côte-des-Neiges, Montréal, Québec H3W 1W5, Canada; Département de psychologie, Université de Montréal, Montréal, Québec H3C 3J7, Canada

WALTER HUBER   Department of Neurology, Technical University (RWTH), D-5100 Aachen, Federal Republic of Germany

YVES JOANETTE*   Laboratoire Théophile-Alajovanine, Centre de Recherche du Centre hospitalier Côte-des-Neiges, Montréal, Québec H3W 1W5, Canada; Faculté de Médicine, Université de Montréal, Montréal, Québec H3C 3J7, Canada

MAUREEN W. LOVETT   Division of Neurology, Department of Pediatrics, The Hospital for Sick Children, Toronto, Ontario M5G 1X8, Canada

RAYMOND MOLLOY   Aphasia Research Center (116 B), Boston V.A. Medical Center, Boston, Massachusetts 02130, USA

ERNEST M. MROSS   Department of Psychology, University of Colorado at Boulder, Boulder, Colorado 80309-0345, USA

GREGORY L. MURPHY   Department of Cognitive and Linguistic Sciences, Brown University, Providence, Rhode Island 02912, USA

JEAN-LUC NESPOULOUS   Laboratoire Jacques Lordat, Section des Sciences du Langage, Université de Toulouse-Le Mirail, 31058 Toulouse Cedex, France

LORAINE OBLER   Program in Speech and Hearing Sciences, Graduate Center, City University of New York, New York, 10036-8099, USA

RICHARD PATRY   Département de linguistique et de philologie, Faculté des arts et des sciences, Université de Montréal, Montréal, Québec H3C 3J7, Canada

CSABA PLÉH, Department of Psychology, University of Budapest, H-1052 Budapest, Hungary

ANDRÉ RENAUD   Laboratory of Applied Cognitive Science, and Department of Educational Psychology, McGill University, Montréal, Québec H3A 1Y2, Canada

HELENE SABO-ABRAMSON   Department of Neurology, Cornell University Medical College, New York, New York 10021, USA

SUSAN DE SANTI   Program in Speech and Hearing Sciences, Graduate Center, City University of New York, New York 10036-8099, USA

HANNA K. ULATOWSKA   University of Texas at Dallas, Callier Center for Communication Disorders, Dallas, Texas 75235, USA

RUTH WODAK   Department of Linguistics, University of Vienna, A-1090 Vienna, Austria

*Editor.

Introduction

This book was motivated by a symposium we organized for the Twenty-Fourth Annual Meeting of the Academy of Aphasia in Nashville in October 1986. The main goal of this symposium, entitled "The Effect of Brain Damage on Discourse Ability," was to highlight the importance of studying the consequences of brain damage on connected speech, or discourse. To date, the contribution of modern neurolinguistics to our understanding of brain-language relations has been made primarily at the word or the sentence level by reference to linguistic processes such as those implicated in phonology, syntax, or lexical semantics. However, there has been a recent growth of interest in language deficits at the *suprasentential* level, a trend first apparent in the description of developmental speech and language disorders. This shift in emphasis brings us closer to what natural communication consists of: sets of sentences that, as a group, convey an idea, a story, or a mood. A full understanding of brain-language relations as well as the effects of brain damage on communication requires that research also focus on discourse-level processes and their impairment. This book will continue and expand the effort begun with the Academy of Aphasia symposium. We will illustrate in detail the nature, relevance, and importance of research in this area. In addition to the participants in the symposium (H. Gardner, P. Goulet, W. Huber, J.-L. Nespoulous, and R. Patry), several additional authors were invited to contribute chapters on the basis of their interest and contributions in this field.

The book is divided into two sections. The first provides in accessible terms a theoretical framework to analyze discourse-level deficits in brain-damaged populations. This framework spans several related fields—linguistics, pragmatics, philosophy, and cognitive psychology—and, as such, may be unfamiliar to many neuropsychologists and neurolinguists. We believe that increased contact with work in these related fields will help readers understand the issues motivating present and future research in discourse and will provide investigators with added perspective on their own research efforts.

Each chapter in the second section focuses on empirical work. This portion of the book illustrates how neurolinguistic studies currently being carried out have made use of the theoretical issues raised in the first section. Among other things, these reports illustrate how issues in discourse comprehension and production have been addressed using different impaired populations and different research styles.

One criterion we tried to use in choosing the different contributors was the potential connection between the empirical chapters and the theoretical chapters. This goal could only be partly achieved, since the full range of empirical studies suggested by the theoretical chapters has not been implemented and the empirical chapters as a group draw on a very wide range of theoretical traditions, only some of which could be included in the first section of the book. Still, the juxtaposition of theoretical and empirical treatments will illustrate how the same broad issues apply across a variety of research settings. In what follows we point out some of these connections between theoretical and empirical chapters.

Chapter 1 introduces Section I with a general introduction to the linguistic analysis of discourse. These authors show that discourse was not a popular topic among linguists before the 1970s. This dearth of interest suggests one explanation for the relative underrepresentation until recently of discourse-level analyses in neurolinguistics. This chapter relates to nearly all the other chapters of this book, whether theoretical or empirical, in that it provides the historical context needed to understand the place of each of the different theoretical and empirical approaches within the general areas of text grammar and discourse analysis.

Chapter 2 complements the linguistic discussion provided by Chapter 1 and provides an overview of the psychology of language as it applies to discourse. This chapter stresses conversation, inference, and social phenomena that affect situated discourse. Of particular interest are the concepts such as speech acts and the distinction between speaker meaning and sentence meaning, which have been borrowed from philosophy. As with the first chapter, this chapter is relevant to nearly all of the empirical chapters. For the most direct link with empirical studies, refer to Chapter 5.

Chapter 3, along with Chapter 4, reviews discourse-level representations and the processes that operate on these representations. Chapter 3 provides an accessible introduction to this highly relevant, although quite complex, branch of discourse. The focus is on the Kintsch and van Dijk model, many features of which have already been incorporated into empirical studies. Representative applications of the Kintsch and van Dijk model are described in Chapters 6 to 9.

Chapter 4, just like Chapter 3, describes a comprehensive framework for the analysis of representations and processes most relevant to discourse. The focus of this chapter is the model developed by Carl Frederiksen and his colleagues which, together with the Kintsch and van Dijk model, provides the most widely used schemes for text analysis. In addition to a summary of this major body of work, the authors suggest how their model can be applied to neuropsychological investigations of discourse ability.

Chapter 5 is the first chapter in Section II. This chapter reviews a series of studies of how damage to the right hemisphere impairs comprehension of brief narratives and of nonliteral utterances such as indirect requests and sarcasm. The authors have organized their discussion around the types of inferencing required to move beyond what is explicitly stated to achieve an understanding of a speaker's point. The discussion of these inference processes is closely tied to the work from psycholinguistics and philosophy reviewed in Chapter 2. One feature of the work described in Chapter 5 is that the processes relevant to narrative and discourse comprehension are examined apart from those needed for phonology, syntax, and lexical semantics. The primary patient population in this research consisted of stroke patients whose right-hemisphere brain damage produced communication deficits but not aphasia. Chapter 5 also discusses the state of evidence for whether discourse comprehension deficits can be localized to the right hemisphere.

Chapter 6 describes a large study of how right-hemisphere brain damage affects comprehension and retelling of an extended narrative in the form of a story. As in the research discussed in Chapter 5, the work reported in Chapter 6 separates the study of discourse from the study of aphasic deficits by assessing performance in a nonaphasic population. The theoretical basis for this work comes from the linguistic analysis of connected text at several different levels as reported in Chapter 3. Chapter 6 uses the framework provided by text analysis to provide theoretically based descriptions of stimulus material and of the selective impairments exhibited in the responses of many of the patients tested. Another important feature of this chapter is its approach to a major empirical problem, the heterogeneity of deficits within an impaired population.

Chapter 7 summarizes several studies of the discourse abilities of left-brain-damaged, aphasic patients and of right-brain-damaged, nonaphasic patients. By definition, aphasic patients exhibit marked disorders of language at the word and sentence level. One important feature of this series of studies, together with the work described in Chapter 8, is that the discourse deficits of aphasic patients are not simple extensions of their impairments at other levels of linguistic description, but require separate treatment. These analyses draw on theoretical distinctions such as outlined in Chapter 3.

Chapter 8, like Chapter 7, reviews a large body of work that complements traditional analyses of aphasic language performance at the word and sentence level. It summarizes the abilities of different types of aphasic patients and discusses how severity of impairment affects discourse performance. The analyses described in this chapter incorporate several theoretical distinctions such as that between procedural and narrative discourse and several others discussed in Chapter 3.

Chapter 9 contrasts with the others in this section in that it describes discourse deficits observed in children rather than adults. It summarizes a number of studies performed with children who had sustained brain damage due to different etiologies, including hemispherectomy. One general finding, which reinforces the importance of studying developmental populations, is that the symptoms observed in children are often quite different from what one would predict on the basis of the literature on adult populations. What this chapter shares with many of the other empirical reviews is a grounding in the work on story grammars and other linguistic analyses of discourse, such as outlined in Chapter 3.

Chapter 10 describes discourse impairments of patients with dementia of the Alzheimers type. These patients exhibit different profiles of cognitive deficits from those associated with stroke patients and thus suggest different aspects of discourse competence for study. The focus of this chapter is on bi- and multilingual speakers' use of their different languages. One question is whether impaired speakers obey the linguistically based rules governing the mixing of different languages in the same utterance: for example, whether switching from one language to another in midsentence violates word order constraints in either language. Another, more social question concerning code switching is whether speakers shape their discourse production to suit their listeners. Speakers should not, for example, switch languages when conversing with a monolingual listener.

Chapter 11, like Chapter 10, examines a social aspect of discourse performance. The specific focus is how discourse style varies as a function of gender and how these differences are affected by the presence of aphasia due to left brain damage and by aphasia therapy. This study represents a first step in using the effects of brain damage to further our understanding of the many differences and similarities between the sexes and of socialization processes in general.

The varied nature of the chapters included in this book reflects the character of current work in this area. In undertaking this project, we have emphasized a theme that cuts across this heterogeneity—the role of theory drawn from related fields. With this book we also hope to inform people working in related fields about the relevance and promise of research with impaired populations to the understanding of the functional organization of the brain for communication.

Acknowledgments. Many thanks to Colette Cerny for her invaluable contribution to the management of this enterprise. This book would not have been possible without the support of the Conseil des recherches médicales du Canada (PG-28) and of the Fonds de la recherche en santé du Québec (Y. Joanette) and of NIH grants NS 11408 and 06209 and the Research Service of the Veterans Administration (H. Brownell).

The order in which our names appear was decided on the basis of a coin toss. This was a fully collaborative effort between the two of us. We thank Colette Cerny and Cathy Desmarais for having performed this delicate operation.

YVES JOANETTE
HIRAM H. BROWNELL

Section 1
Theoretical Perspectives

1
Discourse Analysis in Linguistics: Historical and Theoretical Background

Richard Patry and Jean-Luc Nespoulous

Historical Background: Discourse and the Prevailing Approaches to Language Analysis in Linguistics

How can one explain the very late concern in linguistics' contemporary history for discourse analysis, a topic pertaining so obviously to its field of inquiry? More specifically, what made possible the nearly complete exclusion of discourse-level phenomena in linguistics before the 1970s? The explanations for this strange situation involve the prevailing conceptions of linguistic science and, consequently, the nature and scope of the issues perceived as relevant to language.

Since the 1950s, the two prevailing approaches to language have been structuralism and Chomskyan theory. Although these approaches present, respectively, many different views about language analysis (the discussion of which is beyond the scope of this chapter), they share a central feature that is largely responsible for the unfortunate state of the field of discourse analysis before the 1970s. Following the well-known distinction established by Saussure between *langue* and *parole*, both the structuralist and the Chomskyan approaches are (almost) exclusively preoccupied by phenomena pertaining to the realm of *langue*. These researchers are interested in the internal functioning of grammars seen as nearly closed systems, that is, as systems defined and discussed as largely independent of contingencies observed in everyday language use. Researchers look for regular mechanisms, processes, or rules, especially in the fields of phonology and syntax. The keywords for both these fields are: *units, positions, distributions, relations*, and *changes*. For example, in syntax, Bolinger (1952) studies word sequencing in sentences and finds that sentential adverbs show different contrastive possibilities in English according to their position in a clause.

1. Why did you *abruptly* back away?
   Why did you back away *abruptly*?

According to the author, the first sentence asks essentially "Why did you back away at all?", while the second asks "Why, having decided to back away, did you do it abruptly?" Thus, the first sentence can be contrastive, but only as a whole.

2. Why did you *abruptly back away?*
   Why didn't you courteously *accept* as I wanted you to?

On the other hand, the second sentence is contrastive in either part (back away or abruptly), depending on the location of stress assignment in one of its particular utterances.

3. Why did you *back away* abruptly when I told you to *dart forward* abruptly?
   Why did you back away *abruptly* when I said to do it *gradually?*

This sample of analysis taken from syntax illustrates the radically structural approach of language study prevailing during this period.

Quite obviously, discourse is difficult to categorize within such a framework. Perceived from such a perspective, it is, in fact, characterized by many fuzzy edges that make the possibility of its successful study seem very dubious. First, the study of discourse is closely related to the study of meaning. Second, it is a multileveled object of study. Third, it rests on contextual evidence. Fourth, it is subject to individual (speaker to speaker) variation. Finally, discourse analysis implies a beyond-the-sentence approach. This last requirement was surely the most puzzling for linguists of this period, for whom the sentence was the absolute boundary of language study. Because of all these undesirable characteristics, discourse has been thus generally dismissed as a nonlinguistic entity by a whole generation of linguists.

The Precursors to Current Approaches to Discourse: Working Against the Stream

Paradoxically, during this period when discourse was not a popular topic, important initiatives were nevertheless undertaken in discourse-level analysis. These individual efforts, scattered throughout the century, are noteworthy because they directly underlie the subsequent investigation of questions specific to discourse. This section will review briefly some of the most important of these contributions. The major features of this historical background are summarized in Table 1.1, which specifies the aera(s) in which author or theoretical movement to be reviewed contributed most directly to the emergence of present-day linguistic investigation of discourse-level processes.

Some Innovative Structuralist Approaches

Vladimir Propp was a Russian scholar especially concerned with the analysis of folktales. His major contribution, produced very early in the century (1928) is, in fact, the first contemporary attempt to build up a framework—a version of structuralism in the present case—really suited for discourse study. This "structural" framework provides systematic and exact procedures for discourse analysis and leads to important insights, particularly on two major points. Propp demonstrates structural regularities across narratives, especially in character features,

TABLE 1.1. Historical background.

Authors	Area(s) of contribution
V. Propp (structuralism)	Narrative structure analysis, models based on episodes (story grammars)
E. Benveniste (structuralism)	Discourse type study and cohesion
Prague School (functionalism)	Pragmatics and thematic progression
M.A.K. Halliday (functionalism)	Study of syntax in the perspective of systemic grammar, cohesion (later)
CH. Bally (stylistics)	A systematic account of stylistic features in (ordinary) discourse and the study of modalization
J.L. Austin	Pragmatics — speech acts

and also in types and sequencing of episodes.[1] These findings were of great relevance at the time. They demonstrated that folktales contain structural organization made up of basic "functions," as he called them. Thus, Propp's works greatly helped to overcome linguists' general reluctance to deal with discourse analysis and influenced many later thinkers, among the most prominent of whom are the French anthropologist C. Levi-Strauss and the renowned semiotician A.J. Greimas.

Benveniste (1966) contributed to the identification of more particular phenomena. Specifically, he examined discourse-level processes in very restricted areas where the linguist could count on the help of, at least, partial "grammatical support." Guided by this cautious attitude, Benveniste contributed a great deal to the analysis of two particular questions. First, on the basis of verbal tense distribution in French discourse samples, he identified two fundamental discourse types: *discours* (discourse) and *récit* (narrative). The first type is defined as being "subjective," that is, its realization implies an active participation and integration of the speaker in his own performance (e.g., opinion letters, personal diaries, or criticism). The second type, in contrast, is defined as being "objective." In this case, the speaker is not actually "included" in her linguistic performance. She reports facts and events in which she has no direct participation (e.g., storytelling or scientific writing). This fundamental distinction based on formal linguistic evidence served as a starting point for subsequent research on discourse typology, and it has, more recently, been extended, particularly in the works of Combettes (1975) and Simonin-Grumbach (1975).[2]

Benveniste's second major contribution was an original analysis of the French pronominal system. He identified a functional distinction in discourse between

---

[1] This dimension of discourse study has been further explored in the contemporary framework of story grammar. See section titled "Macrostructure and Procedural Analysis."

[2] This topic of discourse typology has also prompted interesting studies by Longacre (1983), Lundquist (1983), and Dimter (1985).

first- and second-person pronouns and those of third-person pronouns. He also observed a feature common to all three types of pronouns considered as lexical units: outside discourse, in which pronominal forms have no semantic content of their own (except for grammatical specifications), as opposed to nouns and verbs, for example, which have (at least partly) stable semantic components, either in context or considered in isolation as members of the language lexicon. Since discourse is what creates pronominal semantic reference, Benveniste closely examined this structural level in order to make this observation relative to a functional difference between pronouns in the first three grammatical persons.

Another important contribution is that of the Linguistic Circle of Prague, which was founded in 1926 by Czech, Russian, and French scholars grouped around V. Mathesius. Among the most renowned of other linguists were, for example, Nikolai Troubetzkoi, Roman Jakobson, and Karl Bühler. The Prague school constituted one of the most influential movements in linguistics during the first half of the century. One of the basic claims of the movement was to promote, in accordance with Franz Boas and Ferdinand de Saussure, a synchronic approach to language analysis as a reaction against the radical diachronic perspective of comparative linguistics. The major feature characterizing the Prague school's theoretical contribution to linguistics is "functionalism." Following this basic concept, researchers studied language structures according to their function in the linguistic system. This approach was also applied in phonology (Martinet, 1962; Jakobson, 1963), syntax (Tesniere, 1965), and the study of the lexicon (Coseriu, 1976).

Although this model has been applied to all the major fields of language analysis, we will limit our discussion here to the most relevant issue for discourse analysis. This development in functionalism is known as "functional sentence perspective." According to this approach, the content of a sentence was analyzed according to how the information was distributed in it. At one end, the neutral part of the sentence with regard to information was called the "topic," or "theme." It was considered as the starting point of the sentence, what the listener already knew, what the sentence was about. On the other hand, the more informative part was called "comment," or "rheme," and it supplied the new information unknown to the listener.[3]

4. Paul's brother / had a deck built on the back of his house.
    TOPIC   COMMENT

---

[3]The contribution of Henri Weil (1887) is often mentioned in connection with this functional sentence perspective proposed by the Prague school. Weil is associated with comparative linguistics (the only theoretical movement in linguistics at this period) and studied syntax and word order in different languages. He showed no particular concern for discourse-level questions or for the functional dimensions of language study, but discussed the latter indirectly by proposing a notion according to which "thought relations," and not only grammatical rules, are important for word order in the analysis of syntax.

This example illustrates the basic application of a notion that has been subject to many theoretical and methodological refinements over the years (Daneš, 1974; Palek, 1968; Firbas, 1966). Functional sentence perspective must not be confused with syntax or semantics. The analysis of information distribution, or "communicative dynamism," constitutes a third level in the analysis of sentences and differs strikingly from the two other levels in, at least, one important respect. The notion of information cannot be defined satisfactorily in the analysis of a particular instance of a sentence if the surrounding context is not considered; that is, the analyst cannot establish which part of the sentence will be the most informative without taking into account the knowledge already available to the listener on the matter, whereas analysis of syntax and (propositional) semantics are most generally performed without any need to refer to contextual evidence. This particular characteristic relates functional sentence perspective very closely to the realm of "communication" and consequently to discourse-level processes, for the specific study of which the framework of "thematic progression" was created. This framework integrates the basic findings of the Prague school for isolated sentences but also adds the investigation of "thematic transitions" across sentences in discourse. This approach leads to evidence of many relevant discourse-level properties and is used in recent contributions (Combettes, 1983; Clark and Haviland, 1979; van Dijk and Kintsch, 1983).

M.A.K. Halliday's contribution encompasses nearly all the major traditional areas of the discipline: syntax, phonology, semantics, and general linguistics, and also extensive work on discourse-level processes. In this section, we review briefly his early contribution in the "systemic grammar" framework, primarily oriented toward the analysis of syntax (1970). Systemic grammar, being primarily concerned with the mechanisms of selection underlying sentence production, offers an interesting perspective for the study of intersentential relationships and individual style, among others, in discourse analysis. In the following section, his recent analysis dealing directly with discourse will be discussed.

The framework of systemic grammar, proposed by Halliday during the 1960s, goes back to the notion of "system" as defined by the renowned British scholar John Firth and was also largely influenced by the functionalist perspective described in the preceding section. According to Firth, a system consists of a set of mutually exclusive options that come into play at some point in a linguistic structure. Consequently, a systemic grammar emphasizes the analysis of the various choices that one makes (consciously or unconsciously) in deciding to utter a particular sentence out of the infinite number of sentences that one's language makes available. The central component of the grammar is a chart of the full set of functions available in constructing a sentence, with a specification of the relationships existing between choices. Thus, systemic grammar offers an explanation of syntactic structure phenomena, whereas a Chomskyan description of syntax, for example, contains these options but shows no particular concern for them in the interpretation it proposes of these facts.

Ch. Bally was a colleague of Ferdinand de Saussure and contributed, in collaboration with other researchers and students, to the publication of the master's opus, *Le cours de linguistique générale*. He is also the founder of *stylistique de la langue* (stylistics of language) (1905), and his conception of the topic differs strikingly from that of scholars who follow classical rhetoric.[4] Unlike these scholars, Bally did not focus his study on literature. Instead, he proposed to investigate the subjective content expressed by speakers in everyday language. Another original feature of his study was an interest in subjective meaning expressed by word-level elements common to all language users. An interesting example of this approach is a sentence-level analysis in which he identified, in the same utterance, some parts referring to external objective facts of the world and others expressing the speaker's attitude toward these facts (1942). According to Bally, as illustrated in sentence 5, the former part of the sentence is the "dictum" and the latter the "modus." He grouped the various manifestations of these constructs under the generic label of "modalization."

5. I think / that the five o'clock train for Chicago will be late.
   MODUS   DICTUM
          X = the five o'clock train for Chicago will be late.
   I have good reasons to believe that X is true.

This example illustrates the most explicit form of modalization, that is, the modus and the dictum are expressed by different clauses ordered hierarchically. Bally studied the various forms of modalization and the corresponding syntactic patterns by which these parts are joined in sentences. This contribution to the field of stylistics has been integrated with more recent research in discourse analysis, which has lead to a basic and essential distinction between *énoncé* (statement) and *énonciation* (enunciation). This phenomenon is also of great interest in neurolinguistics. One can indeed generally observe a radical dissociation between referring (dictum) and modalizing (modus) content in the speech performances of brain-damaged subjects, the latter being often far less impaired than the former, which sometimes remains intact. The explanation of this phenomenon constitutes a challenging question for neurolinguistics and is discussed extensively in Nespoulous (1980, 1981) and Nespoulous and Lecours (1987).

The Contribution of Philosophy of Language

Educated in the tradition of Oxford, J.L. Austin, a British philosopher, was inclined to study meaning in context and, consequently, to undertake language

---

[4]The beginning of classical rhetoric goes back to the fifth century B.C. and is associated with the teachings of Empedocles in Syracuse. This movement had no scientific ambitions (at least not before the Renaissance, when it specialized progressively in the study of literature). It was a "prescriptive" approach, that is, it showed someone different ways of using language in order to communicate adequately and was oriented toward practical purposes. Despite the fact that classical rhetoric bears no direct connection with the questions currently asked in linguistics about discourse, it is a very important contribution to the broader perspective of "communication study," a field of which it was the sole investigator for nearly 2000 years.

study without dissociating it from its communicative setting. He did not confine his investigation to the exclusive question of truth values or meaning interpretation but, instead, integrated this problem into a broader one structured along three major lines: (1) the study of semantic content in utterances, (2) the study of the relationships between the utterance and the speaker, and (3) the communicative effect of utterances according to combinations of different values for the two preceding categories. The process resulted in a taxonomy of "illocutory forces" (1962).

6. I'm going down to my office to write this tedious report.

This sentence, for example, expresses a sequence of actions that a particular unknown speaker intends to perform in what seems to be a not too distant future. This kind of descriptive utterance has no particular communicative effect and is evaluated by Austin as having locutory force, that is, a basic informative function with regard to the addressee.

7. I promise you that I will be home for five o'clock.

In comparison with the preceding utterance, Sentence 7 exhibits many distinctive properties. According to Austin, such utterances do not only express an intended action, but are actions by themselves. In other words, when a speaker produces a similar utterance, he performs an action at the same time, hence the label "performatives" that Austin gave to these speech acts. Second, this relation between the utterance and the speaker is stronger or tighter in performatives, because by these utterances, the speaker takes on himself the responsibility of performing an action through language use. As a consequence of the preceding point, these utterances are thirdly characterized by a stronger communicative effect (illocutionary force) on the addressee and, finally, the semantic analysis of performatives cannot be realized adequately without taking into account elements from the surrounding context. Austin's work has been an inspiration to his contemporaries, and his most renowned follower is certainly J. Searle (1969). With regard to the specific area of discourse analysis, Austin's contribution directly underlies the recent developments in pragmatics.

The Emergence of Discourse as a Field of Inquiry

Around 1970, structuralism was losing momentum while the Chomskyan approach to language, already accepted as a more interesting framework, was gaining more and more influence. This prevalence of the Chomskyan approach must be stressed with regard to what followed, because a general body of criticism directed against the Chomskyan model's limitations led to the first contemporary theoretical attempt to investigate discourse-level phenomena in linguistics: text-grammar.

Text-Grammar

This movement, which originated primarily in Germany (Kummer, 1972; Kiefer, 1977), studied connected sentences guided (at least in the beginning) by an extended version of generative grammar, which was originally designed for sentence analysis. The basic Chomskyan rule for the analysis of sentences was then

8. $S = NP + VP$

in which S represents sentence, NP is nominal phrase, and VP is verbal phrase. Text-grammarians proposed to reformulate this rule as follows:

9. $S = S + S \ldots (n)$

in which the possibility of recursive repetitions of the sentence is represented by the last part of the formula. From this new starting point, generative grammar could describe not only sentences in isolation but also strings of sentences belonging to the whole of a discourse production. This approach proved very interesting for the study of some sentence-level phenomena that were difficult to explain without the help of the surrounding linguistic context. Examples of such phenomena include anaphoric pronouns, sentential adverbs, sentential stress assignment, and ambiguous structures.

The initial statement of text-grammar analysis was, however, rapidly challenged by the innovative contribution of van Dijk (1972). This contribution contained many stimulating reflections, but the most important, that which is still considered today as one of the major turning points in the recent history of discourse analysis, is the distinction the author proposed between micro and macrostructures.[5] van Dijk argued that text-grammar, as initially conceived, based its analysis on surface-level material constituting discourse and that a step-by-step analysis of contiguous sentences (microstructure) could not adequately explain the true nature of discourse. At a higher level, discourse constitutes a whole, a communicative unit and, according to van Dijk, its realization by discrete and successive linguistic material should be governed by an underlying plan[6] that directly influences the selection of particular options within the body of discourse, for example, lexical units and verb tenses. van Dijk stated that to provide an adequate framework for discourse study, text-grammar must also take this macrostructural level into account. van Dijk's proposal influenced subsequent research in text-grammar (e.g., Petöfi, 1975; Petöfi and Rieser, 1973) as well as in other areas of discourse analysis.

However, this proposal, together with other efforts to bring the text-grammar approach closer to topics central to discourse, was not enough to insure text-grammar's longevity. As linguistics formulated new questions about discourse, text-grammar became less and less attractive for three major reasons. First, the explanatory power of text-grammar was limited by an inherent contradiction; this

---

[5]See Chapter 3 for a more detailed presentation of this concept.

[6]Further developments in this area are presented in the section titled Macrostructure and Procedural Analysis.

approach aimed eventually to explain discourse-level processes but was built on a theoretical construct designed for sentence analysis. Second, text-grammar was never really concerned with dynamic aspects of discourse production and comprehension, which are at the heart of recent psycholinguistic research on discourse. Finally, inspired by formal logic in the analysis of semantics, text-grammar progressively developed a heavy and daunting formalism that was not easily accessible and not always justified.

In hindsight, it can be said that text linguistics tried to apply formal apparatuses too early, perhaps because in general the role of formalization in theory construction was grossly overrated. Also, everybody tried to use formalism without reconsidering whether this was really appropriate. (Rieser, 1978, p. 15)

The Development of Questions Specifically Related to Discourse

During the same period and using essentially the same linguistic evidence, other researchers, who cannot be grouped under a common heading, followed a radically different approach. Influenced by work on text-grammar and the contributions of their predecessors, these scholars developed an approach that was completely independent of generative grammar and, to some extent, contrary to its aims. They directed their efforts toward the establishment of a linguistics of communication in which language would be conceived as something dynamic and consequently analyzed with regard to users and social settings.

A synthesis of the questions progressively worked out in order to identify relevant fields of interest in this innovative linguistic approach to discourse study is presented in Table 1.2. The rest of this chapter presents a discussion of these topics.

TABLE 1.2. Discourse-level questioning and domains.

Fundamental questions	
1. What are the characteristics constantly observed in successful (communicative) discourse?	
Questions	Corresponding fields
2. Do some linguistic markers (of the lexical level) contribute directly and systematically to the semantic continuity of discourse?	Cohesion
3. Do some aspects of semantic continuity in discourse exist that are not directly realized by linguistic elements of word level?	Coherence
4. What is the semantic structure and organization of linguistic material underlying discourse production and comprehension?	Macrostructure
5. What exactly are the cognitive processes at work during discourse production or comprehension and how do they interact?	Procedural analysis
6. Is it possible to identify reasonably plausible relations between linguistic content and the contextual setting of discourse?	Pragmatics
7. What are the characteristics of linguistic communicative acts involving at least two participants at the same time?	Conversational analysis

TABLE 1.3. Fundamental properties of discourse.

Remote	Intermediate	Surface
Unity	Coherence	Cohesion
Intentionality		
Appropriateness		
Topicality		
Informativeness		

Fundamental Characteristics

The study of fundamental characteristics of discourse was primarily governed by two major arguments derived from observation. First, adequate and communicative discourse differs formally from an unrelated collection of sentences. Second, native speakers of a given language, regardless of their education or language skills, can spontaneously distinguish between the extremes of coherent and incoherent passages. Thus, researchers in the field of discourse assumed that if it can be recognized so easily, discourse must have specific properties, distinctive features of its own. These characteristics were assumed to override discourse types or individual style of speech and to be invariant markers of meaningful and successful communication.

Influenced by structuralism, linguists tried to identify these properties at the sentence level. Since the common denominator of every adequate discourse is that it is realized using linguistic material, they looked for correlations between linguistic and communicative levels: how does discrete linguistic material contribute to the communicative act as a whole (a question often referred to in the literature as the study of the relation between discourse and grammar). This question is of great interest and remains a central topic in discourse analysis, but investigation showed that discrete linguistic features identified as necessary are not sufficient to insure the adequacy of discourse performance. Also, most of the fundamental properties defined up to now are remote from the surface structure of discourse, and their precise linguistic content is difficult (or even impossible) to ascertain. The most commonly accepted of these fundamental properties of discourse are given in Table 1.3 and have been established on the basis of work by Charolles (1978), Nevert et al. (1980), De Beaugrande and Dressler (1981), and Patry (1986).

Surface and intermediate properties, respectively, represent cases in which the underlying semantic structure of discourse is directly realized (1) by word-level elements, and (2) by means that are less systematically accounted for by word-level components. Their respective characteristic properties, "cohesion" and "coherence" will be discussed at length in the following sections.

Remote properties with regard to the surface structure of discourse represent the major characteristics observed in adequate language performances. The property of "unity" embodies the observation that, at a communicative level, adequate discourse is perceived as a whole and not as simply a collection of sentences. "Intentionality" specifies that it must contain a *message*; that is, communication must have a transparent purpose for the addressee. Discourse must also be performed in accordance with the communicative setting, at an appropriate register (not too formal and not too colloquial), and taking into account the addressee's knowledge of the topic. These requirements are those of "appropriateness." The last two properties are implications or specifications of intentionality. In addition to conveying a clear communicative intent as a general requirement, "topicality" adds the need for discourse to bear on an identifiable topic, and "informativeness" goes further by requiring that discourse contain a reasonable amount of information, excluding sequences of tautologic repetitions as noncommunicative performances.

These features are unquestionably relevant and necessary components in an attempt to characterize the fundamental properties of discourse. However, they are remote from the surface structure and consequently very difficult to associate with any particular linguistic material in a discourse. This gap between the linguistic content of discourse performance and fundamental properties implies that the latter are not readily amenable to empirical investigation, in spite of numerous efforts in that direction during recent years. This state of affairs is one of the most important limitations on the evolution of discourse analysis as a scientific domain. It underlies to some extent nearly all the important questions raised by recent research and is the keystone of developments in the different areas of the field, which are different ways of trying to bridge the gap, as we will see in the following sections.

Coherence and Cohesion

Macro-continuity of discourse is achieved by coherence. This analysis points to semantic relations not directly realized by word-level entities and represents the content of a discourse as the expression of facts and events according to two major approaches. The first looks for the occurrence of logical relations, an important means by which *texture* is created in discourse without the systematic support of word-level units.

10. The piece of evidence you produced for the trial doesn't look like a social diary. Most of the engagements are in the evening but quite a lot of them are eleven in the morning and three thirty in the afternoon, and that sort of time.

The second sentence of this pair is the "cause" of the first. In this piece of language, the *consequence* is expressed first: "the fact that the diary is not a suitable piece of evidence for a trial" and is followed by the *cause*: "the engagements it contains are not scheduled at appropriate hours of the day." This kind of logical relation between sentences is not expressed by any particular words but is a relation occurring between the facts expressed by the two sentences.[7] They constitute

---

[7]These logical relations can also be expressed in discourse by connectors such as because, thus, or while.

a major contribution to discourse texture, an addressee who, for some reason, cannot establish these logical relations adequately will hardly be able to identify what the communication is about.

Second, these relations are also studied in terms of the degree of "explicitness" linking together different facts. "Overt coherence" occurs when the type of logical link between some facts can be established directly from the propositional content of utterances, whereas "covert coherence" describes a link involving inferences. These two types of coherence relations are illustrated in sentence 11.

11. Lost in the forest, we finally came to a hunter's shack.
    OVERT COHERENCE
    Happily, there was someone in to help us find our way back.
    COVERT COHERENCE
    Happily, white smoke came out of the chimney.

        .

        .

        .

        INFERENCES
        (a) There is someone in the hunter's shack or nearby.
        (b) Being lost, we can ask this person our way back.

Discourse-level phenomena based more narrowly on information explicitly coded in the surface structure of speech performance show cohesion. According to Halliday and Hasan (1976), it consists of semantic ties between word-level entities across sentence boundaries, that is, continuity is provided by relations between referents and notions in discourse. As a general formula, cohesion occurs when the interpretation of a word depends on the semantic content of another one in the flow of discourse. More specifically, two different types of cohesive device are unanimously recognized in studies of this topic (Gutwinski, 1976; Ola-Östman, 1978; Patry, 1986).

The first one is grammatical and includes referring elements of closed lexical sets such as, for example, personal, possessive, or demonstrative pronouns and conjunctions. Grammatical cohesion is illustrated in the following pair of sentences in which the pronoun *it* in the second sentence is related by a semantic tie (identity of reference) to the phrase *the story* in the first utterance.

12. The story is becoming more complicated, dear friend.
    It began by the diatribes of some overcurious wayfarers and now an entirely different trail emerges.

The second type of cohesive device is lexical and refers to the semantic relations created by open lexical classes, that is, nouns, verbs, and adjectives, and realized in discourse by word repetition, synonymy, or antonymy, for example. In the following illustration, the phrase *the man* of the second sentence is coreferential with *the inspector* of the first utterance. This identity of reference between two different lexical forms is possible in discourse because both items stand in relation of "hyponymy": that is, the cohesive occurrence (*the man*) is the lexical head of a paradigm that includes *the inspector*. The major difference between them is that *the man* is semantically less specific and can act as a coreferent of more specific lexical items of the same paradigm in discourse.

13. What Charles told *the inspector* was quite confused.
    It really seemed that he had drawn *the man* down there only to lure him away from the garden.

As lexical cohesion is based on the least determined elements in the lexicon, it is far more difficult to analyze than grammatical cohesion, both for purposes of determining the description of this process and for explaining its occurrence in the dynamic analysis of a specific speech production.[8]

Coherence and cohesion share many common features. They are both fundamental to semantic, interpropositional relations, which themselves are crucial to discourse adequacy. These two aspects of discourse, now distinguished in the literature, initially were both treated as one domain—coherence, as discussed by Bellert (1970) and Charolles (1978). As explained previously, the main difference between coherence and cohesion is that the latter is concerned with word-level semantic relations while the former studies higher-discourse processes not always realized by linguistic material. The linguistic aspect of coherence, so to speak, was first brought in a systematic and very convincing account by Halliday and Hasan (1976) and, since then, the boundaries of both these areas have become clearer to linguists even if some marginal conflicting data remain.

Cohesion is the step-by-step construction of discourse continuity based on the sequential enunciation of propositional frames. Coherence, as defined in recent contributions such as those of Charolles (1983) and van Dijk and Kintsch (1983), is a general principle governing the interpretation of human actions. Its scope is very broad, and its relevance to discourse analysis represents only one among a wide range of applications. Coherence is not especially concerned with language but primarily with the analysis of strings of facts and events, whatever the medium by which they are expressed. In discourse analysis, this perspective accounts for many phenomena, independent of linguistic knowledge, that contribute to discourse understanding. This type of evidence is often called "everyday knowledge," or "world knowledge" in the literature.

Thus, coherence and cohesion are now two distinct aspects of discourse whose existence and separate status are thoroughly justified. However, they also show a subtle interplay in discourse, and there are some cases in which both linguistic and nonlinguistic knowledge are involved at the same time.

14. You see, *Lucy*, they are going off from Paddington, said Shirley. Piles and piles of luggage. I don't call that a holiday. Nor do I, said *the yes-girl*.

In this example, the use of a definite article and the topic position of the phrase *the yes-girl* are clear linguistic indications of coreference with *Lucy*. In addition

---

[8]For an extensive discussion of this topic, see Patry and Menard (1985) and Patry (1986).

to this source of knowledge, the addressee must however resort to extralinguistic knowledge if she wishes to establish why precisely *Lucy* is called a *yes-girl*!

Macrostructure and Procedural Analysis

Linguistic analysis of discourse must extend beyond defining the characteristics of speech performances. Producing or understanding discourse requires, first, an underlying semantic plan, in the same way as, for example, a syntactic deep structure is postulated for sentences. Second, it also requires a mixture of linguistic and nonlinguistic knowledge, since both are simultaneously involved in discourse production and comprehension. Finally, to give a complete account of these dynamic processes, one must specify the roles of supporting cognitive abilities (memory, planning, attention). The first aim is the major concern of macrostructure, while the second and the third are those of procedural analysis.[9]

The proposal that a semantic plan underlies discourse has received much attention in linguistics during the last decade. This area of discourse analysis began with the general study of macrostructure, but rapidly developed in three major specialized areas: narrative, macrostructure, scripts, and scenarios and, finally, story-grammars.[10]

An adequate narrative contains a certain amount of structure and organization, as just discussed. Moreover, the linguistic content of discourse generally includes some passages of various length (phrases, clauses, or sentences) that have an important function for higher-level processes in discourse understanding. According to the literature (Kintsch, 1975 and 1976; van Dijk, 1979; Glenberg et al., 1987), these passages may have four major functions in discourse.

The linguistic material referred to in Table 1.4 has a macrostructural status in discourse. It coincides with or reveals some aspects of discursive semantic structure. It is also an important guide for the listener in that it facilitates the integration of information and the building up of a unified representation of discourse. The relevance of these macrostructural passages for discourse comprehension has been confirmed by much experimental research as, for example, in Kieras (1978), Vipond (1980), and Guindon and Kintsch (1984).

---

[9]Macrostructure and procedural analysis are made up of two very different levels of investigation closely entwined in most discussions of these topics. First, they involve what we may call "procedural models" as those presented in Tables 1.4 and 1.5 that express a reflection by which researchers try to identify the components of verbal operations and their internal organization. Second, these schemas are often accompanied by comments pertaining to the analysis of psycholinguistic processes, a very different matter more closely related to the performance of an actual speaker than to the analysis of an abstract verbal production. Thus, *the reader must* distinguish carefully these levels of argumentation in the literature.

[10]For a discussion of scripts and scenarios, see especially Schank and Abelson (1977) and Abelson (1981) and for a presentation of story-grammar's framework, see Mandler and Johnson (1977).

TABLE 1.4. Macrostructure.

Summarizing:	By its specific content and location, the passage recapitulates a whole development.
Anticipating:	This represents the reverse of the preceding. In this case, the passage precedes the development and facilitates its integration.
Explaining:	The content of the passage explains the full meaning of a preceding development.
Topic orientation:	A passage indicates a change or a particular orientation for the following development.

Discourse is not only an abstract construct or a static performance confined to paper or tape and available on request to the linguist. There is also a sense in which a discourse constitutes a particular event in the life of a single individual at a certain point of time.

Discourse is studied in this perspective by procedural analysis, a field of research that has expanded rapidly during recent years and for which an adequate review would require a complete study. This topic raises several new questions.

According to de Beaugrande and Dressler (1981), on-line discourse production is an "actual system" made of options selected in a "virtual system." What procedural analysis asks is how these choices are made and how they are harmonized in a unified communicative structure. This is a difficult question. Since descriptive syntactic frameworks already at hand, such as Chomskyan generative grammar (Chomsky, 1982) or the lexical-functional grammar of Kaplan and Bresnan (1982), are not at all suited to this type of investigation, new models for language analysis must be built.

Another dimension of this perspective is the identification of the principal steps according to which discourse is produced or understood. de Beaugrande and Dressler (1981) have proposed the following divisions (see Table 1.5).

Table 1.5 contains two major subdivisions demarcated by a dashed line. The upper part specifies procedural steps in which language is not involved and,

TABLE 1.5. Procedural analysis.

Planning
    Pursuing a goal through text
Ideation
    Providing control centers for productive, meaningful behavior
Development
    Expanding, specifying, elaborating ideas obtained and
    searching stored knowledge spaces

- -

Expression
    Searching for natural language expression
Parsing
    Putting the expression into grammatical dependencies

roughly speaking, it deals with the formation and conceptual planning of the communicative act. The lower part is directly concerned with the linguistic content of discourse. This table and its subdivisions suggest an interplay among three main components: language, world knowledge, and cognitive abilities. The explanation of their synergic action and of their relationships is certainly one of the most challenging questions facing contemporary discourse analysis.

Table 1.5 also raises the question of the sequencing of these operations in on-line discourse performance. Does the speaker execute them serially? According to the literature (Winograd, 1975; Walker, 1978; Brady and Berwick, 1983), the nature of these operations is "interactive" rather than "modular", that is, they would be activated all at the same time from the beginning of the process, with quick shifts of emphasis throughout the procedure according to the specific needs of definite operations.

Finally, one of the most central questions raised by the on-line study[11] of discourse is that of the relationships between production and comprehension of discourse. A simple and straightforward hypothesis would be that these processes are the reverse of one another, that is, production would be the top-down direction and comprehension the bottom-up one according to Table 1.5. But two fundamental observations undermine this simple view. First, discourse production obviously implies bottom-up processes, which are especially perceptible in self-repair, corrections, and modalizing comments on the speaker's own performance (e.g., "Oh, excuse me, I didn't mean that!"). And, on the other hand, it is now well known that discourse comprehension is not only a receptive and passive process, that the addressee—while "understanding"—formulates (top-down) hypotheses and expectations with regard to the further development of what has already been said. Thus, discourse production and comprehension are thought to be fairly different processes (even if they certainly share fundamental properties) and are currently examined separately in most recent procedural studies.

Pragmatics and Conversational Analysis

Communication is based not only on language but also on a social interaction between individuals. This particular aspect of discourse has other requirements besides formal adequacy. For example, a piece of discourse addressed to a listener must contain a reasonable amount of information (enough at least to justify the communicative act); it must be formulated in accordance with the type of social relation the speaker has with the listener (e.g., friend, office colleague, or superior); the content of the communicative act must exhibit a sufficient degree of explicitness; and, finally, the information transmitted by a discourse must be in accordance with the knowledge already available to the addressee about the topic at hand. These requirements are very difficult to handle satisfactorily in approaches concerned with formal language properties. They are nonetheless

---

[11]For further exploration of these psycholinguistic processes, see especially Marslen-Wilson and Tyler (1980).

TABLE 1.6. Conversational analysis.

Opening section
Identification, purpose
First topic slot
Introduce subject matter
Topic shift (1 _____ N)
Change subject matter
Preclosing section
Agreement to stop the exchange
Closing section
Final turn pass

extremely important for a complete analysis of discourse characteristics and are studied in the field of pragmatics.

The definition of the scope of contemporary pragmatics goes back to the work of Charles Morris (1938). Morris distinguished three fundamental areas for language study: syntax, semantics, and pragmatics, the last being defined as the study of the relations between "signs" and "users." This orientation defined pragmatics as a linguistic field different from syntax and semantics and contributed to the further elaboration of well-articulated questions and convincing analyses, such as those of Austin (1962), Grice (1975), and Goffman (1976).[12]

One of the most interesting contexts in which to see pragmatics at work is the analysis of conversation to which we will now turn for the rest of this development.

Conversation is another topic that linguists neglected for a long time. The first contemporary studies in this field were carried out in ethnomethodology (Hymes, 1962; Ervin-Tripp, 1972; Garfinkel, 1972; Turner, 1974) and proved that conversation was a valuable scientific object of study. They demonstrated, in particular, that conversation was characterized by a reasonable amount of structure and organization. On the specific question of "turn-taking," Ervin-Tripp (1979) showed that as a general rule, one can identify a proportion of about 5 percent of a given conversation during which participants speak at the same time. This small overlap observed in turn-taking suggests, at a basic level, that conversation is not a random process and that is must certainly be characterized by rules or conventions. The efforts of the last decade in this field were directed toward the identification of this supposed structure and gave fruitful results. Following recent literature (Goodwin, 1981; Planalp and Tracy, 1980; Tracy, 1982), we propose the following general formalization of conversational structure (see Table 1.6).

In the opening section, participants express their will to communicate (by salutations or identification of one of them in the context of a phone call). This is also the step during which one of the participants generally takes the initiative to give

---

[12]See Chapter 2 for a discussion of similar notions in a psycholinguistic context.

an orientation or a purpose to the verbal exchange. She proposes, in fact, the first topic to be discussed, one that will be developed in the second section. These first two steps are crucial for the success of communication, and the participant who takes the lead must be careful to make both the orientation and the first topic of the conversation perfectly explicit.

Topic shift is the most important and complex process involved in conversational analysis. It occurs when one of the participants (not necessarily the one who took the lead in the first two steps) wants to introduce another topic and abandon the discussion of the one already at hand. This operation will be properly realized inasmuch as the four basic following requirements are satisfied: the participant who wishes to undertake a topic shift in conversation must (1) inform the other participant(s) of a desire to abandon the discussion of the topic at hand, (2) receive the agreement of the other participant(s) to do so, (3) introduce the new topic for discussion, and (4) establish the relevance or the absence of relevance of this topic to the preceding one(s). The omission of one of these procedures may mislead the other participant(s) with regard to the speaker's intentions and jeopardize communication, as observed by Vuchinich (1977).

The last two steps of Table 1.6 concern the termination of a conversation. In the preclosing section, the participants agree by a series of appropriate exchanges that they want to abandon the discussion of the current topic and that they do not want to introduce a new one. Finally, they proceed with the final turn pass, which generally consists of salutations, greetings, or commitment to further exchanges.

This rather schematic survey has shown enough of conversational structure to establish its relevance to the study of pragmatics. All the steps involved in conversation require close attention of each participant to the other(s) in order to give and receive information; moreover, this information is not always expressed through verbal channels alone, but also by mimicry, gestures, eye movements, or posture, for example. Thus, conversation is certainly the linguistic context in which the relation between signs and users finds its fullest extension.

Discourse Analysis and Neurolinguistics

In this chapter, we have presented the particular questioning raised in linguistics by discourse-level study. We have also established why the prevailing approaches to language initially put a brake on the development of this questioning and afterward how they have influenced its evolution. Finally, we have presented the process by which this questioning has been progressively transformed into several areas of study, which we briefly reviewed in turn. This review showed clearly that discourse analysis is an expanding research domain and that the models proposed in its different areas have not yet reached an advanced stage of formalization, as can be seen in syntax and phonology, for example. However, in spite of the obvious deficiencies that should be filled, this approach provides a framework rigorous enough for an adequate investigation of completely unexplored linguistic phenomenon to date.

The innovative perspective of this approach in language study gave rise to a deep interest in neurolinguistics, a field in which discourse-level studies are more and more numerous as the years go by. Discourse-level study raises, in fact, original and fascinating questions in the analysis of brain-damaged speech performance and stimulated the development of new research directions in neurolinguistics during the last decade. The final development of this chapter proposes a summarized account of three important new research directions prompted by discourse-level study in neurolinguistics.

Brain-Damaged Subjects and Communication

Linguistic discrete tasks submitted to brain-damaged subjects give us some information about the subject's "linguistic knowledge." These tasks serve, for example, to determine the subject's ability to name different objects, to assess the production or comprehension of complex syntactic material, or to evaluate the subject's phonological ability by using words of various compositions with regard to sound arrangement, frequency, and length.

This kind of information is undoubtfully very useful in clinical as well as research activities. However, for the brain-damaged individual as for the normal individual, language use is not an exhibition of linguistic competence but a behavior primarily oriented toward communication. In normal conditions, the ordinary use of language in natural settings has as a major goal to make contact with other individuals.

This important perspective of language use must be taken into account in the linguistic assessment of brain-damaged subjects (Holland, 1978; Hutchinson and Jensen, 1980; Feyereisen and Al, 1988), all the more so since "communicative competence" is not a straightforward consequence of linguistic competence: a brain-damaged subject with minor problems at language levels is not necessarily a better communicator than someone who has more important language difficulties. Communication ability is obviously based on an adequate formulation of propositional material, but moreover includes the appraisal of particular features such as motivational factors, strategic use of strong points in linguistic competence, attitude toward social intercourse, and knowledge of interactional conventions. These aspects of communicative competence must be analyzed very cautiously, because they show a great deal of variation from subject to subject (normal or brain damaged) and give rise to a wide range of individual "discursive styles" in which it is often difficult to make a clear distinction between normal individual features and abnormal behavior. These aspects of communicative competence can be best dealt with by resorting to conversational analysis and pragmatics.

In this book, communicative competence will be the topic of a detailed discussion in Chapter 2, and it will be more or less directly developed in every chapter of the empirical section.

Brain-Damaged Subjects and Types of Discourse Problems

Since discourse is a multileveled object of study, its production or comprehension implies the simultaneous activation of various components: phonology, lexicon, syntax, the elaboration of macrostructure, the establishment of cohesion and coherence links, and so on. In this perspective, the identification of "deviance(s)" in a speech performance is only the first step of a complex analysis at the end of which it will be necessary to determine precisely the specific features of the observed problem(s) in discourse.[13] Four major different explanations can be proposed to characterize the problems observed in discourse.

First, an observed deviance can be caused by the transposition in discourse of propositional-level problems such as, for example, anomia, semantic or phonemic paraphasias, and different problems at syntax level (Patry, 1988). Second, it can be caused by discourse-level problems in establishing "local coherence" links, as defined by van Dijk and Kintsch (1983): that is, difficulties with the management of coherence or cohesion relations between adjacent propositions (Huber and Gleber, 1982; Lesser, 1986; Ripich and Terrell, 1988). Third, deviance in discourse can be explained by "global coherence" problems in macrostructure's elaboration, planning, or maintenance (Engel-Ortlieb, 1981; Remacle and Francois, 1986; Liles, 1987). Finally, discourse can be characterized by "pragmatic" deviance, being adequate in every linguistic and discourse-level respect, but irrelevant with regard to the situation in which it takes place (Nespoulous, 1980; Sandson et al., 1986). The first and the last categories are of particular concern for the study of discourse production, whereas the second and the third are of equal interest to the analysis of discourse production or comprehension.

All the domains of discourse analysis are obviously concerned by this challenging research direction, and they all try in the area of their specific questioning to go deeper into the characterization of discourse "abnormality." However, these questions are of great complexity, and a complete understanding of their content and implications requires both important theoretical advances and empirical work.

Brain-Damaged Subjects and Discourse-Level Problems Interpretation

A problem in one of the aspects of linguistic competence is generally interpreted as a difficulty in the mastery (in production or comprehension) of a language structuration level's grammar. But what is the signification of discourse-level

---

[13]In the final development of this chapter, we deliberately avoid the use of the term "impairment." This term is generally used in neurolinguistics to refer to very specific and definite deficits in different areas of linguistic competence. Problems encountered in discourse being more "holistic" and less amenable to extensive definition (in the actual state of the field), we prefer to qualify them by the term "deviance."

problems? The question under examination in this development is of great topical interest in recent neurolinguistic contributions and concern the nature of the underlying deficit, which is manifested by abnormalities observed in discourse performance.

As discourse production and comprehension depend partly on the synergic activation of linguistic competence components, its abnormality can be of informative value with regard to the functioning of these components, as was indicated in the first category identified in the preceding development. This relationship between discourse and linguistic competence is unquestionable, but it is only indirect for two principal reasons.

1. Because this relationship is not "necessary" (i.e., some problem in linguistic competence does not systematically make discourse deviant). However, the converging effect of more than one linguistic deficit affects discourse adequacy to various extents on a very broad scale of which it is actually impossible to propose a theoretically governed account.
2. As presented in the two last categories of the preceding development, there are discourse deviances in the definition of which formal linguistic features have no place at all. Thus, what kind of problem does discourse deviance reveal if language problems account only for a restricted set of data?

An hypothesis insistently proposed during the last years in neurolinguistic contributions consists in the interpretation of discourse deviance as a manifestation of underlying deficits in the functioning of cognitive abilities as memory, attention, and planning (Joanette et al., 1986; Brownell et al., 1983; Lovett et al., 1986). It is in fact reasonable to conceive, for example, that a memory problem in brain damage can be of consequence for referential continuity or macrostructure elaboration, and that an attentional deficit can cause breaks and inappropriate topic shifts in conversation.

However, the investigation of this hypothesis is far from simple because the two types of processes involved in this questioning are extremely complex on their own, and that the building of a conceptual bridge between them raises additional difficulties for the investigation of which important theoretical and methodological advances are needed.

The questioning of this research direction is discussed to various extents in nearly all the chapters of this book.

This presentation of the major domains of discourse analysis and of the most topical research orientations in neurolinguistics provides a synthesis of a new and expanding development of contemporary linguistic research. The actual state of the art and the future advances of this new perspective in language analysis will bring about a better understanding of what makes possible and what hinders human communication.

References

Abelson, R. (1981). Psychological status of the script concept. *American Psychologist, 7*, 715–729.

Austin, J.L. (1962). *How to do things with words*. Oxford: Oxford University Press.

Bally, CH. (1905). *Traité de stylistique francaise*. Paris: Klincksieck.

Bally, CH. (1942). Syntaxe de la modalité explicite. *Cahiers Ferdinand de Saussure, 2,* 3–13.

Bellert, I. (1970). On a condition of the coherence of texts. *Semiotica, 4,* 335–363.

Benveniste, E. (1966). *Problèmes de linguistique générale*. Paris: Gallimard.

Bolinger, D. (1952). Linear modification. *Publications of the Modern Language Association of America, Vol. 67* (pp. 1117–1144).

Brady, M., & Berwick, R. (1983). *Computational models of discourse*. Cambridge, Mass.: MIT Press.

Brownell, H., Michel, D., Powelson, J., & Gardner, H. (1983). Surprise but not coherence: Sensitivity to verbal humor in right hemisphere patients. *Brain and Language, 18,* 20–27.

Charolles, M. (1978). Introduction aux problèmes de la cohérence des textes. *Langue Francaise, 38,* 7–41.

Charolles, M. (1983). Coherence as a principle in the interpretation of discourse. *Text, 3,* 71–97.

Chomsky, N. (1982). *Some concepts and consequences of the theory of government and binding*. Cambridge, (Mass.): MIT Press.

Clark, H.H., & Haviland, S.E. (1979). Comprehension and the given-new contract. In R.O. Freedle (Ed.), *New directions in discourse processing*. Norwood, N.J.: Ablex.

Combettes, B. (1975). *Pour une grammaire textuelle*. Nancy: CRDP.

Combettes, B. (1983). *Pour une grammaire textuelle: La progression thématique*. Paris: Duculot; Bruxelles: A. De Beock.

Coseriu, E. (1976). L'étude fonctionnelle du vocabulaire: Précis de lexématique. *Les Cahiers de Lexicologie, XXIX,* 5–23.

Daneš, F. (Ed.) (1974). *Papers on functional sentence perspective*. The Hague: Mouton.

de Beaugrande, R., & Dressler, W. (1981). *Introduction to textlinguistics*. New York: Longman.

Dimter, M. (1985). On Text classification. In T.A. van Dijk (Ed.), *Discourse and literature*. Amsterdam: John Benjamins.

Engel-Ortlieb, D. (1981). Discourse processing in aphasics, *Text, 4,* 361–383.

Ervin-Tripp, S. (1972). On sociolinguistic rules: Alternation and co-occurrence. In J.J. Gumperz & D. Hymes (Eds.), *Directions in sociolinguistics: The ethnography of communication*. New York: Holt, Rinehart and Winston.

Ervin-Tripp, S. (1979). Children's verbal turn taking. In E. Och & B. Schieffelin (Eds.), *Developmental pragmatics*. New York: Academic Press.

Feyereisen, P., Barter, D., Goosens, M., & Clarebaut, N. (1988). Gestures and speech in referential communication by aphasic subjects: Channel use and efficiency. *Aphasiology, 2,* 21–33.

Firbas, J. (1966). On defining the theme in functional sentence analysis. *Travaux linguistiques de Prague, 2,* 267–280.

Garfinkel, H. (1972). Remarks on ethnomethodology. In J.J. Gumperz & D. Hymes (Eds.), *Directions in sociolinguistics*. New York: Holt, Rinehart and Winston.

Glenberg, A., Meyer, M., & Lindem, K. (1987). Mental models contribute to foregrounding during text comprehension. *Journal of Memory and Language, 26,* 69–83.

Goffman, E. (1976). Replies and responses. *Language in Society, 5,* 257–313.

Goodwin, C. (1981). *Conversational organization: Interaction between speakers and hearers*. New York: Academic Press.

Grice, H.P. (1975). Logic and conversation. In P. Cole & J.L. Morgan (Eds.), *Syntax and semantics 3: Speech acts*. New York: Academic Press.

Guindon, R., & Kintsch, W. (1984). Priming macropropositions: Evidence for the primacy of macropropositions in the memory for text. *Journal of Verbal Learning and Verbal Behavior, 23,* 508–519.

Gutwinski, W. (1976). *Cohesion in literary texts*. The Hague: Mouton.

Halliday, M.A.K. (1970). Language structure and language function. In J. Lyons (Ed.), *New horizons in linguistics*. Middlesex: Penguin Books.

Halliday, M.A.K., & Hasan, R. (1976). *Cohesion in English*. London: Longman.

Holland, A. (1978). Factors affecting functional communication skills of aphasic and non aphasic individuals. San Francisco, Paper Presented at the American Speech and Hearing Association Convention.

Huber, W., & Gleber, J. (1982). Linguistic and non linguistic processing of narratives in aphasia. *Brain and Language, 16,* 1–18.

Hutchinson, J.M., & Jensen, M. (1980). A pragmatic evaluation of discourse communication in normal and senile elderly in a nursing home. In L. Obler & M. Albert (Eds.), *Language and communication in the elderly*. Lexington, Mass.: Lexington Books.

Hymes, D. (1962). The ethnography of speaking. In T. Gladwin & W.C. Strutevant (Eds.), *Anthropology and human behavior*. Washington, D.C.: Anthropological Society of Washington.

Jakobson, R. (1963). *Essais de linguistique générale*. Paris: Editions de Minuit.

Joanette, Y., Goulet, P., & Nespoulous, J.L. (1985). Right hemisphere cognitive processing involved in narrative discourse. Copenhagen, Paper Presented at the Eighth European Conference of the International Neuropsychological Society.

Kaplan, R.M., & Bresnan, J. (1982). Lexical-functional grammar: A formal system for grammatical representation. In J. Bresnan (Ed.), *Mental representation of grammatical relations*. Cambridge, Mass.: MIT Press.

Kiefer, F. (1977). Review of studies in text grammars. *Journal of Pragmatics, 1,* 177–193.

Kieras, D.E. (1978). Good and bad structure in simple paragraphs: Effects on apparent theme, reading time and recall. *Journal of Verbal Learning and Verbal Behavior, 17,* 13–28.

Kintsch, W. (1975). *The representation of meaning in memory*. Hillsdale, N.J.: Lawrence Erlbaum Associates.

Kintsch, W. (1976). Bases conceptuelles et mémoire de texte, *Bulletin de Psychologie*, "La mémoire sémantique," 327–334. Special Issue edited by Endel Tulving.

Kummer, W. (1972). Outlines of a model for a grammar of discourse. *Poetics, 3,* 29–56.

Lesser, R. (1986). Comprehension of linguistic cohesion after right brain-damage. Veldhoven, Paper Presented at the Ninth Annual Conference of the International Society of Neuropsychology.

Liles, B. (1987). Episode organisation and cohesive conjunctives in narratives of children with and without language disorder. *Journal of Speech and Hearing Research, 30,* 185–197.

Longacre, R. (1983). *The grammar of discourse*. New York: Plenum.

Lovett, M.W., Dennis, M., & Newman, J. (1986). Making reference: The cohesive use of pronouns in the narrative discourse of hemidecorticate adolescents. *Brain and Language, 29,* 1–28.

Lundquist, L. (1983). *L'analyse textuelle: Méthode, exercices*. Paris: Cedic.

Mandler, J., & Johnson, N.S. (1977). Remembrance of things parsed: Story structure and recall. *Cognitive Psychology, 9,* 111–151.

Marslen-Wilson, W., & Tyler, L. (1980). The temporal structure of spoken language understanding. *Cognition, 8,* 1–71.

Martinet, A. (1962). *A functional view of language.* Oxford: Clarendon Press.

Morris, C. (1938). Foundations of the theory of signs. In O. Neurath, C. Carnap, & C. Morris (Eds.), *International Encyclopedia of Unified Science.* Chicago: University of Chicago Press.

Nespoulous, J.L. (1980). De deux comportements verbaux de base: Référentiel vs modalisateur. De leur dissociation dans le discours aphasique. *Cahiers de psychologie, 23,* 195–210.

Nespoulous, J.L. (1981). Two basic types of semiotic behavior: Their dissociation in aphasia. In P. Perron (Ed.), *The neurological basis of signs in communication processes.* Toronto: Toronto Semiotic Circle.

Nespoulous, J.L., & Lecours, A.R. (in press). Pourquoi l'aphasique peut-il dire: "Je ne peux pas le dire" et pas "Elle ne peut pas la chanter"?: De l'intérêt des dissociations verbales dans l'étude du comportement verbal des aphasiques. To appear in A.R. Lecours et al. (Eds.), *Le parler des parlers.*

Nevert, M., Nespoulous, J.L., & Lecours, A.R. (1980). Approches psycholinguistiques du discours du psychotique. In *Communiquer demain,* Proceedings of the International Conference of French Speech Pathologist.

Ola-Östman, J. (Ed.) (1978). *Cohesion and semantics.* Abo: Publication of the Research Institute of The Abo Akademi.

Palek, B. (1968). *Cross-reference: A study from hyper-syntax.* Prague: Charles University Press.

Patry, R. (1986). *Le lexique dans l'analyse de la cohésion linguistique: Aspects problématiques et perspectives d'applications,* doctoral dissertation, University of Montreal.

Patry, R. (in press). Analyse de niveau discursif de la déviance dans le discours continu de sujets aphasiques: Lexique et syntaxe ou incohérence. Chapter to appear in A.R. Lecours, M. Nevert, & L. Branchereau (Eds.), *Parler des parler.*

Patry, R., & Ménard, N. (1985). Spécificité du lexique dans l'analyse de la cohésion: Problématique et perspectives d'applications. *Bulletin of the Canadian Association of Applied Linguistics, 7,* 167–178.

Petöfi, J. (1975). Modalité et topic – Comment dans une grammaire textuelle à base logique. *Semiotica, 15,* 121–170.

Petöfi, J., & Rieser, H. (1973). (Eds.) *Studies in text grammar.* Dordrecht: Reidel.

Planalp, S., & Tracy, K. (1980). Not to change the topic but . . . a cognitive approach to the management of conversation. In D. Nimmo (Ed.), *Communication yearbook 4.* New Brunswick, N.J.: Transaction Books.

Propp, V. (1928). *Morphology of the folktale.* Philadelphia, American Folktale Society 1958; original Russian edition, 1928.

Remacle, N., & Francois, F. (1986). Organisation et mémorisation du récit chez trois personnes âgées hospitalisées. *Cahiers de l'institut linguistique de Louvain, 12,* 151–166.

Rieser, H. (1978). On the development of text-grammar. In W. Dressler (Ed.), *Current trends in text linguistics.* Berlin: De Gruyter.

Ripich, D., & Terrell, B. (1988). Patterns of discourse cohesion and coherence in Alzheimer's disease. *Journal of Speech and Hearing Disorders, 53,* 8–15.

Sandson, J., Albert, M., & Alexander, M. (1986). Confabulation in aphasia. *Cortex, 22,* 621–627.

Schank, R., & Abelson, R. (1977). *Scripts, plans, goals and understanding.* Hillsdale, N.J.: Erlbaum.

Searle, J. (1969). *Speech acts*. Cambridge: Cambridge University Press.

Simonin-Grumbach, J. (1975). Pour une typologie du discours In J. Kristeva (Ed.), *Langue, discours et société*. Paris: Editions du Seuil.

Tesniere, L. (1965). *Eléments de syntaxe structurale*. Paris: Klincksieck.

Tracy, K. (1982). On getting to the point: Distinguishing "issues" from "events"; an aspect of conversational coherence. In M. Burgoon (Ed.), *Communication yearbook 5*, New Brunswick, N.J.: Transaction Books.

Turner, R. (Ed.) (1974). *Ethnomethodology: Selected readings*. Harmondsworth: Penguin.

van Dijk, T.A. (1972). *Some aspects of text grammars*. Mouton: The Hague.

van Dijk, T.A. (1979). *Macrostructure*. Hillsdale, N.J.: Lawrence Erlbaum Associates.

van Dijk, T.A., & Kintsch, W. (1983). *Strategies of discourse comprehension*. New York: Academic Press.

Vipond, D. (1980). Micro and macro processes in text comprehension. *Journal of Verbal Learning and Verbal Behavior, 19*, 276–296.

Vuchinich, S. (1977). Elements of cohesion between turns in ordinary conversation. *Semiotica, 20*, 229–257.

Walker, D. (Ed.) (1978). *Understanding spoken language*. Amsterdam: North-Holland.

Weil, H. (1887). *The order of words in the ancient languages compared with that of the modern languages*. Boston: Ginn; original French edition, 1844.

Winograd, T. (1975). Frame representation and the declarative procedural controversy. In D. Bobrow & A. Collins (Eds.), *Representation and understanding*. New York: Academic Press.

2
The Psycholinguistics of Discourse Comprehension

GREGORY L. MURPHY

The advent of modern psycholinguistics can be traced to the work of Noam Chomsky in his ground-breaking studies of syntax (Chomsky, 1957, 1965). Chomsky's theories proposed that language was a highly complex system of rules represented in the mind by a grammar, a device that can generate all the sentences of a language without generating any sentences that are not in the language. Psychologists, excited by the proposal that people are endowed with such complex mental structures, which could be precisely formulated, followed this lead by investigating whether people possess the particular linguistic rules suggested by Chomsky and his followers (e.g., Miller and Isard, 1963; Savin and Perchonock, 1965; see Fodor, Bever, and Garrett, 1974, for a complete review). One interesting characteristic of this research tradition is that its hypotheses generally applied to individual sentences. Since the grammar generates individual sentences based on strictly formal principles, it does not take into account the relations between sentences in a discourse or how the sentences relate to the setting in which they are uttered. For example, early psycholinguistic experiments investigated whether passive sentences require more processing than active sentences (since passive sentences required the use of more rules, according to the grammar); whether sentences with negative elements in them are more difficult to understand; whether interrogative sentences are more difficult than affirmative sentences; and so on. In each of these cases, experiments could test these hypotheses by comparing isolated sentences in a timed task. There was no need for the sentences to be part of a story or to be spoken by an actual speaker in a naturalistic situation. In fact, such additions would have been considered confounding variables that would prevent a clean test of the hypothesis.

This approach to psycholinguistics has formed an important part of our knowledge of how people process sentences. However, recent work has turned to questions involving *situated discourse*: instead of investigating how people understand isolated sentences, this work has investigated how sentences in a discourse must be related to each other and to the setting in which they are produced. For example, the activity of telling a story puts constraints on a speaker and gives cues to a listener that are different from those of giving instructions or a speech. The same sentence when spoken by me to my daughter could have very different significance when spoken by my daughter to her best friend. In short, situated discourse has principles and problems that are not apparent in studies of disembodied, isolated sentences. In some cases, the results found for isolated sentences may even change when more realistic discourse is investigated. This chapter will not focus on these cases, however, but will review some of the main principles and findings of the psychology of understanding situated discourse. Because other chapters in this volume discuss issues of discourse coherence and textual structures (see Chapters 1, 3, and 4), this chapter will focus on conversations, inference, and social phenomena that arise in situated discourse.

The chapter will begin by discussing the general principles of conversation and other discourse situations. Much of this work derives from linguistics and philosophy rather than psychology. After these principles have been presented, the chapter will discuss specific examples of psycholinguistic studies that have provided evidence for them.

General Principles

Perhaps the simplest null hypothesis to use as a point of departure is the view that characteristics of the speaker and situation are irrelevant in an account of understanding. One possible such viewpoint is to conceive of conversation as a logical argument. On this view, the primary purpose of conversation is to express true propositions about the world. The listener's task is to recover the propositions from the utterance and to use various rules to combine the propositions in order to draw inferences. This viewpoint is not as farfetched as it may seem, as modern theories of semantics are based on extended logics (e.g., Dowty, Wall, and Peters, 1981), and logic has a long history as an explanatory tool of language and reasoning. Of course, we know that people make faulty inferences sometimes and that they fail to make some valid inferences. However, we can partially save the logical view by allowing rules of inference other than the traditional ones. Also, we may admit that people use "missing premises" that do not appear in the discourse but that affect their understanding. Indeed, when one thinks of many uses of language—writing an essay, telling a story, or giving instructions—the logical metaphor has considerable plausibility. Although many writers may have realized the limitations of such a model, it is a useful one to take as a contrast to the views that we will review in this chapter.

Recent writings on the philosophy of language have attacked the premises of such a view. They have suggested that human language is not merely a means of representing true assertions, but rather a system of communicative acts. Thus, the theory of *speech acts* (Austin, 1961; Searle, 1969) argues that language is a system that includes a variety of acts, such as requesting, marrying, vetoing, threatening, promising, and greeting, as well as asserting. Of course, most of these acts have no place in a logical model, which only represents propositions (typically expressed by assertions).

Furthermore, this emphasis on speech acts raises a host of new questions. Consider what one needs to know in order to perform the speech act of promising (see

Searle, 1969, Ch. 3). To start with, one needs to know the grammar of the language, including the meaning of the word *promise*. However, this is hardly sufficient to be able to make a well-formed, sincere, successful promise. For example, suppose that I were to tell someone "I promise not to fly to the moon before dinner." On the face of it, this would seem to be a successful promise, since I have taken on an obligation to do something and in fact intend to do it. However, it is a very bizarre promise, in that I should only promise to do things that the addressee does not expect me to do. Or I could say "I promise to punch you in the nose," with a sincere intention to do so. However, this is not a real promise, but rather a threat, since you do not wish me to punch you in the nose (let's assume).

In short, making a successful promise requires the speaker not only to know the grammar of English but also to know various facts about the addressee and his or her desires and beliefs. Sometimes the addressee's desires and beliefs can be inferred just by virtue of general properties of human beings (e.g., no one wants to be punched in the nose), but others require quite specific knowledge of the addressee (Richard wants to go skating on Tuesday but not Thursday). This sort of knowledge is not restricted to the speech act of promising. It can be found in the very basic act of referring to something (described shortly) and in the more exotic cases of vetoing or marrying, in which knowledge of institutional structures and rules is required (e.g., only certain people can perform marriages, and only in the context of certain rituals with complex preconditions).

Interestingly, the speech act that an utterance expresses is not always evident in a surface analysis of that utterance. For example, one might think that assertions are marked by indicative sentences, that commands and requests are marked by the imperative, and so on. There are two problems with this view. First, there are many more kinds of speech acts than there are categories of sentence mood to differentiate them (Gibbs, 1984). For example, the difference between promising, threatening, and warning cannot be detected in formal aspects of sentence structure, but must take into account the sentence's content. Second, there are cases of mismatches between the surface meaning of a sentence and the speech act that is carried out. The best known case of this is the *indirect speech act* (Searle, 1975). Consider the sentence "Can you tell me the time?" On the surface, it is a request for information about your abilities—a request to tell me what you can and cannot do. Clearly, however, its function could be to request you to actually tell me the time. At the dinner table, "This soup needs salt" may be a comment on the food, but it may also be an indirect request to have someone pass the speaker the salt. In indirect speech acts there is a direct speech act that is apparent on the surface (e.g., the question about someone's abilities or the comment on the food) and an indirect speech act (e.g., a request) that the speaker intends in addition to or instead of the direct speech act.

Indirect speech acts are important for our purposes because they are often understood only in the context of a particular situation. When the head chef tastes the soup and says "This soup needs salt," she is not asking someone to pass the salt but is instead perhaps rebuking the sous-chef who made it. When talking to a small child, "Can you tell me the time?" may be a direct question about the child's abilities. Thus, people's ability to understand indirect speech acts depends both on their analysis of the sentence and their ability to integrate it into the situation appropriately.

The philosopher Paul Grice (1957) codified the distinction I am drawing here by contrasting *sentence meaning* with *speaker meaning*. According to Grice, sentence meaning is the meaning of a sentence that is constant across all its occurrences. One heuristic to help one pick out the sentence meaning is Katz's (1977) anonymous letter criterion. Imagine that I were to pick up a letter on the street with no address on it. Inside, there is a single sheet of paper with the sentence "This soup needs salt" written on it. The meaning that I could extract from that sentence could only be due to the sentence itself, and this is its sentence meaning. Speaker meaning, however, is the meaning that is actually intended by a speaker when uttering the sentence. Speaker meaning may carry considerable additional information over the sentence meaning, because of the previous discourse and the situation in which it is uttered. For example, if I say to my wife, "Isn't it time to go?" I am certainly asking for information about the time (the sentence meaning). But I may also be conveying meanings such as "We're late" or "Hurry up!" even though these are not properties of the sentence itself (i.e., not part of sentence meaning). In some cases, speaker meaning even seems to contradict the sentence meaning, as in ironic sentences such as "You're a fine friend!"

In this chapter, we will strictly be investigating issues of speaker meaning, since it is speaker meaning that listeners are attempting to extract from a conversation. That is, listeners have little interest in the inherent properties of the sentences they hear—they are primarily interested in what message the speaker is attempting to communicate. Of course, there is little doubt that speaker meaning greatly depends on the sentence meaning. However, there is some doubt as to whether sentence meaning is ever actually computed by understanders as a prelude to computing speaker meaning (Gibbs, 1984). Let us begin now to examine how speakers do come to understand speaker meaning.

Cooperativity in Conversation

If we view communication on a logical model, understanding corresponds to compiling a list of logical formulas. With every succeeding sentence, we add another formula to our list. In some cases, we will wish to make inferences based on this list. For example, if I have heard the sentences "The blue cat is on the mat" and "The mat is in front of the door" then I can infer that the cat is blue and that the cat is in front of the door. Certainly, some of our understanding does involve such logical or plausible inferences (Clark, 1977). However, there are many inferences that people draw in conversation that seem to be quite different from the one just described. For example, Grice (1975) gives this example of writing a letter of recommendation for a student: "Dear Sir, Mr. X's command of English is excellent, and his attendance at tutorials has been regular. Yours, etc." The inference that the recipient of this letter would likely draw is that Mr. X is unsuitable for the position he is being considered for. However, one cannot find

TABLE 2.1. The conversational maxims of Grice (1975).

Quantity
  Make your contribution as informative as is required.
  Do not make your contribution more informative than is required.
Quality
  Do not say what you believe to be false.
  Do not say that for which you lack adequate evidence.
Relation
  Be relevant.
Manner
  Avoid obscurity of expression.
  Avoid ambiguity.
  Be brief (avoid unnecessary prolixity).
  Be orderly.

such information anywhere in the letter, nor can it be supplied by any simple "hidden premises."

Grice (1975) describes a number of such inferences that listeners draw easily but that cannot be found in the sentence's meaning. In order to explain such inferences, which he calls *implicatures*, Grice proposed a Cooperative Principle of conversations: "Make your conversational contribution such as is required, at the stage at which it occurs, by the accepted purpose or direction of the talk exchange in which you are engaged." In short, Grice is proposing that speakers actively cooperate with their listeners in producing sentences that the listeners will easily understand and that will be appropriate to the speech activity they are engaged in. The Cooperative Principle can be supplemented by Grice's four Conversational Maxims, which give more specific advice to speakers (see Table 2.1). These maxims form the basis for virtually all current theory in discourse analysis and linguistic pragmatics (see Levinson, 1983).

The Gricean maxims provide a basis for conversational participants to draw inferences. If listeners assume that speakers are following cooperative rules, then they can make inferences that logical analysis of the sentence would not allow. For example, the maxims of Quantity and Relevance (see Table 2.1) suggest that the letter of recommendation given previously is uncooperative: the writer has not provided sufficient, relevant information for the prospective employer. However, if we maintain our assumption that the recommender is being cooperative, we can draw a new inference, that there is nothing positive to be said about the student's academic career, and so the recommender has purposely said nothing. Similarly, if Ann has just told Betty that she did not discourage Carol from buying a hideous sweater, Betty's statement "You're a fine friend!" seems to violate the maxim of Quality. However, in order to retain our assumption that Betty is speaking cooperatively, we can reinterpret her statement as being ironic, as literally meaning "You're a rotten friend!"

Examination of even one conversation would show that much of our linguistic communication takes place through implicature. That is, much of a speaker's message is not directly said, but is understood through inference. Readers may think that the recommendation or ironic examples given are rather exotic. But most examples of implicatures are so mundane that we hardly notice that there is an inference involved. Consider the following example (from Grice, 1975):

A: I'm out of gas.
B: There's a gas station around the corner.

Listeners assume that B believes that this gas station is open, that has gas, and that it will sell the gas to them. Of course, B's utterance does not actually say these things, but if he did not intend them, his statement would violate the Maxim of Relation (there is no point in telling A about closed gas stations in this situation). Thus, listeners interpret B as in fact intending these implicatures. Consider another example (also adopted from Grice):

A: Where is Alice going?
B: To France somewhere.

We assume that B does not know any more precisely where Alice is going. If she did, then the Maxim of Quantity would require her to be more specific. Since she was not more specific, listeners draw an inference about how much she knows.

In summary, the Conversational Maxims provide listeners with a way to draw inferences in conversation that is not based on traditional rules of logic. Suppose that a speaker utters a statement that is not obviously true, or not obviously relevant, or the like. Rather than accepting the speaker's intentions as being synonymous with the sentence meaning, the listener attempts to draw an implicature. This implicature should show that the speaker's contribution is relevant, truthful, and so on, after all. Finding the correct implicatures can require world knowledge (e.g., knowing what letters of recommendation normally look like or what gas stations do), knowledge of the speaker (e.g., Betty is supposed to be friends with Carol), and linguistic conventions (e.g., ironic intonation).

The Gricean approach to conversation has been very influential. However, it does not yet fully explain how listeners come to the interpretations of sentences that they do. One addition to the conversational maxims is the notion of *mutual knowledge*. In order to achieve full cooperation in communication, the speaker must know quite a bit about the listener. Of course, in some situations, speakers have little knowledge about their audience, as in public speaking or when meeting someone new at a party. However, even here, one may often assume that the addressees are adult, fluent speakers of the native language and are informed members of the community. For example, if I were to meet someone at a reception following a colloquium at Brown University, I would assume that this person was familiar with the material presented in the colloquium and with the major characters and issues of Brown University, of Rhode Island, and of the country. Although I may know little about this person's personal life and interests, I can probably refer to the previous presidential election, to the major news story of the day or to campus events and personages.

In other situations, mutual knowledge may be more extensive. My brother and I share mutual knowledge about some of our pasts, about relatives, and about limited aspects of our present lives. However, we do not share mutual knowledge about each other's careers, except in a very general way. My colleagues and I have almost the reverse pattern: we know a great deal about each other's everyday lives, careers, and professional matters, but very little about each other's pasts, relatives, and so on.

Why is mutual knowledge important? It is important because it is one of the main determinants of what speakers can say and what listeners can understand. That is, people who are well versed in some topic talk about it very differently from those who know little about it, and they talk differently when speaking to other experts than when speaking to novices. More specifically, as we have already noted, speakers do not speak in perfectly connected, logical arguments; rather, they leave much up to the listeners to infer. However, if the listeners do not have the appropriate knowledge, they cannot draw the necessary inferences. For example, a child who knows little about job qualifications and recommendations might interpret Grice's letter as a favorable recommendation. Accordingly, when we speak to children, we are much more explicit about some things than when we speak to adults.

How do speakers and listeners know what knowledge they have in common? Clark and Marshall (1981; see also Clark and Murphy, 1982) mention three main sources of mutual knowledge. The first, community membership, says that people who are members of the same community can assume that they share the knowledge common in that community. Communities may be quite large (North Americans) or quite small (nurses in the cardiac ward of a particular hospital). The second source of mutual knowledge is physical copresence. If some object or event is physically present during a conversation, it is safe to assume that the speaker and listener share the knowledge of it. The third source, linguistic copresence, refers to the previous conversation that these participants have been involved in.

Community membership was illustrated in the example of the colloquium reception. There, I was a member of some of the same communities as the person I met, and my speech could assume only knowledge prevalent in those communities. An illustration of physical copresence might be found in understanding references such as "the desk" in "Please put the papers on the desk." If there is a desk in the room, the speaker can assume that the addressee can locate it perceptually and understand the reference.

Of course, communication also occurs long distance, in writing, telephone, or radio. Here, physical copresence is virtually eliminated and any mutual knowledge must be established through community membership and linguistic copresence, that is, by explicit mention. For example, most ellipsis takes advantage of mutual knowledge through linguistic copresence (Clark and Murphy, 1982): A: "Do you want to go to the movies?" B: "Sure." A and B share the knowledge of the previous conversation, and this knowledge is necessary to understand the elliptical sentence "Sure." The same utterance in part of a completely different conversation would not be interpreted as "I want to go to the movies," but as something entirely different. In other cases, a speaker may refer to something quite remote in the conversation.

Mutual knowledge is important, as I have said, because speakers could not provide cooperative contributions without knowing a considerable amount about their audience. But mutual knowledge is not simply a matter of the speaker knowing what the listener also knows—the listener must know what it is that the speaker knows about him or her. That is, mutual knowledge does not refer to knowledge that the speaker and listener just happen to have in common. It refers to the knowledge that each knows that they have in common. (I am simplifying considerably here. See Clark and Marshall, 1981, for a more complete account.) For example, imagine that two Tibetan farmers met on the way to the marketplace. If they have never met before, it would be uncooperative for one of them to use the expression "He struck out," since it is unlikely that a given Tibetan farmer knows baseball terminology. This is true even if both do in fact know baseball terminology, since neither knows that the other is familiar with it. Now imagine that both farmers have been following American baseball and, further, that one of the farmers knows that the other has been following baseball, but that the second farmer is still completely ignorant about the first. If the first farmer uses the expression "He struck out," the second farmer would be puzzled. Although he has this phrase in his lexicon, he would not know what the first farmer meant by it, since he assumes that the first farmer knows nothing about baseball. As Clark and Marshall (1981) show with even more elaborate examples, the listener must have considerable knowledge of what the speaker knows, and especially what the speaker knows about the listener, in order to be certain of understanding.

Simply sharing knowledge is not sufficient, because of the cooperative nature of conversation. Listeners interpret speakers' utterances by assuming that they are trying to speak in terms that they can understand. But if the listeners do not know what the speakers know about them, this assumption becomes difficult to put into practice. The three sources of information given earlier provide mutual knowledge in a complete sense: if speaker and listener know that both are members of some community, for example, then they not only share knowledge, they believe that the other shares their knowledge and believe that the other knows that they share knowledge, and so on. Although mutual knowledge may seem rather abstract, its importance will be illustrated in the section on reference.

Conversational Rules

The preceding discussion dealt with general rules of cooperation in conversation. However, there are also more specific rules that govern particular parts of conversational interactions. A simple example would be a greeting. When meeting an acquaintance after an extended absence, one should greet the acquaintance by saying an appropriate greeting ("hi," "hello," "how are you?," "hey there," etc.), and the acquaintance should return the greeting with another greeting. Other kinds of conversational rules dictate how to begin and end conversations, how to take turns in conversations, how to interrupt speakers, and the like.

Because of space constraints, this chapter cannot describe such conversational rules. However, it should be clear that these rules arise not out of constraints on individual sentences but rather on how sentences must be related to each other as part of a conversational activity. One important consequence of this is that a sentence that appears in different parts of a conversation could have different functions in each part. For example, "empty" statements such as "Well, that's the way it goes" and "Such is life," when uttered at the end of a story indicate something like "That's the end of the story," even though their sentence meanings say nothing of the kind (Schegloff and Sacks, 1973). But such statements in other parts of a conversation might not have such a function.

Speakers who learned a language without learning the conventions of conversations would be incompetent conversationalists. In fact, Gumperz (1982) has argued convincingly that cross-cultural communication often suffers from exactly this problem. That is, different languages and cultures often have different techniques for greetings, making points in conversations, making offers or compliments, ending stories, and so on. Because these techniques are often not taught as part of language instruction, interactions involving two or more cultures are often awkward, or worse. Such problems suggest that listeners are sensitive to conversational conventions and use them to help structure speakers' messages. Examples of such rules are described by Gumperz (1982), Sachs, Schegloff, and Jefferson (1974), and Schegloff and Sacks (1973).

Politeness

One of the main activities that conversationalists engage in is to preserve social relations of various kinds. Again, the model of conversation as a logical argument leads to an emphasis on the content of conversation, that only the propositions expressed by a sentence are important. Conversational analysis shows, on the contrary, that the precise way in which utterances are expressed is important. In particular, different forms can differ greatly in how polite they are perceived as being. "Get out of here" and "We would like to discuss this in private" may achieve the same effect on an addressee's behavior, but certainly differ in important social messages being transmitted. Similarly, "That jerk is coming" and "Ms. Smith is coming" might describe the same situation, but they surely differ in the attitude being expressed towards Ms. Smith.

One of the most influential analyses of politeness derives from Goffman's (1967) work on face preservation. A person's face is the sum of the positive attributes that he or she claims. Face, then, is a publicly presented image that may or may not correspond to reality. However, in order for social interactions to progress normally, Goffman argues that we often accept others' faces even when we doubt their veracity. Partly, this is a matter of mutual back scratching; if I accept your dubious claims, then you will have to accept mine. This is also partly a matter of convenience to allow a conversation to take place. For example, if we are discussing modern art, and you attempt to give the impression of being an expert on contemporary painting, I may not challenge this claim—even if I believe it to be false—because if I do, you will lose face and perhaps end the conversation. At best, the conversation will end up being about your claims to expertise rather than about art. Finally, for me to destroy someone else's face can itself result in loss of face on my part. My image as a kind, tactful person will be tarnished, perhaps causing others to avoid me. (And, of course, our back-scratching relationship being lost, you may choose to now attack my face.)

For these and other reasons, Goffman argues that speakers are motivated to preserve the faces of others involved in an interaction. Face preservation requires us to be careful about how we speak.

When a person volunteers a statement or message, however, trivial or commonplace, he commits himself and those he addresses, and in a sense places everyone present in jeopardy. By saying something, the speaker opens himself up to the possibility that the intended recipients will affront him by not listening or will think him forward, foolish, or offensive in what he has said . . . . Furthermore, by saying something the speaker opens his intended recipients up to the possibility that the message will be self-approving, presumptuous, demanding, insulting, and generally an affront to them or to their conception of him . . . . (Goffman, 1967, pp. 37–38)

Face preservation, then, is a matter primarily for the speaker to watch out for. But such considerations suggest that listeners must be attending to such matters themselves. That is, when listening to you, I am (among other things) trying to decide whether you are acting in a foolish or self-approving way, and I am making sure that you are not saying something that will show that you do not respect my face. If you do, then I may challenge you on it.

Once again, the matter of politeness is one that does not arise in the anonymous letter situation, but only as a part of real conversations with specific people taking part. What is polite when talking to your grandmother is not appropriate when talking to a student, a friend, or a spouse. And what is polite at a ball game is not necessarily polite in a formal dinner, at home, or in the classroom. Politeness, then, depends on both the setting and the participants involved. Part of knowing what is polite is knowing the conventions governing that situation. Another part is knowing enough about the other participants to be able to avoid situations that they will regard as threatening, in poor taste, or otherwise objectionable. These variables will be illustrated in the case studies of the following section.

Specific Topics

Definite Reference

Many of the issues raised in the first part of this chapter can be illustrated in the topic of definite reference. In definite reference, speakers use an expression to pick out objects or events in the world so that the listener can also pick them out. In indefinite reference, the speaker is introducing to the conversation a new object or event. Definite noun phrases in English are preceded by the definite article "the," whereas indefinite noun phrases are preceded by either the indefinite article "a" or by nothing (for plurals).

In the simple definition just given, the complexity of definite reference from the point of view of the speaker can already be seen. For example, how does the speaker know whether to use the definite or indefinite article? In many cases, speakers can follow the rule that whatever has not been mentioned in the conversation must receive the indefinite article the first time it is mentioned, and the definite article thereafter. However, there are many examples that seem to violate this. For example, in a newscast, a reporter may use the phrase "the president" without previously introducing this person into the discourse. In my classroom, I may refer to "the window" without a previous mention. Apparently, the speaker can assume that the listener has in some sense already introduced these objects into the conversation, even though they have never been explicitly mentioned. Equally important, listeners know when they hear such expressions that a new object is not being introduced, even though no president or window has been previously mentioned. Apparently, mutual knowledge is crucial in determining this usage.

This problem is a simple one compared with the central problem of definite reference, which is how the speaker chooses a referring expression that picks out just the right object for the listener. We can deceive ourselves as to how difficult this problem is. For example, Bertrand Russell interpreted "The king of France is bald" to mean that there is one and only one king of France and he is bald. Similarly, the reporter who says "The president shouted a few comments while walking to his helicopter" may be depending on the fact that there is only one president of the United States. But most definite reference does not involve descriptions that pick out a unique object. For example, references to "the window, the book, the tables, the car," and so on are ubiquitous in speech and writing, yet these phrases in and of themselves hardly pick out unique objects.

A beginning at an answer to this question was provided by Olson (1970), who introduced the notion of a *referent array*. The reason that a reference such as "the window" can be successful is that listeners do not attempt to find one window out of all the windows in the world; instead, they attempt to find it in a smaller set of objects, the referent array. The referent array may consist of perceptibly present objects, for example. If there is one object in the array that fits the description in the reference, then listeners will understand the reference to apply to that object. In fact, Olson presented subjects with a variety of referent arrays and showed how their reference decisions depended on both the description and the array.

This view, however, does not provide a sufficient explanation of definite reference. First is the question of how speakers and listeners define the referent array. Unlike psychology experiments, natural discourse does not necessarily provide a well-defined array of objects. Certainly, there is often a set of perceptually present objects that speakers can refer to, but conversations often refer to things that are not present at the moment. Even worse, stories and novels use definite reference considerably even though the writer and reader may share no perceptual information. In short, although Olson is probably correct that listeners consider only a subset of possible referents, we must still determine how they narrow down the very large number of possibilities to a smaller number.

A second problem is that speakers often do not maintain an unambiguous referring expression over an entire conversation (Krauss and Weinheimer, 1964). For example, I may start by referring to something as "the blue book on the second shelf" but from then on refer to it as "the book," even though there are many other books perceptually present to me and the listener. Since these other perceptually present objects should be contained in the referent array, it is unclear how people understand such references.

Clark and Marshall (1981) provided a more detailed explanation of how speakers produce and listeners understand definite references. They argued that speakers produce referring expressions that they believe that the listener can uniquely identify based on their mutual knowledge. Mutual knowledge, therefore, provides the key as to where the referent array comes from (in fact, we will no longer need to speak of such an array). In reference, only the material that the speaker and listener know that they share will be relevant. So, in saying "the window," I cannot be referring to any arbitrary window, because my addressee would not understand such a reference. The addressee, also realizing this, will not consider all possible referents of the phrase, but only the objects that we have mutual knowledge of. In some situations, there will be only one such object, making reference quite easy.

By invoking mutual knowledge, we are not simply renaming the referent array. Recall that mutual knowledge arises from three primary sources: community membership, perceptual copresence, and linguistic copresence. Thus, in determining what "the window" could refer to, a listener need only determine whether there is some general knowledge that she needs to invoke for this particular speaker (e.g., both teach in the same room), whether there is some window present that she could be referring to, or whether she has already mentioned some window in the conversation.

In some cases, there may be a number of possible objects that fit the description even within the domain of mutually known objects (e.g., there are two windows present). How does the listener "uniquely determine" which object is being referred to? One general answer is salience. If one window is closer, larger, or has been most recently mentioned, it probably corresponds to the one that is now being referred to. Clark, Shreuder, and Buttrick (1983) had subjects interpret ambiguous references such as "this flower," used to refer to a scene with a number of flowers in it. Subjects consistently chose the most salient of the flowers (the brightest colored or largest) in the picture as the referent. Another source of information is the rest of the sentence that contains the definite noun phrase. For example, in the sentence "The president addressed Congress today," the president of the United States is being referred to. However, in "The president met with student protestors," the president of a university is probably being referred to. Thus, listeners use not just the referring expression itself but the entire sentence (and previous discourse) in picking the referent out of mutually known objects.

How can we explain the phenomenon in which references change with repeated use? Krauss and Weinheimer (1964; see also Clark and Wilkes-Gibbs, 1986) found that first references to unfamiliar objects were often quite lengthy. With repeated reference, the length of the noun phrase decreased to one or two words, even though the actual referent array remained constant. This increasing efficiency is possible because the listener and speaker develop a history of referring expressions that becomes part of their mutual knowledge. For example, when I refer to only one of the books in my office as "the book," this may be successful because I have already picked out this book more explicitly, making it more salient than any other book in the office. Of course, it might not be more salient for a neutral observer but only for the specific listener who has shared the prior conversation with me.

In summary, in order to explain the delicate choice of referring expressions that speakers make and the difficult decisions that listeners make in interpreting them, we are forced to consider what the speaker and listener mutually know. Reference, then, depends only in part on the literal meaning of the words in the referring expression. It depends greatly on other knowledge that is evoked in the discourse situation.

Reference also raises problems of politeness. As mentioned earlier, the expression "Ms. Smith" may pick out the same person as "that jerk," but the two differ greatly in other characteristics. Sociolinguists have studied in some detail the politeness rules of *address*, that is, the name speakers used in talking to someone (Brown and Ford, 1961; Brown and Gilman, 1960; Paulston, 1976). However, they have paid less attention to politeness when referring to other people. This question is a somewhat more complicated one, because at least three people are involved: the speaker, the addressee, and the referent. Politeness must take all three into account.

Assume that I want to refer to someone named Jane Smith who is not present in the conversation. First, I must choose a referring expression that accurately portrays my relation to Jane Smith. If she is a famous public figure whom I have never met, then it would be presumptuous of me to refer to her as "Jane." But if we are close friends, it would be more acceptable for me to use the first name. Second, I must take into account the relationship between the addressee and referent. If I am friends with Jane Smith, but the addressee is not, it might be considered one-upmanship for me to refer to her as "Jane" in that situation. That is, it would be rubbing in the fact that I am friendly with her, when the addressee is not. Third, I must use a referring expression that will express a suitable relationship in the eyes of the addressee. If Jane Smith is a very important person, and the addressee is rather conservative, then he or she may expect me to use a title in referring to her, such as "President Smith" or "Dr. Smith," regardless of how well I think I know her. To use a more informal expression could cause friction in the conversation.

In a series of experiments, Murphy (1988a) showed that speakers were sensitive to such factors in choosing references to people. They switched from "Jane" to "Dr. Smith" in just the situations that this analysis suggested they should. These results can be explained by Goffman's (1967) theory of face preservation: in each case, the speaker must attempt to present an image that is acceptable in the eyes of the addressee. If I try to take on a better face than I deserve (e.g., I do not really know Jane Smith, even though I refer to her as "Jane"), then doubt will be cast on other positive qualities that I claim for myself. Equally importantly, the speaker must preserve the addressee's face. If I use a referring expression that emphasizes that I hold a more intimate relationship with Jane Smith than the addressee does, I am causing him or her to lose face, creating a rift in our relationship. Assuming that speakers attempt to preserve the face of conversational participants, any such controversial references should be avoided. Of course, this theory assumes that listeners are attuned to such subtle social factors, or else speakers would not take such care in their choices of reference.

To summarize, definite reference depends on situated discourse in a number of ways. In order to choose a referring expression, speakers take into account the exact knowledge that they share with their listeners, and listeners do the same in interpreting the reference. Furthermore, in choosing polite references, speakers take into account quite specific knowledge about the addressee, the referent, and their relationship. Clearly, neither of these phenomena appear in the anonymous letter situation.

Understanding Speech Acts

In some cases, the speech act that a speaker intends is directly conveyed by the sentence uttered. For example, the previous sentence is a simple declarative sentence, and it corresponds to the speech act of an assertion. Similarly, the interrogative sentence "What time is it?" corresponds to a request for information. But, as mentioned earlier, many speech acts are performed indirectly, such that the conveyed meaning is not apparent in the sentence form. How do listeners get from the sentence that is actually spoken to the final meaning?

Linguists and philosophers have given standard explanations of why indirect speech acts have the meanings they do (Gordon and Lakoff, 1971; Grice, 1975; Searle, 1975), and we can turn this linguistic analysis into a psychological explanation of how people interpret these utterances. When listeners first hear a sentence, this explanation goes, they construct a literal, direct interpretation of it. Let us call this meaning *M1* (after Clark, 1979). Then they attempt to integrate this sentence into their understanding of the discourse as a whole. However, if this integration is difficult or if the speaker seems to be violating the cooperative principle, then the listener will attempt to construct another interpretation that does not have these problems. This second interpretation, *M2*, would be the indirect interpretation of the sentence.

For example, imagine that a stranger stops me outside my office and asks "Do you have a watch?" When I first hear this sentence, I construct the interpretation that the speaker is asking information about whether I own a watch. However, this direct interpretation (M1) is problematic: it is irrelevant to any activity I am involved in, and it is inappropriate for a stranger to ask me about my personal belongings. Therefore, I must consider other interpretations that the speaker might have in mind. Since the main function of watches is to tell the time, and since it would be appropriate for a stranger to ask me the time, I construct an indirect interpretation of this utterance (M2), namely that the speaker is requesting me to tell him or her the time.

This model of understanding has a number of advantages. First, it suggests that listeners focus on the most obvious interpretations, constructing more difficult interpretations only if the first interpretation fails. Second, it explains when listeners will and will not interpret a sentence indirectly. And third, it explains why it is that listeners seem to pay attention to both the direct and indirect meanings (Searle, 1975). That is, when someone asks me "Do you have a watch?" I may answer "Yes, it's 3:30." But where did the answer "Yes" come from? It is a response to the direct speech act, the question about my watch. A request for the time by itself does not produce the answer "Yes" (i.e., if someone asked me "What time is it?" I would not answer "Yes, it's 3:30."). In many cases, people seem to answer *both* the direct and indirect request, suggesting that they must have constructed both interpretations.

Unfortunately, this model also has a number of problems. It is not always the case that the psychological processing of some construction follows the same path as its linguistic derivation, as psycholinguists found in early studies of syntax (Fodor et al., 1974). Just because indirect speech acts can be analyzed as modifications of direct speech acts does not mean that subjects understand them by first constructing a direct meaning and then constructing an indirect meaning. For example, when someone asks me "Can you tell me the time?" I have no sensation of considering the direct meaning "Do you have the ability to tell me the time?" Rather, it is the request to tell the time that I am aware of. Such introspective evidence is hardly conclusive, but it can be combined with more principled arguments. If a certain linguistic form is commonly used to indicate indirect requests, it would be peculiar if listeners were to consistently misinterpret those requests at first to be something else. That is, after people have heard "Can you do X?" a few thousand times to mean "Please do X," it seems hard to believe that they are "fooled" into thinking that it is a question about their abilities. In fact, Shatz (1978) found that preschool children understand such questions as requests and cannot interpret them as direct questions at all, suggesting that even children have found some way of bypassing the direct meaning.

This hypothesis has been put to empirical test. Clark and Lucy (1975) asked subjects to evaluate various kinds of requests. They did this by presenting a request along with a picture in which the request might have been fulfilled. Subjects had to read the request and, as quickly as they were able, decide whether the request was fulfilled in the picture. Thus, this method required only that subjects understand M2. Clark and Lucy found, first, that direct requests were easier to respond to than indirect requests. They also found that the exact form of the request was important, even though the conveyed meaning was constant. That is, varying the surface meaning (M1) affected how difficult the request was to interpret. Both of these results provided evidence for the hypothesis that subjects computed and used the direct meaning during interpretation.

Gibbs (1979) replicated Clark and Lucy's results. However, he then added a condition in which a request was a natural part of a larger story instead of being presented in isolation. In this situation, the previous results reversed: subjects were faster in understanding the indirect meaning than the direct meaning of sentences such as "Must you open the window?" Furthermore, the direct request "Do not open the window" was no easier to process than its indirect counterpart. In short, Gibbs's results suggest that when indirect requests are in an appropriate context, subjects have ready access to the indirect meaning, and that they do not necessarily require more processing than direct requests. When the same sentences are presented in isolation, a quite different pattern of results obtains.

It might be premature to conclude that listeners do not attend to the direct meaning of sentences in normal conversations. For example, we still have to explain why it is that responses to indirect requests often include an answer to the direct question as well (e.g., "Do you have a watch?" "*Yes I do*, it's 3:30."). Also, as we will see, politeness phenomena depend on the direct meaning. Clark (1979) attempted to provide a more complete explanation of how indirect requests are understood. He argued that speakers do not have the same intentions toward all indirect requests: depending on the situation, they intend only M1, only M2, or both M1 and M2. It is the listener's job to figure out which of these situations holds.

Clark's study used the novel technique of calling up area businesses and making various requests for information. By varying the form and content of the request and examining the responses listeners gave to each request, he was able to demonstrate how different variables affected which interpretations were understood (or, at least, responded to). In some cases, the listeners would respond only to M1 or M2, whereas in others, they would respond to both. Some of the factors he discovered were as follows. English has a number of conventional forms for making requests, such as "Can you do X?" or "Would you do X?" Similar forms such as "Are you able to do X?" or "Are you willing to do X?" are less conventional. The more conventional the form, the more likely listeners were to ignore M1 and to respond to M2. Also, English contains special markers, such as "please," which indicate M2 is intended. Another factor is whether M1 is plausible in that situation. If I go to a hot dog stand that has four signs advertising hot dogs and ask "Can I get a hot dog, please?" chances are that I do not truly intend to question whether hot dogs can be bought there. In such cases, listeners tend to ignore M1.

At one extreme, such as the hot dog vendor example or "Can you do X?" requests, the listener may never process M1. At the other extreme, when the request is in an unconventional form and somewhat implausible, the listener may think that M1 is intended but not be sure about M2. The reader may have noticed that there is something paradoxical about this reasoning. I have suggested that whether listeners attend to M1 depends on factors such as whether M1 is plausible. But this seems to require that listeners analyze M1 in order to decide whether to analyze M1. This paradox cannot be completely avoided, because of the evidence that properties of M1 determine whether it will be encoded (Clark, 1979; Gibbs, 1979, 1986b). One escape from this paradox is to suggest that some characteristics of M1 may be derived without a full analysis. Gibbs (1986b) suggests that indirect requests may be understood in part like idioms, in that some of their meaning may be directly accessed without a word-by-word analysis.

Thus, listeners may get rough ideas about M1 and M2 at early stages of processing and may use these ideas to direct their later processing.

There is probably more to be said to specify just how listeners interpret indirect speech acts. In particular, more studies that examine the time course of their comprehension are needed. Also, it should be noted that, although this discussion has focused strictly on requests, there are many other kinds of indirect speech acts besides indirect requests. Most of these have not yet been intensively studied.

This discussion raises the question of why there are indirect requests at all. That is, in principle, "Do not close the window" should be easier to understand than "Must you close the window?" Wouldn't life be easier if all speech acts were made directly? The most obvious answer of why there are indirect requests is that they are more polite than direct requests. However, this is perhaps surprising, in that indirect requests are perceived to be requests, after all. That is, in saying "Must you close the window?" the speaker is not hiding the fact that he or she is making a request, and so it is puzzling that it seems to be more polite.

Brown and Levinson (1977) helped to solve this puzzle in a detailed analysis of the politeness of requests. They point out that making a request is a face-threatening act. One aspect of people's face is their desire to fulfill their goals without interference. In asking someone to do something for you, you are imposing your will on the other person, denying that person to have complete freedom in his or her actions. Furthermore, making a request threatens the speaker's own face, in that a refusal reflects badly on the requester. However, as just noted, indirectness does not really hide the fact that the requester is indeed asking the addressee to do something, so why is it more polite?

Brown and Levinson argue that indirect requests give speakers more options to refuse the request. For example, in asking "Can you do X?" the speaker is overtly giving the addressee the possible out, "No, I can't." Instead of putting the addressee in an all-or-none situation, the indirect request suggests some acceptable alternatives to complete compliance, for example, protesting inability to fulfill the request. If the addressee does respond "No, I can't," this does not have the effect of a flat refusal, since the speaker suggested such a possibility in the request. Similarly, "Would you do X?" suggests that the addressee need do X only if he or she wishes to; "Will you do X?" has a similar meaning; and "Could I ask you to do X?" gives the addressee even more options. Thus, indirect requests are more polite by virtue of giving the addressee an "out" from either flatly denying the request or being pressured to do it.

In their study of requests in English, Clark and Schunk (1982) found that listeners' perceptions of request politeness are as this analysis predicts. They found that the politeness of a request depended on how many options the request gave to the addressee. For example, the indirect request "Can you do X?" does not give as many options as "Would you mind doing X?" does. The first gives the listener the option of protesting inability, but the second gives the broader option of protesting lack of desire. That is, "Would you mind . . ." suggests that the addressee's desires are important and that the speaker is not trying to infringe upon them. "Can you . . . ," on the other hand, suggests that so long as it is within the addressee's abilities, he or she should perform the requested act. In fact, subjects judged the requests that gave the requested party the most options to be the most polite.

Clark and Schunk's examples point out that one can also form quite impolite indirect requests by taking away options that the listener might have had. For example, the request "Shouldn't you answer the door?" does not just request that the addressee open the door—it suggests that the addressee has an obligation to do so. Since obligations are restrictions on one's future behavior, requests of this sort were judged to be quite impolite.

I have spent so much time on indirect requests because they illustrate many of the issues involved in understanding situated discourse. They show how the precise linguistic form of a request can affect how people understand it and its social acceptability. However, the relation of the request to the context—both linguistic and nonlinguistic—was also seen to be quite important. Experiments that used isolated sentences found different results from those that used sentences in context. Also, issues of politeness and comprehensibility arise in situated discourse that do not arise in the anonymous letter situation (and in many psychology experiments).

Other Topics

Because of space limitations, it has not been possible to discuss all, or even most, of the topics that arise in situated discourse. In this section, I will only mention a few additional topics, primarily to let the reader know that they are subjects of psychological investigation.

First, it must be noted that the linguistic field of *pragmatics* attempts to account for many aspects of how linguistic meaning depends on the conversational participants and situation. In addition to the issues just discussed, standard topics in pragmatics include *deixis*, the use of "pointing" words such as "this" and "that," whose meaning depends intrinsically on the context. Less obvious examples of deixis include the pronouns "I" and "you," as well as temporal terms and tenses. Pragmatics also addresses the issue of how sentences must be related in order to form acceptable sequences in a discourse. These and other matters are discussed in Levinson's (1983) standard text.

One prominent topic of psychological research is metaphor construction and comprehension. Metaphors are another case in which the conveyed meaning differs from the literal meaning of the sentence. For example, in a metaphor like "That surgeon is a butcher," the conveyed meaning is not that the surgeon has a shop in which he or she sells meat. Rather, it is taken as a comment on the doctor's surgical skills. Theories of metaphor have been proposed that are similar to the accounts already discussed for indirect speech acts. It has been suggested that listeners must first construct a literal meaning, compare it to the context, and then construct metaphorical meanings that might be more appropriate. However, just as in indirect speech acts, empirical results have challenged this theory—it seems that in some cases, the metaphorical interpretation is psychologically the primary one (Glucksberg, Gildea, and Bookin, 1982; Ortony, Schallert, Antos, and Reynolds, 1978).

A related topic is that of idioms. Again, the surface meanings of phrases such as "kick the bucket" are not their intended meanings. But because idioms are frozen expressions, it also seems likely that they have prestored interpretations such that listeners do not have to compute the meaning each time they hear the phrase, but only need to retrieve the stored interpretation. In fact, experiments have shown that it is difficult for listeners to interpret idioms in a nonidiomatic way (Gibbs, 1986a; Ortony et al., 1978).

Finally, a topic that has only begun to receive attention is innovative language. Newspapers, books, and conversations are filled with novel uses of language that the speakers and writers create on the spot. Among these are nouns used as verbs ("the delivery boy porched the newspaper"), compound noun phrases ("family planning delivery services"), eponymous adjective ("very San Francisco"), and pro-act verbs ("do the lawn"). These cases are interesting in part because they depend so heavily on the context in which they are uttered. Using the word "porch" as a verb can have a very large number of meanings (put something on a porch, put a porch on a house, draw a picture of a porch, etc.), depending on the sentence and discourse in which it occurs. Because such innovations have been little investigated, there is less to conclude now about how people understand them. However, the first attempts to investigate them can be found in Clark (1983), Clark and Gerrig (1983), Gerrig (1989), and Murphy (1988b).

Although it has not been possible to discuss these topics in any detail, no doubt the reader will see that they are similar in some respects to the "case studies" that I did discuss in detail: in many cases, the interpretation that one might give of these constructions in isolation is not the interpretation that they receive in actual discourse. Furthermore, instead of being unusual constructions that are very difficult to understand, they are fairly common and normally pose no apparent problems for comprehension.

Morals and Conclusions

The moral of the story has already been mentioned a number of times. To repeat: many interesting psycholinguistic phenomena arise only when real people talk to other real people in real situations. Psychology experiments using simplified settings and disembodied texts can tell us important facts about the comprehension of language. However, they may be misleading in two respects. First, they may ignore factors and phenomena that do not arise in such settings. Crucial issues such as reference and indirect and nonliteral speech cannot be fully explored in the anonymous letter situation. Second, their results may actually be incorrect in some other situations. For example, Gibbs's (1979) experiment showed strikingly different patterns of results for isolated requests and requests that occurred as parts of stories. His later work (Gibbs, 1986b) has shown that speakers design their requests quite precisely for a given context. When identical requests were placed in different settings, readers found them much more difficult to understand. Thus, even for questions that can be stated in terms of isolated sentences (e.g., "Do indirect requests require more processing than direct requests?"), the answer to the question may depend on discourse variables. [Olson and Filby (1972) give a similar example for the syntactic issue of whether passive sentences are more difficult to process than active ones.]

A less obvious moral has to do with linguistic analyses. It is important to have a linguistic analysis of some structure or form as a starting point for understanding how people would process such structures. Without a theory of syntax, it would be difficult even to embark on the question of what makes sentences more or less complex. And without a theory of pragmatics or of politeness, it would be difficult to create an account of how some utterances are understood in context and why some are appropriate whereas others are not. However, it is important not to take the linguistic analysis — even a correct one — to be necessarily accurate as an account of how people process language. Processing theories are concerned with the actual mental processes that people go through in order to understand some piece of language, whereas linguistic theories attempt to give the most elegant, economical account of the structure of a language. For better or for worse, people's mental processes and representations do not seem to confine themselves to the elegant rules and representations of linguistics.

This lesson has been shown in early studies of syntactic processing (Fodor et al., 1974) as well as in the previous examples. The analysis of indirect speech acts taken from Searle (1975) and Gordon and Lakoff (1971) seems to be a roughly correct one. It provides an explanation of why some questions can be indirect requests and others cannot, and that explanation is integrated into an overall theory of language. However, the results of Clark (1979), Gibbs (1979), and others have argued that people do not go through the same processes as the linguistic analysis does. In the end, they may come to the same answer as the linguistic explanation, but they do not restrict themselves to the variables of that explanation, nor do they follow the steps that it goes through. People depend on imperfect but salient information; they learn to skip some steps through practice; they attend to other factors that interest them. In sum, the linguistic analysis of some form, even one that incorporates "context" into its explanation, is only a starting point for explaining how people understand that form.

To conclude, then, the ultimate goal of this line of research must be to use linguistic theory to develop psychological accounts both of purely grammatical processing and of contextual processing in order to arrive at a complete explanation of the comprehension of situated discourse.

Acknowledgment. The writing of this chapter was supported by NIMH grant MH 41704.

References

Austin, J.L. (1962). *How to do things with words*. Oxford: Oxford University Press.

Brown, P., & Levinson, S. (1978). Universals in language usage: Politeness phenomena. In E. Goody (Ed.), *Questions and politeness* (pp. 56–324). Cambridge: Cambridge University Press.

Brown, R., & Ford, M. (1961). Address in American English. *Journal of Abnormal and Social Psychology, 62*, 375–385.

Brown, R., & Gilman, A. (1960). The pronouns of power and solidarity. In T.A. Sebeok (Ed.), *Style in language* (pp. 253–276). Cambridge, Mass.: MIT Press.

Chomsky, N. (1957). *Syntactic structures*. The Hague: Mouton.

Chomsky, N. (1965). *Aspects of the theory of syntax*. Cambridge, Mass.: MIT Press.

Clark, H.H. (1977). Inferences in comprehension. In D. LaBerge & S.J. Samuels (Eds.), *Basic processes in reading: Perception and comprehension*. Hillsdale, N.J.: Erlbaum.

Clark, H.H. (1979). Responding to indirect speech acts. *Cognitive Psychology, 11*, 430–477.

Clark, H.H. (1983). Making sense of nonce sense. In G.B. Flores d'Arcais & R. Jarvella (Eds.), *The process of understanding language* (pp. 297–331). New York: Wiley.

Clark, H.H., & Gerrig, R.J. (1983). Understanding old words with new meanings. *Journal of Verbal Learning and Verbal Behavior, 22*, 591–608.

Clark, H.H., & Lucy, P. (1975). Understanding what is meant from what is said: A study in conversationally conveyed requests. *Journal of Verbal Learning and Verbal Behavior, 14*, 56–72.

Clark, H.H., & Marshall, C.R. (1981). Definite reference and mutual knowledge. In A.K. Joshi, B.L. Webber, & I.A. Sag (Eds.), *Elements of discourse understanding* (pp. 10–63). Cambridge: Cambridge University Press.

Clark, H.H., & Murphy, G.L. (1982). Audience design in meaning and reference. In J.-F. Le Ny & W. Kintsch (Eds.), *Language and comprehension* (pp. 287–299). Amsterdam: North-Holland Publishing.

Clark, H.H., Schreuder, R., & Buttrick, S. (1983). Common ground and the understanding of demonstrative reference. *Journal of Verbal Learning and Verbal Behavior, 22*, 245–258.

Clark, H.H., & Schunk, D.F. (1982). Polite responses to polite requests. *Cognition, 8*, 111–143.

Clark, H.H., & Wilkes-Gibbs, D. (1986). Referring as a collaborative process. *Cognition, 22*, 1–39.

Dowty, D.R., Wall, R.E., & Peters, S. (1981). *Introduction to Montague semantics*. Dordrecht: D. Reidel.

Fodor, J.A., Bever, T.G., & Garrett, M.F. (1974). *The psychology of language: An introduction to psycholinguistics and generative grammar*. New York: McGraw-Hill.

Gerrig, R.J. (1989). The time course of sense creation. *Memory & Cognition, 17*, 194–207.

Gibbs, R.W. (1979). Contextual effects in understanding indirect requests. *Discourse Processes, 2*, 1–10.

Gibbs, R.W. (1984). Literal meaning and psychological theory. *Cognitive Science, 8*, 275–304.

Gibbs, R.W. (1986a). Skating on thin ice: Literal meaning and understanding idioms in conversation. *Discourse Processes, 9*, 17–30.

Gibbs, R.W. (1986b). What makes some indirect speech acts conventional? *Journal of Memory and Language, 25,* 181–196.

Glucksberg, S., Gildea, P., & Bookin, H.A. (1982). On understanding nonliteral speech: Can people ignore metaphors? *Journal of Verbal Learning and Verbal Behavior, 21,* 85–98.

Goffman, E. (1967). On face-work. In E. Goffman, *Interaction ritual: Essays on face-to-face behavior* (pp. 5–45). New York: Pantheon Books.

Gordon, D., & Lakoff, G. (1971). Conversational postulates. In *Papers from the Seventh Regional Meeting* (pp. 63–84). Chicago: Chicago Linguistic Society.

Grice, H.P. (1957). Meaning. *Philosophical Review, 66,* 377–388.

Grice, H.P. (1975). Logic and conversation. In P. Cole & J.L. Morgan (Eds.), *Syntax and semantics, Vol. 3: Speech acts* (pp. 41–58). New York: Academic Press.

Katz, J.J. (1977). *Propositional structure and illocutionary force.* New York: Crowell.

Krauss, R.M., & Weinheimer, S. (1964). Changes in reference phrases as a function of frequency of usage in social interaction: A preliminary study. *Psychonomic Science, 1,* 113–114.

Levinson, S.C. (1983). *Pragmatics.* Cambridge: Cambridge University Press.

Miller, G.A., & Isard, S. (1963). Some perceptual consequences of linguistic rules. *Journal of Verbal Learning and Verbal Behavior, 2,* 217–228.

Murphy, G.L. (1988a). Personal reference in English. *Language in Society, 17,* 317–349.

Murphy, G.L. (1988b). Comprehending complex concepts. *Cognitive Science, 12,* 529–562.

Olson, D.R. (1970). Language and thought: Aspects of a cognitive theory of semantics. *Psychological Review, 77,* 257–273.

Olson, D.R., & Filby, N. (1972). On the comprehension of active and passive sentences. *Cognitive Psychology, 3,* 361–381.

Ortony, A., Schallert, D.L., Reynolds, R.E., & Antos, S.J. (1978). Interpreting metaphors and idioms: Some effects of context on comprehension. *Journal of Verbal Learning and Verbal Behavior, 17,* 465–477.

Paulston, C.B. (1976). Pronouns of address in Swedish: Social class semantics and a changing system. *Language in Society, 5,* 359–386.

Sacks, H., Schegloff, E.A., & Jefferson, G. (1974). A simplest systematics for the organization of turn-taking for conversation. *Language, 50,* 696–735.

Savin, H.B., & Perchonock, E. (1965). Grammatical structure and immediate recall of English sentences. *Journal of Verbal Learning and Verbal Behavior, 4,* 348–353.

Schegloff, E.A., & Sacks, H. (1973). Opening up closings. *Semiotica, 8,* 289–327.

Searle, J.R. (1969). *Speech acts: An essay in the philosophy of language.* Cambridge: Cambridge University Press.

Searle, J.R. (1975). Indirect speech acts. In P. Cole & J.L. Morgan (Eds.), *Syntax and semantics, Vol. 3: Speech acts* (pp. 59–82). New York: Academic Press.

Shatz, M. (1978). On the development of communicative understandings: An early strategy for interpreting and responding to messages. *Cognitive Psychology, 10,* 271–301.

3
Text Analysis: Macro- and Microstructural Aspects of Discourse Processing

ERNEST F. MROSS

The study of discourse comprehension has enjoyed a great surge in interest in recent years. Investigators in a wide variety of fields such as psychology, artificial intelligence, linguistics, philosophy, education, and the neurosciences have come to realize the importance of developing an understanding of language comprehension as a tool for understanding the workings of the mind. On the one hand, there are the philosophers, logicians, and mathematicians who are interested in formal semantics or the study of formal systems (e.g., Barwise and Perry, 1983; Montague, 1974; Seuren, 1985). This chapter is not concerned with this emphasis on representation in terms of a formal descriptive system. On the other hand, many researchers are interested in describing natural language as a means of communication, both in terms of its structure and its use as a communicative device. Linguists, for example, are concerned with analyses at the sentential level; however, a substantial amount of work has been done recently on larger portions of discourse in an area of study sometimes referred to as discourse analysis (Brown and Yule, 1983). Computer scientists, for example, are interested in building working computational language systems (Allen, 1987). Psychologists, in particular, are interested in both the representations and the *processes* involved in language comprehension.

The reason that psychologists and others interested in text comprehension are concerned with representation is because there are many different tasks people can do with a text. For example, they can recall it, summarize it, paraphrase it, answer questions about it, or even translate it into a different language. Investigators in the study of language need a way of dealing with the meaning of the text in order to devise theories that describe and explain the multitude of things that people can do with texts. A common thread among these investigators is their use of propositional representations. This chapter initially discusses the suitability of this format for representing discourse. Then a particular model of text comprehension is covered, that of van Dijk and Kintsch (1983). The van Dijk and Kintsch model consists of a three-level representation scheme, and each level is discussed in turn. The model's application to various empirical phenomena (e.g., short-term memory constraints and effects of knowledge structures) is presented throughout.

Propositional Representations

Several theories have been described in the (mostly psychological) literature, all of which may be suited for different purposes (Anderson and Bower, 1973; Frederiksen, 1975, 1977, 1979; Kintsch, 1974; Kintsch and van Dijk, 1978; Graesser and Goodman, 1985; Meyer, 1975, 1985; Norman and Rumelhart, 1975; Schank, 1972; van Dijk and Kintsch, 1983). All of these bodies of work are based on representations that are basically propositional in nature [but see Perrig and Kintsch (1985) and Weaver and Kintsch (1987) discussed later]. But just as there is no absolute meaning of a text, there is no one "correct" representation for a text. What is of interest is the purely psychological phenomenon of meaning resulting from the interaction of text and comprehender. A reader has certain more or less specific goals and some amount of knowledge which she brings to the text. In addition, a text's writer has certain goals and assumptions about how much knowledge the typical reader would be bringing to the reading of the text. These entities interact to yield the "meaning" of a text. Thus, for different purposes, different forms of representation are then more suitable.

Researchers may be interested in different aspects of the interaction, and thus it is important that they use the representation that best satisfies *their* goals. For example, some researchers are interested in the inferences a person can make from a text (Schank, 1972), whereas others are concerned with the causal coherence of a text (Trabasso, Secco, and van den Broek, 1984), while still others are concerned with what people can recall after reading a text (Kintsch and van Dijk, 1978; Meyer, 1975). Each model tries to describe the salient aspects of this interaction, according to its own purposes. This is not to say that all models are equally good at achieving their goals. It is just that the abundance of language problems of interest at this point still requires a number of different representations.

Based on ideas originally discussed in formal semantics and logic, these various propositional representational schemes consist of either a graphic network or a list-based representation. For practical reasons, a list-based representation is easier to work with when studying longer texts. A proposition is, for the most part, a shorthand for representing the elementary meaning of a simple sentence. In Kintsch's system (1974), propositions are case based (after Fillmore's case-grammar, 1968) and consist of a predicate with one or more arguments. Some examples of predicates (in English) in this system are verbs, modifiers, and sentential connectors. For example, the verb "throw" may take three arguments, corresponding to the agent (i.e., the thrower), the goal (i.e., the receiver of what is thrown), and the object (i.e., what is thrown). Thus the sentence "Chuck threw the ball to Debbi" can be represented as the proposition: (THROW, agent:CHUCK, goal:DEBBI, object:BALL). Propositions can also be embedded within other propositions as a way of providing greater descriptive power. Thus the sentence "The ring is very valuable" can be represented thus: (VERY, (VALUABLE, RING)).

There is a great deal of evidence for the psychological reality of propositional representations, of which just a few of the relevant studies will be mentioned here. For example, there are cued recall studies showing that a word from the same proposition is a more effective recall cue than a word from a different proposition of a sentence (Lesgold, 1972; Wanner, 1975). There are also free recall studies that demonstrate that propositions tend to be recalled holistically, in an all-or-none manner (Anderson, 1980; Goetz, Anderson, and Schallert, 1981; Graesser, 1981; Kintsch, 1974). In addition, there is evidence that reading rate for sentences and what can be recalled from them depends on the number of propositions that make up those sentences (Forster, 1970). Kintsch and Keenan (1973), for example, had subjects read sentences of approximately equal length, but varying in the number of propositions the sentences contained. When subjects were done reading a sentence, they pressed a button and then tried to recall the gist of the sentence. Reading time for propositions encoded into memory (based on the recall test) increased by about 1.5 seconds for each proposition recalled. However, Graesser, Hoffman, and Clark (1980) argued that this estimate of encoding time was inflated due to the fact that the sentences used by Kintsch and Keenan confounded the number of propositions with the number of new arguments introduced. Graesser et al. (1980) replicated Kintsch and Keenan's (1973) result of a linear relationship between reading time and recall of propositions, but found that, after controlling for the number of new arguments statistically, subjects needed only slightly more than 100 milliseconds to encode new propositions.

Perhaps the best evidence for the psychological reality of propositions comes from Ratcliff and McKoon (1978). They employed an item recognition priming technique that has proven to be an important methodological contribution in itself. Their procedure was as follows. Subjects were presented sentences for study. After the study period, subjects were given a recognition test that went as follows. A list of words was presented to the subjects, one by one, and the subject decided whether or not each word came from a studied sentence by pressing a "yes" or a "no" key. Their results indicated that if a subject saw a word from a studied sentence and responded "yes," the response time to another word from the same proposition was 100 milliseconds faster, as compared to words that were not from the same proposition. More important, this 100 millisecond priming effect for words from the same proposition was found to be significantly greater than the 91 millisecond effect observed when the two words came from different propositions but the same sentence. This finding was truly an intra-proposition priming effect, and not due to such factors as surface distance, which was controlled by the investigators. For example, one of their sentences was:

1. The mausoleum that enshrined the tzar overlooked the square.

Ratcliff and McKoon showed that "square" primed "mausoleum" more than it primed "tzar," even though "tzar" occurred physically closer in the sentence. The sentence consists of the two propositions (OVERLOOKED, MAUSOLEUM, SQUARE), and (ENSHRINED, MAUSOLEUM, TZAR), and thus one can see that this result obtained because "mausoleum" and "square" came from the same proposition.

These studies provide a great deal of support for the use of propositions as a representational format in text comprehension. However, for researchers interested in text comprehension, a representational system is incomplete without a specification of the processes that operate on that representation. It should also be noted that while some of the arguments to be developed here could be made within the context of some of the propositional representation models mentioned earlier, only the Kintsch and van Dijk model (Kintsch and van Dijk, 1978; van Dijk and Kintsch, 1983) will be discussed in detail. It has been applied to a variety of phenomena and thus is one of the most comprehensive models in scope.

The Kintsch and van Dijk Model

The Kintsch and van Dijk model provides discussions of representation intimately tied in with discussions of the processes that operate on that representation. In addition, the model has an important assumption about the *strategy*-based nature of discourse processing. The goal of discourse processing is to construct the best possible mental representation as efficiently as possible. Since the reader-text interaction often takes place in an environment of only partial information, powerful strategies must be used to compensate for this incompleteness.

Before the details of the Kintsch and van Dijk model are explored, a brief overview will be provided as an aid to the reader. An important assumption of Kintsch and van Dijk is that theirs is a buffer model, and incorporating limited-capacity, short-term memory constraints on processing is a prime feature of the model. A couple of studies pertinent to this topic will be discussed shortly. Another important assumption of the model is that text ultimately ends up being represented at three different levels. The first level of representation, which will not be discussed in any great detail, is that of the surface or verbatim trace. This is the memory for the particular words and surface structure of a discourse, which rapidly decays over time. The second level of representation is that of the text base. This is the structure where the meaning of the text is represented. The text base consists of two parts, corresponding to local and global information, which Kintsch and van Dijk call the microstructure and macrostructure of a discourse, respectively. Finally, the third level at which discourse is represented is called the situation (or mental) model. It is at this level that world knowledge is used most extensively. In addition to the different levels of representation of text postulated by Kintsch and van Dijk, the various forms of knowledge organization, such as scripts, frames, and schemata, in use during text comprehension fall under the heading of superstructures in the model, and these will be discussed where appropriate.

The Text Base

The text base is the resulting structure that is formed as a person reads a text. There are two types of information contained in the text base corresponding to local and global information. Kintsch and van Dijk hypothesized that a reader comprehends a text in cycles, with a cycle corresponding roughly to a sentence or clause. The propositions of the text are entered into a limited-capacity, short-term buffer (or short-term memory, STM). Then the propositions in STM are checked for argument overlap, or co-reference, and those deemed to be important for maintaining the coherence of the text are held over in STM, while the others are replaced with new input.

Fletcher (1981) provided empirical support for the buffer component of the Kintsch and van Dijk model. He performed two experiments, one using a cued recall procedure, the other using a probe recognition procedure. In both experiments, subjects read short passages clause by clause and were interrupted at some point for an STM test. On the cued recall test, a previously read content word from the text was presented and the subject was asked to respond with the content word that followed it in the text. In the probe recognition procedure, the subject was asked at the point of interruption to verify whether or not a short probe (i.e., a proposition) had appeared in the passage. The cues used in the cued recall experiment were the probes used in the recognition experiment. The explicit predictions with regard to particular propositions were obtained from the Miller and Kintsch (1980) computer simulation of the Kintsch and van Dijk (1978) model. Fletcher's results showed that propositions that were predicted to be in STM were responded to more quickly and more accurately as compared to propositions not predicted to be in STM. In addition, these same propositions were shown to be better recall cues in the cued recall task.

The Miller and Kintsch (1980) computer simulation used the "leading-edge strategy" of Kintsch and van Dijk (1978) to predict which propositions should be held over in STM. This is a strategy based on a compromise between recency and importance. Importance is defined in terms of the structural properties of the propositional text base (Kintsch, 1974). Propositions that share the properties of recency and importance are assumed to contribute to the coherence of a text, but the leading-edge strategy is by no means the only (or even the best) strategy that one might devise. To this end, Fletcher conducted another pair of studies in which he compared different strategies.

Fletcher (1986) compared several different strategies for the allocation of STM during comprehension. For example, some of the strategies he compared were ones based on plans and goals, the discourse topic, and the discourse structure, to name a few. Fletcher (1986) used two types of texts, stories (e.g., the fable "The Tortoise and the Crow") and news articles, in order to see if alternative memory allocation strategies proved differentially effective for these rather different types of texts. In the first experiment, verbal protocols were collected from subjects who were asked simply to report any thoughts that occurred to them as they read, sentence by sentence, several texts of each type. In a second experiment, reading times and recall data were collected from different subjects for the same texts. Fletcher used the different memory allocation strategies to predict which propositions should be in STM during each processing cycle. He then computed the correlations between these predictions and the propositions evoked in the think-aloud task, and between the predictions and reading time per proposition recalled (a readability measure, after Miller and Kintsch, 1980). To sum up briefly, the strategy that best described subjects' verbal reports and their reading time per proposition recalled was a strategy based on the plans and goals of the characters. This held true for both types of texts. Fletcher hypothesized that this was due to the importance of causal connections in a strategy based on deducing a character's plans and goals. A number of researchers have argued that causal coherence plays a critical role in text comprehension (Black and Bower, 1980; van den Broek, 1988; Keenan, Baillet, and Brown, 1984; O'Brien and Myers, 1987; Trabasso et al., 1984; Trabasso and Sperry, 1985; Trabasso and van den Broek, 1985), and a post-hoc analysis by Fletcher of the texts he used showed that causal connections occurred quite liberally in them.

In an ideal world the needed propositions are held over in STM but, practically speaking, this is often an imperfect process. Thus readers must conduct long-term memory (LTM) searches to fill in missing information. What results from this process is the text base, consisting of a connected, partially ordered list of propositions. The connections determine, in part, the coherence of the text. Only semantic coherence is at issue here; other forms of coherence (e.g., syntactic, structural) are described elsewhere (Halliday and Hasan, 1976; van Dijk, 1972; for a review see de Beaugrande, 1980).

The Microstructure

The microstructure is that part of the representation that contains the local information corresponding to the individual words and their relationships in the text. Local coherence is based on argument overlap (co-reference). Propositions that share common arguments are said to be related, according to Kintsch (1974) and Kintsch and van Dijk (1978). It is a simple view, as those authors readily admit, but it has been shown to be quite powerful when applied to a variety of comprehension phenomena. The advantages to this view of coherence are mainly objectivity and the ease with which the system can be used. The disadvantage is that other types of relationships (e.g., causal ones) are ignored.

Despite the disadvantages of this simple view of coherence, there have been numerous demonstrations of the psychological importance of co-reference among propositions (Haviland and Clark, 1974; Kintsch and Keenan, 1973; Kintsch, Kozminsky, Streby, McKoon, and Keenan, 1975; Manelis and Yekovich, 1976). For example, Haviland and Clark (1974) demonstrated that a sentence that shared a referent with a preceding sentence was read faster than a sentence that had no specific shared referent. Sentence pairs 2 and 3 are taken from Haviland and Clark (1974). The sentence "The beer was warm" was read faster in sentence 2 than in sentence 3 because of the shared argument in sentence 2.

TABLE 3.1. Fragment of an episode from a short story and the corresponding text base[a]

Text	Text base
This Landolfo, then, having made the sort of preliminary calculations merchants normally make, purchased a very large ship, loaded it with a mixed cargo of goods paid for out of his own pocket, and sailed with them to Cyprus. (The episode continues with a description of how this endeavor finally resulted in Landolfo's ruin.)	1(PURCHASE,agent:L,object:SHIP) 2(LARGE,SHIP) 3(VERY,2) 4(AFTER,1,5) 5(CALCULATE,agent:L) 6(PRELIMINARY,5) 7(LIKE,5,8) 8(CALCULATE,agent:MERCHANT) 9(NORMAL,8) 10(LOAD,agent:L,goal:SHIP,object:CARGO) 11(MIXED,CARGO) 12(CONSIST OF,object:CARGO,source:GOODS) 13(PAY,agent:L,object:GOODS,instrument:MONEY) 14(OWN,agent:L,object:MONEY) 15(SAIL,agent:L,object:GOODS,goal:CYPRUS)

[a] Modified from Kintsch (1976).

2. George got some beer out of the car. The beer was warm.
3. George got some picnic supplies out of the car. The beer was warm.

To retain coherence in sentence 3, readers must make a bridging inference, in effect, that beer must have been part of the picnic supplies.

Another demonstration of the importance of co-reference comes from Kintsch et al. (1975). Kintsch et al. presented subjects with texts that were controlled both for number of words and number of propositions. The texts in one case contained many references to the same seven or eight concepts, while the other texts contained fewer references to approximately twice the number of concepts. The texts with many references to fewer concepts were read faster by subjects and, when reading time was controlled by the experimenter, the fewer-concept texts were recalled better. Thus, argument repetition facilitates processing.

A very brief example of how one begins to construct the propositional text base of a text will be described here, based on rules originally described in Kintsch (1974) and elaborated on in Bovair and Kieras (1981, 1985), Turner and Greene (1978), and Turner (1987). For much more complete instruction in how to propositionalize a text, these other sources should be consulted. Bovair and Kieras are mainly concerned with technical (expository) prose, whereas the Turner papers are concerned with a wider variety of prose, and issues of semantics. The Bovair and Kieras system is simpler and is preferred if it is sufficient for one's needs.

As stated earlier, local coherence in the Kintsch and van Dijk model is based on argument overlap (co-reference). (Note that local coherence is distinct from global coherence, which will be discussed in the section entitled "The Macrostructure.") Each proposition in a text base must share an argument with at least one other proposition. This is a necessary but not sufficient condition of coher-

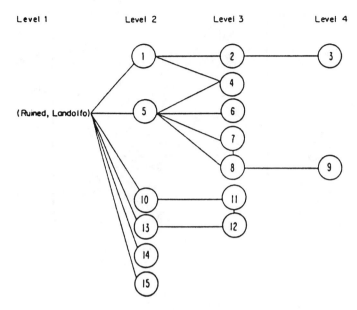

Level 1   Level 2   Level 3   Level 4

FIGURE 3.1. The text-base hierarchy for the fragment of text shown in Table 3.1. Propositions are indicated only by their number; shared arguments among them are shown as connecting lines. (After Kintsch, 1976.)

ence. Individual propositions are represented hierarchically. One or more propositions form the superordinate position in the hierarchy. Propositions that share arguments with the superordinate proposition(s) form the second level. Propositions that share arguments with propositions at the second level, but none at the first level, form the third level in the hierarchy. Any remaining levels are similarly defined.

A brief example will demonstrate how to construct the propositional text base and hierarchy for a given text. In Table 3.1, a sentence from a story from Boccaccio's *Decameron* is reprinted together with the corresponding propositional text base. Each proposition is written on a separate line and given a reference number to make it easier to work with. The initial proposition is P1(PURCHASE, agent:LANDOLFO, object:SHIP). The second proposition's predicate is the modifier "large," and thus the second proposition is P2(LARGE, SHIP). The third proposition is an example of an embedded proposition, since "very" modifies "large ship" and not just "large" [and thus the third proposition is P3(VERY, P2)]. The remaining propositions follow from this.

Figure 3.1 depicts the hierarchical representation of this part of the text base. The sole superordinage (level 1) proposition is (RUINED, LANDOLFO), which does not appear in the analyzed sentence. It is represented here because it is the topic of the episode to which the example sentence belongs. This proposition contains only one argument (i.e., LANDOLFO), and all propositions containing this argument are assigned to level 2 of the text base. Thus proposition 1

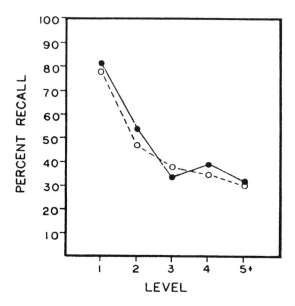

FIGURE 3.2. Recall probability as a function of the level of a proposition in the text base hierarchy. The data are for seventy-word paragraphs about history (filled circles) and science (open circles). (After Kintsch et al., 1975.)

(PURCHASE, agent:LANDOLFO, object:SHIP) is assigned to level 2 because it contains the argument LANDOLFO. Proposition 2 is assigned to level 3 because it repeats an argument (SHIP) appearing in proposition 1. All other propositions are assigned to a level in the hierarchy in the same objective manner.

There are some important things to note about this procedure. Only the microstructure has been represented here, except for the superordinate proposition (RUINED, LANDOLFO), which comes from the macrostructure. (The macrostructure is the representation concerned with the main ideas or overall organization of the text, and it will be discussed shortly.) In addition, the text itself appearing in Table 3.1 is only one possible paraphrase that could be generated from this list of propositions. Of concern is the underlying meaning of a text and, once that is represented, the surface structure is not of particular interest. This basically means that there are many ways to say the same thing.

There is at least one implication of the hierarchical representation scheme for psychological processing. These hierarchical levels (or similar ones) have been shown to be excellent predictors of recall (Britton, Meyer, Hodge, and Glynn, 1980; Kintsch and Keenan, 1973; Kintsch et al., 1975; Manelis, 1980; Meyer, 1975; Yekovich and Thorndyke, 1981). That is, the higher in the hierarchy for a particular text a proposition appears, the more likely it is that that proposition will be recalled. This finding is commonly referred to as the "levels" effect, and an example of this phenomenon is depicted in Figure 3.2. The Kintsch and van Dijk model provides a straightforward explanation for why superordinate propositions are recalled better. By definition, subordinate propositions repeat the arguments of higher-level propositions. If one assumes that when a person processes a subordinate proposition she must identify the repeated argument with the argument originally introduced, then this is in some way an implicit reprocessing of the superordinate proposition. The higher-level propositions are implicitly processed more often and thus are recalled better.

The Macrostructure

The term "macrostructure" was introduced by van Dijk (1972) as a name for the abstract semantic description of the global content of a discourse. The macrostructure is that part of the text base that represents the main ideas in the text, corresponding to notions such as theme, gist, topic, or upshot. In the previous section on the micro-structure of a text, the notion of local coherence was defined as the relationships between propositions as exhibited by a sequence of sentences. Global coherence is a more general phenomenon and is a property of whole discourses, or larger portions of discourse. Of concern is the semantic coherence, just as before, but this time it is of the discourse as a whole. There are other global structures, for example, scripts (Schank and Abelson, 1977), and the narrative schema (or story grammar; see Mandler and Johnson, 1977; Rumelhart, 1975; Stein and Glenn, 1977; Thorndyke, 1977), but these structures are more a description of the overall form a discourse *may take* and are *not* a representation of the semantic content of a particular discourse. These types of knowledge structures are referred to as superstructures by van Dijk and Kintsch (1983). Although these superstructures are relevant to varying degrees during macrostructure formation, they will be discussed in more detail later.

The macrostructure, by definition, consists of semantic units and is based on the meanings of the sentences of a text. Because the meanings of the sentences are represented as propositions, the macrostructure must itself consist of propositions, that is, macro-propositions. Kintsch and van Dijk (1978; van Dijk and Kintsch, 1983) have hypothesized three macro-rules that operate recursively on the micro-propositions to yield the macro-propositions. The macro-rules relate sequences of propositions at the local level to higher-level sequences of propositions, in so doing yielding the global meaning of a discourse. Because the macro-rules are recursive, they may apply repeatedly, each time yielding an even higher level of macrostructure. Thus the macrostructure consists of a partially ordered list of propositions, arranged in a hierarchy, just like the microstructure.

The macro-rules as defined by van Dijk and Kintsch (1983) are:

1. *Deletion*. Given a sequence of propositions, delete each proposition that is not a presupposition for another proposition in the sequence.
2. *Generalization*. Given a sequence of propositions, replace the sequence by a proposition that is entailed by each of the propositions of the sequence.
3. *Construction*. Given a sequence of propositions, replace it by a proposition that is entailed by the joint set of propositions of the sequence.

These are essentially reduction rules, allowing propositions to be deleted entirely or allowing sequences of micro-propositions to be replaced with a single macro-proposition. The deletion macro-rule simply consists of the deletion of nonessential detail. The generalization macro-rule specifies when a concept can be replaced by its superconcept, for example:

4. We heard a raccoon in the bushes. → We heard an animal in the bushes.

The construction rule specifies when a joint set of propositions can be replaced by single proposition, as in the case of a description of a scripted activity, for example:

5. David entered the building, sat down, and ordered lunch. → David went to a restaurant.

It is extremely important to note that exactly what constitutes a macro-proposition is very task and situation dependent. The notion of a macro-proposition was originally defined as that representation containing the gist information. However, what is considered gist information may be quite varied for different people under different circumstances. The goals and the knowledge that a reader brings to the task will determine in large part what kinds of gist information (i.e., macro-propositions) are extracted from a particular text. This is not due to a lack of objectivity on the part of the macro-rules, however. It is due to a lack of control over what a particular reader's goals are and the amount of knowledge he brings to the task. A theory of macrostructure should be able to predict some prototypical macrostructures for some basic reading goals, or verify post hoc what happened in a particular case.

Although application of the macro-rules is still poorly understood, this does not mean that no progress is being made in the area of macrostructure formation. For example, recent evidence supports the notion that macro-processing takes place on-line (Geleta and Yekovich, 1986; Guindon and Kintsch, 1984; Lorch, Lorch, and Matthews, 1985; Mross, 1988). Some of these investigators have made use of procedures described earlier in this chapter (Ratcliff and McKoon's item recognition procedure, 1978; Fletcher's probe procedure, 1981) in attempts to delineate the processes involved in on-line macroprocessing.

Superstructures

Many types of discourse are quite conventionalized. These conventions are captured in the van Dijk and Kintsch model by abstract cognitive structures termed "superstructures." Superstructures guide and facilitate the ongoing text comprehension process. If the comprehender recognizes the particular superstructure to which a discourse conforms, this can allow for greater understanding and/or recall of that discourse. These structures operate in some sense as "outlines" for the global semantic content (or macrostructure) of a discourse. They are, according to van Dijk and Kintsch (1983, p. 237), the "macrosyntax corresponding to the macrosemantics."

A superstructure exists for almost every discourse type. Thus one may speak of rhetorical, poetical, narrative, and argumentative superstructures, for example. There also exist superstructures for many text types, such as newspaper articles and scientific articles. These superstructures may function at different levels and over a different scope. For example, a newsstory superstructure may only function at the surface level, such that one expects a boldface headline at the beginning that functions as the first or highest macro-proposition. This structure has nothing to say about the length or scope of the newsstory, since it may vary anywhere from a few sentences to much longer. This is in contrast with a narrative superstructure, which is semantic in nature and categorizes the information content of a story. In addition, a narrative superstructure's scope is different also, as one expects more than a few sentences because a story is implicitly textual in nature.

What is most interesting here is how superstructures function in terms of psychological processes. As stressed earlier, discourse processing is strategic in nature, and it is important to attempt to specify the nature of these strategic processes. There are many strategies a person has available for recognizing and using such superstructures. Some of the types of information that function as input to these strategies consist of cultural, social context, and pragmatic information. Cultural information is the broadest category. All communication takes place with the participants as members of a specific culture, and with this comes certain general constraints on the form and content of the discourse. At a less broad level, the social context of the discourse also serves to put constraints on the discourse. The most ubiquitous example is that of everyday conversation. The age, status, and amount of shared knowledge of the participants function as bounds to what is and what is not acceptable with regard to the content, style, and even length of a conversation. Perhaps the most important type of information for strategic use of superstructures is that of pragmatic information. Because the intent is to communicate, pragmatic information can override all else.

There is a large amount of data pertaining to certain types of superstructures just discussed. Without a doubt, the narrative superstructure has been the focus of the most empirical work. Only one of the relevant studies and its conclusions will be elaborated on here. One of the well-known facts about the narrative superstructure, or story schema, is that it can be described as having a "canonical form." From this one can specify the allowable transformations that can take place. Kintsch, Mandel, and Kozminsky (1977) had subjects read and summarize simple stories in either their canonical form or with the paragraphs randomly reordered. This random reordering had no effect on the summaries, as subjects in both cases gave quite good ones. In addition, the scrambled stories were always summarized in canonical form. One might be tempted to conclude that the story schema had no effect, since both groups summarized the stories quite well. However, additional evidence suggests that the story schema can, in some situations, exert a strong effect on subjects' performance. Subjects took much longer to read the scrambled stories, implying that additional processing was required by them. Also, Kintsch et al. (1977) reported that the story that had the least correspondence to a story schema was summarized the poorest in its reordered form.

Thus, the story schema effect is strong enough to allow people to overcome the inherent difficulties of understanding a text consisting of randomly ordered paragraphs. Other investigators have found evidence along similar lines (Bartlett, 1932; Johnson and Mandler, 1980; Kintsch and Greene, 1978). In the domain of descriptive texts, Kintsch and Yarbrough (1982) and Meyer, Brandt, and Bluth (1980) demonstrated convincing superstructure effects.

The Mental Model of the Situation

The text base that results from comprehending a text is essentially only the information directly contained in the words and sentences of the text. However, there is an increasing variety of empirical results that are difficult, if not impossible, to explain without reference to some additional construct. Thus, in addition to the micro- and macrostructures (i.e., the text base) of a text, van Dijk and Kintsch hypothesize that readers construct a structure referred to as the situation model. Other authors have popularized the term "mental model" (Gentner and Stevens, 1983; Johnson-Laird, 1983) in attempts to get at much the same thing as van Dijk and Kintsch. The van Dijk and Kintsch (1983) notion of a situation model is quite similar to the Gentner and Stevens' mental model idea, although Johnson-Laird's use of the term is more restrictive. To remain consistent with van Dijk and Kintsch's terminology the term "situation model" will be used, with the understanding that this is essentially the same thing as a mental model.

One of the first studies exhibiting the need for an additional representational level is that of Bransford, Barclay, and Franks (1972). More recently, Fletcher and Chrysler (in press), Garnham (1981), Glenberg, Meyer, and Lindem (1987), Morrow, Greenspan, and Bower (1987), Perrig and Kintsch (1985), Schmalhofer and Glavanov (1986), Weaver and Kintsch (1987), and Zimny (1987) have all found evidence supporting the existence of (indeed, the need for) an additional representational level in discourse processing.

A representative set of results was reported by Schmalhofer and Glavanov (1986). They investigated the different types of information people obtained from studying a few paragraphs from a programmer's manual of the high-level programming language LISP. Following van Dijk and Kintsch (1983), Schmalhofer and Glavanov hypothesized that people form representations of three types of information: verbatim, propositional, and situational. They then manipulated the degree of propositional and situational processing by giving their subjects different study goals. One group of subjects was told they would be asked to give a summary of the text they had read (the text summarization group). Another group of subjects was told they would be asked to write and verify LISP expressions (the knowledge acquisition group). After studying the portion of the programmer's manual, both groups were given sentences to verify. By manipulating the type of information contained in the to-be-verified sentences and looking at the accuracy of responses to them, it was possible to assess the relative contributions of each level of representation to performance on the verification task. Schmalhofer and Glavanov found that more propositional (i.e., strictly text-based) information was remembered by the text summarization group, while the knowledge acquisition group remembered situational information better. Thus the text summarization subjects were better able to answer questions about information that actually appeared in the text. However, when it came to *using* the information described in the text (i.e., verifying LISP expressions), the knowledge acquisition subjects performed better.

Along these lines, a distinction has been made between remembering text and learning from it (Kintsch, 1986; Mannes and Kintsch, 1987). These studies describe instances where simply remembering a text is not enough. If true learning from a particular text is to take place, the development of a situation model must occur. Explorations of the contribution of the situation model to this topic are proving fruitful.

In terms of representational format, situation models can be propositional or nonpropositional in nature. This is in contrast to the text base, which is always propositional. An example where the situation model is most likely nonpropositional is when readers are asked to obtain a knowledge of the spatial layout of a hypothetical town. This was the case in Perrig and Kintsch (1985) and Weaver and Kintsch (1987). Perrig and Kintsch manipulated the structure of a text in such a way that one version would lead to a textually based representation, while the other would lead to a spatially based representation (a mental map). They found that those with the mental maps could infer spatial relations better than the other group while retaining equivalent performance on nonspatial tasks. Weaver and Kintsch showed the same effect, but they did so by manipulating the reader's goals instead of the texts. Weaver and Kintsch also found evidence that readers' recalls were reconstructive in nature—that is, readers "recalled" by looking at their mental map and then describing the map instead of recalling directly from their text base.

The formation of situation models and their subsequent usage is a very important topic on which a great deal of research is being concentrated. This is not surprising, because the situation model is where knowledge use in discourse comprehension is most active. General world knowledge, as well as opinions, attitudes, beliefs, and other sociocultural factors influence and assist in the formation and utilization of a model of the situation. It is a ground rich in potential for empirical and theoretical advancement, and cause for great excitement.

Conclusions

The need for, and the utility of, a comprehensive theory of text comprehension should be self-evident. The first component of such a theory is a system for representing the meaning of the text. While such notions as "the" meaning of a text were thought to be nontenable, the proposition does seem to provide a straightforward and useful representational format. It was stressed that a theory of comprehension is incomplete without a description of the processes that operate on that representation, however. The Kintsch and van Dijk model (van Dijk and Kintsch, 1983; Kintsch and van Dijk, 1978) is such a theory. Their process model has proved useful to researchers interested in things such as STM usage during comprehension, recall of passages of various text types, on-line processing of a local and global nature, and the ways in which world knowledge helps people to understand discourse.

The Kintsch and van Dijk model claims that there are multiple levels of representation that are used for different kinds of information and for different purposes. The level of least interest in this chapter is the surface structure or verbatim trace. The text base, consisting of the microstructure and macrostructure, is another level of representation. The microstructure corresponds to the meaning contained in the words and phrases of the text, while the macrostructure contains the topic- or gist-level information. Finally, the situation (or mental) model is the third level of representation. This is where the comprehender constructs a model of the situation described in a text. One might say that this level is where "true" understanding is represented.

In conclusion, an extensive body of knowledge has accumulated in the literature on discourse comprehension by normal subjects, yielding a powerful tool for application to other areas, such as the communication deficits of various types of patients. In addition, researchers interested in language comprehension in any population would do well to attend to work going on in the areas of discourse analysis and artificial intelligence. These areas have in the past made major contributions to language comprehension and can continue to remain helpful. The study of language comprehension encompasses a true interdisciplinary enterprise, and it is by this method that real progress is being made.

Acknowledgment. The author gratefully acknowledges the helpful comments of Walter Kintsch and Deborah S. Main.

References

Allen, J. (1987). *Natural language understanding.* Menlo Park, Calif.: Benjamin/Cummings.

Anderson, J.R. (1980). Concepts, propositions, and schemata: What are the cognitive units? *Nebraska Symposium on Motivation, 28,* 121–162.

Anderson, J.R., & Bower, G.H. (1973). *Human associative memory.* Washington, D.C.: Winston.

Bartlett, F.C. (1932). *Remembering: An experimental and social study.* Cambridge: Cambridge University Press.

Barwise, J., & Perry, J. (1983). *Situations and attitudes.* Cambridge, Mass.: MIT Press.

de Beaugrande, R. (1980). *Text, discourse, and process.* Hillsdale, N.J.: Erlbaum.

Black, J.B., & Bower, G.H. (1980). Story understanding and problem solving. *Poetics, 9,* 233–250.

Bovair, S., & Kieras, D.E. (1981). A guide to propositional analysis for research on technical prose. Technical Report No. 8, University of Arizona.

Bovair, S., & Kieras, D.E. (1985). A guide to propositional analysis for research on technical prose. In B.K. Britton & J.B. Black (Eds.), *Understanding expository text*. Hillsdale, N.J.: Erlbaum.

Bransford, J.D., Barclay, J.R., & Franks, J.J. (1972). Sentence memory: A constructive versus interpretive approach. *Cognitive Psychology, 3*, 193–209.

Britton, B.K., Meyer, B.J.F., Hodge, M.H., & Glynn, S. (1980). Effect of the organization of text on memory: Tests of retrieval and response criterion hypothesis. *Journal of Experimental Psychology: Human Learning and Memory, 6*, 620–629.

Brown, G., & Yule, G. (1983). *Discourse analysis*. Cambridge: Cambridge University Press.

Fillmore, C.J. (1968). The case for case. In E. Bach & R.T. Harms (Eds.), *Universal of linguistic theory*. New York: Holt, Rinehart, & Winston.

Fletcher, C.R. (1981). Short-term memory processes in text comprehension. *Journal of Verbal Learning and Verbal Behavior, 20*, 564–574.

Fletcher, C.R. (1986). Strategies for the allocation of short-term memory during comprehension. *Journal of Memory and Language, 25*, 43–58.

Fletcher, C.R., & Chrysler, S.T. (in press). Surface forms, textbases, and situation models: Recognition memory for three types of textual information. *Discourse Processes*.

Forster, K.I. (1970). Visual perception of rapidly presented word sequences of varying complexity. *Perception and Psychophysics, 8*, 215–221.

Frederiksen, C.H. (1975). Acquisition of semantic information from discourse: Effects of repeated exposures. *Journal of Verbal Learning and Verbal Behavior, 14*, 158–169.

Frederiksen, C.H. (1977). Semantic processing units in understanding text. In R.O. Freedle (Ed.), *Discourse production and comprehension*. Norwood, N.J.: Ablex.

Frederiksen, C.H. (1979). Discourse comprehension and early reading. In L.B. Resnick & P.A. Weaver (Eds.), *Theory and practice of early reading* (Vol. 1). Hillsdale, N.J.: Erlbaum.

Garnham, A. (1981). Mental models as representations of text. *Memory & Cognition, 9*, 560–565.

Gentner, D., & Stevens, A.L. (1983). *Mental models*. Hillsdale, N.J.: Erlbaum.

Geleta, N., & Yekovich, F.R. (1986). The interactive effect of micro- and macrostructural processing during text comprehension. Presented at the annual convention of the A.P.A., August.

Glenberg, A.M., Meyer, M., & Lindem, K. (1987). Mental models contribute to foregrounding during text comprehension. *Journal of Memory and Language, 26*, 69–83.

Goetz, E.T., Anderson, R.C., & Schallert, D.L. (1981). The representation of sentences in memory. *Journal of Verbal Learning and Verbal Memory, 20*, 369–385.

Graesser, A.C. (1981). *Prose comprehension beyond the word*. New York: Springer-Verlag.

Graesser, A.C., & Goodman, S.M. (1985). Implicit knowledge, question answering, and the representation of expository text. In B.K. Britton & J.B. Black (Eds.), *Understanding expository text*. Hillsdale, N.J.: Erlbaum.

Graesser, A.C., Hoffman, N.L., & Clark, L.F. (1980). Structural components of reading time. *Journal of Verbal Learning and Verbal Memory, 19*, 135–151.

Guindon, R., & Kintsch, W. (1984). Priming macropropositions: Evidence for the primacy of macropropositions in the memory for text. *Journal of Verbal Learning and Verbal Memory, 23*, 508–518.

Halliday, M.A.K., & Hasan, R. (1976). *Cohesion in English*. London: Longman.

Haviland, S.E., & Clark, H.H. (1974). What's new? Acquiring new information as a process in comprehension. *Journal of Verbal Learning and Verbal Behavior, 13*, 515–521.

Johnson, N.J., & Mandler, J.M. (1980). A tale of two structures: Underlying and surface form in stories. *Poetics, 9*, 51–86.

Johnson-Laird, P.N. (1983). *Mental models.* Cambridge, Mass.: Cambridge University Press.

Keenan, J.M., Baillet, S.D., & Brown, P. (1984). The effect of causal cohesion on comprehension and memory. *Journal of Verbal Learning and Verbal Behavior, 23*, 115–126.

Kintsch, W. (1974). *The representation of meaning in memory.* Hillsdale, N.J.: Erlbaum.

Kinstch, W. (1976). Memory for prose. In C.N. Cofer (Ed.), *The structure of memory.* San Francisco: Freeman.

Kintsch, W. (1986). Learning from text. *Cognition and Instruction, 3*, 87–108.

Kintsch, W., & Greene, E. (1978). The role of culture-specific schemata in the comprehension and recall of stories. *Discourse Processes, 1*, 1–13.

Kintsch, W., & Keenan, J.M. (1973). Reading rate as a function of number of propositions in the base structure of sentences. *Cognitive Psychology, 6*, 257–274.

Kintsch, W., Kozminsky, E., Streby, W.J., McKoon, G., & Keenan, J.M. (1975). Comprehension and recall of text as a function of content variables. *Journal of Verbal Learning and Verbal Behavior, 14*, 196–214.

Kintsch, W., Mandel, T.S., & Kozminsky, E. (1977). Summarizing scrambled stories. *Memory and Cognition, 5*, 547–552.

Kintsch, W., & van Dijk, T.A. (1978). Toward a model of text comprehension and production. *Psychological Review, 85*, 363–394.

Kintsch, W., & Yarbrough, J.C. (1982). The role of rhetorical structure in text comprehension. *Journal of Educational Psychology, 74*, 828–834.

Lesgold, A.M. (1972). Pronominalizations: A device for unifying sentences in memory. *Journal of Verbal Learning and Verbal Behavior, 11*, 316–323.

Lorch, R.F., Lorch, E.P., & Matthews, P.D. (1985). On-line processing of the topic structure of a text. *Journal of Verbal Learning and Verbal Behavior, 24*, 350–362.

Mandler, J.M., & Johnson, N.S. (1977). Remembrance of things parsed: Story structure and recall. *Cognitive Psychology, 9*, 111–151.

Manelis, L. (1980). Determinants of processing for a propositional representation. *Memory & Cognition, 8*, 49–57.

Manelis, L., & Yekovich, F.R. Repetition of propositional arguments in sentences. *Journal of Verbal Learning and Verbal Behavior, 15*, 301–312.

Mannes, S.M., & Kintsch, W. (1987). Knowledge organization and text organization. *Cognition and Instruction, 4*, 91–115.

Meyer, B.J.F. (1975). *The organization of prose and its effects on memory.* Amsterdam: North-Holland.

Meyer, B.J.F. (1985). Prose analysis: Purposes, procedures, and problems. In B.K. Britton & J.B. Black (Eds.), *Understanding expository text.* Hillsdale, N.J.: Erlbaum.

Meyer, B.J.F., Brandt, D.M., & Bluth, G.J. (1980). Use of top-level structure in text: Key for reading comprehension in ninth-grade students. *Reading Research Quarterly, 16*, 72–103.

Miller, J.R., & Kintsch, W. (1980). Readability and recall of short prose passages: A theoretical analysis. *Journal of Experimental Psychology: Human Learning and Memory, 6*, 335–353.

Montague, R. (1974). *Formal philosophy.* Cambridge, Mass.: Harvard University Press.

Morrow, D.G., Greenspan, S.L., & Bower, G.H. (1987). Situation models in narrative comprehension. *Journal of Memory and Language, 26,* 165–187.

Mross, E.F. (1988). *Macro-processing in expository text comprehension.* Unpublished doctoral dissertation, University of Colorado, Boulder.

Norman, D.A., & Rumelhart, D.E. (1975). *Explorations in cognition.* San Francisco: Freeman.

O'Brien, E.J., & Myers, J.L. (1987). The role of causal connections in the retrieval of text. *Memory & Cognition, 15,* 419–427.

Perrig, W., & Kintsch, W. (1985). Propositional and situational representations of text. *Journal of Memory and Language, 24,* 503–518.

Ratcliff, R., & McKoon, G. (1978). Priming in item recognition: Evidence for the propositional structure of sentences. *Journal of Verbal Learning and Verbal Behavior, 17,* 403–417.

Rumelhart, D.E. (1975). Notes on a schema for stories. In D.G. Bobrow & A.M. Collins (Eds.), *Representation and understanding: Studies in cognitive science.* New York: Academic Press.

Schank, R.C. (1972). Conceptual dependency: A theory of natural language understanding. *Cognitive Psychology, 3,* 552–631.

Schank, R.C., & Abelson, R.P. (1977). *Scripts, plans, goals, and understanding.* Hillsdale, N.J.: Erlbaum.

Schmalhofer, F., & Glavanov, D. (1986). Three components of understanding a programmer's manual: Verbatim, propositional, and situational representations. *Journal of Memory and Language, 25,* 279–294.

Seuren, P.A.M. (1985). *Discourse semantics.* Oxford: Basil Blackwell Ltd.

Stein, N.L., & Glenn, C.G. (1979). An analysis of story comprehension. In R.O. Freedle (Ed.), *New directions in discourse processing,* Vol. 2. Norwood, N.J.: Ablex.

Thorndyke, P.W. (1977). Cognitive structures in comprehension and memory of narrative discourse. *Cognitive Psychology, 9,* 77–110.

Trabasso, T., & van den Broek, P. (1985). Causal thinking and the representation of narrative events. *Journal of Memory and Language, 24,* 612–630.

Trabasso, T., Secco, T., & van den Broek, P.W. (1984). Causal cohesion and story coherence. In H. Mandl, N.L. Stein, & T. Trabasso (Eds.), *Learning and comprehension of text.* Hillsdale, N.J.: Erlbaum.

Trabasso, T., & Sperry, L.L. (1985). Causal relatedness and importance of story events. *Journal of Memory and Language, 24,* 595–611.

Turner, A. (1987). *The propositional analysis system.* Technical report no. 87-2, Institute of Cognitive Science, University of Colorado.

Turner, A., & Greene, E. (1978). *Construction and use of a propositional text base.* JSAS catalogue of selected documents in psychology, MS 1713.

van den Broek, P. (1988). The effects of causal relations and hierarchical position on the importance of story statements. *Journal of Memory and Language, 27,* 1–22.

van Dijk, T.A. (1972). *Some aspects of text grammars.* The Hague: Mouton.

van Dijk, T.A. (1977). *Text and context.* London: Longman.

van Dijk, T.A. (1980). *Macrostructures.* Hillsdale, N.J.: Erlbaum.

van Dijk, T.A., & Kintsch, W. (1983). *Strategies of discourse comprehension.* New York: Academic Press.

Wanner, E. (1975). *On remembering, forgetting and understanding sentences.* The Hague: Mouton.

Weaver, C.A., & Kintsch, W. (1987). Reconstruction in the recall of prose. *Text, 7,* 165–180.

Yekovich, F.R., & Thorndyke, P.W. (1981). Identifying and using referents in sentence comprehension. *Journal of Verbal Learning and Verbal Behavior, 17,* 265–277.

Zimny, S.T. (1987). *Recognition memory for sentences from discourse.* Unpublished doctoral dissertation, University of Colorado, Boulder.

4
The Cognitive Representation and Processing of Discourse: Function and Dysfunction

CARL H. FREDERIKSEN, ROBERT J. BRACEWELL, ALAIN BREULEUX, and ANDRÉ RENAUD

Natural language discourse, when viewed from a cognitive and psychological perspective, is a manifestation in extended natural language productions of conceptual representations and thought processes. A discourse reflects knowledge (of the writer or speaker as well as the reader or listener), purpose in communicating meaning through language, and the cognitive processes required to produce and comprehend knowledge and represent it as discourse. Thus, to a cognitive psychologist, discourse is viewed in terms of the knowledge and processes that generated it and that are required to understand it.

The analysis of discourse within cognitive research reflects this premise. Any formal structure generated to represent discourse is regarded as an hypothesis about the cognitive representation of the discourse by its producer or by a comprehender. As such, a formal representation of discourse must be theoretically linked to processes of generation or comprehension and tested experimentally against psychological data.

The specification of precise models of discourse processing ability entails an extremely wide range of cognitive operations and representations, including multiple levels of linguistic and semantic representation and processes of structure generation and transformation associated with these different levels and types of representation. Because of its complexity and the range of fundamental abilities and representations it involves, discourse is a fundamental source of information about human cognitive representations and processes. Psychological investigations of discourse abilities have led to advances in our general conception of an "architecture" for human cognition. They have advanced our conception of the organization and structure of temporary memory stores, of types of knowledge and their representation in memory, of reasoning and inference, of learning (i.e., acquisition of new knowledge), and of the use of knowledge to control action in planning and problem solving. All of these psychological processes are implicated in various discourse-processing activities, and their functions may be investigated in discourse-processing tasks.

The research problem is, given the many "layers" of processing and representation involved in discourse processing, to explain how these are routinely exercised and managed in performing normal discourse-processing tasks. Cognitive researchers have made progress in accomplishing this by analyzing discourse processing in terms of a stratified model in which discourse is represented in terms of multiple and independent levels of representation. In addition, researchers have suggested that the processing operations associated with these representations also are modular and parallel. In this type of model component processes interact when the particular type of representational structure on which one process operates is generated as output by another process. Processes also can be managed through the use of high-level plans or strategies that control their application.

Progress in developing such a stratified model has been in three areas: (1) development of formal models of semantic and linguistic representations of discourse at different levels, (2) development of computational models of the specific processes that generate or operate on particular representations, and (3) development of models of plans or control strategies that manage the processing of discourse.

The previous discussion, emphasizing as it does the complexity and range of abilities involved in discourse processing, provides answers to the question of why it is important to study discourse ability in relation to brain damage. From a basic research standpoint, such studies offer two unique advantages.

First, an important way to test any complex psychological model is to provide evidence that particular processes (or functions) specified by the model may become dysfunctional with brain damage. Because of the range of specific functions involved in discourse processing and the ability to trace their operation using discourse-analysis methods, the study of dysfunctions associated with brain damage promises to contribute importantly to the testing of assumptions concerning component cognitive processes and representations.

Second, examining how brain-damaged individuals adjust their processing to overcome the loss of specific functions can provide important information about the nature of interactions among component processes and the role of plans or strategies in managing discourse processing. We rarely have the opportunity to examine how the cognitive system adjusts to compensate for the loss or degrading of performance of an important component process. Thus, studies with patients having well-documented functional deficits can lead to fundamental knowledge about the adaptive properties of the cognitive system.

Both of these research approaches to discourse ability and brain damage can lead to specific diagnoses and treatment methods for the recovery of lost functions or the development of compensating strategies for comprehension, production, and communication.

This chapter introduces researchers in the field of discourse ability and brain damage to models that have been developed in cognitive science to account for discourse-processing ability, and the discourse-analysis and experimental methods that have been used to assess representations and the functioning of component processes. Our specific objectives therefore are: (1) to review the particular representations and component-processing abilities that have been identified in contemporary cognitive theories of discourse processing with reference to comprehension and production; (2) to describe methods of discourse analysis that are based on these models; (3) to describe experimental methods that have been developed to assess an individual's cognitive representations and functioning of component processes in discourse processing; and (4) to discuss cognitive theories of discourse processing from the standpoint of their potential applications to the study of dysfunctions associated with brain damage.

Discourse Comprehension
Stratified Models of Text Comprehension

Researchers in the fields of natural language and discourse comprehension have converged on a conception of the comprehension process as a stratified process involving multiple levels of representation of language and of semantic information. The semantic information associated with discourse has been recognized as including not only that specifically encoded in language structures (propositions) but also that which must be inferred by a reader or listener. Such inferences allow one to understand the larger knowledge structure that is being communicated and how it relates to the situation in which discourse communication occurs. It is reasonably accurate to say that the history of psychological studies of discourse comprehension involved a progression from models that consisted only of processes for the generation of representations of language structures at the sentence level, to models that included processes for the interpretation of discourse in terms of high-level semantic representations or "mental models."

More specifically, this progression involved the addition of levels of representation in approximately the following sequence: (1) models involving only syntactic representations, meaning being associated with the lexical elements of a syntactic representation; (2) models involving the generation of propositional representations; (3) propositional models that include inferential operations applied to propositions to generate new propositions that elaborate, summarize, or relate propositions, and so forth; (4) models that include a process of integrating propositional information into connected semantic network structures, representations that are assumed to constitute the form of declarative knowledge in long-term semantic memory; and (5) models that include the generation of particular types of semantic network representations (i.e., frames, "scripts," or "schemata"). These semantic network structures were assumed to constitute the declarative forms by which our knowledge of the world is represented.

This development of a model of discourse comprehension has benefited from experimental demonstrations that processing at different levels occurs and is necessary in certain situations; advances in semantics and pragmatics within linguistic theory; increasingly precise formal models of semantic representations developed by psychologists, computer scientists, and linguists; and advances in the design of computer systems for natural language and semantic processing. One outcome of this progression is that semantic processing has supplanted syntactic processing as the central phenomenon of comprehension in discourse-

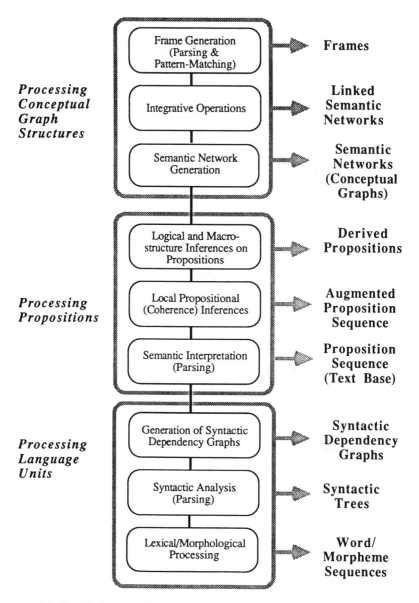

FIGURE 4.1. Stratified model of discourse processing. (Note. From "Monitoring cognitive processing in semantically complex domains" by C.H. Frederiksen and A. Breuleux (1989, in press), In N. Frederiksen, R. Glaser, A. Lesgold and M. Shafto (Eds.), *Diagnostic monitoring of skill and knowledge acquisition*. Hillsdale, N.J.: Erlbaum. Copyright 1989 by Lawrence Erlbaum Associates, Inc. Reprinted by permission.).

processing theory. In the description that follows we will describe the model that is being developed in our laboratory. While we will refer to similar work being undertaken at other laboratories, we will make no attempt at presenting a comprehensive account of work being done by other research groups.

The major levels of representation and processing that have been identified in stratified models of discourse comprehension are depicted in Figure 4.1. These involve representations of:

1. *Linguistic structures.* Word/morpheme sequences, syntactic trees, and syntactic dependency graphs (representing relations across syntactic trees).
2. *Propositions.* Representations of semantic information explicitly encoded in language structures, that is, the so-called text base; and inferred propositions that complete, elaborate, or connect local semantic information in a text (e.g., slot-filling inferences, inferences that resolve anaphoric reference, "coherence" inferences, and derived propositions that result from the application of logical or "macro-structure" rules to derive propositions that represent logical entailments of or generalizations of text propositions).
3. *Conceptual graph structures.* Semantic networks constructed to link propositional information into a connected memory structure; integrated semantic networks that link text-derived semantic information into prior knowledge structures in long-term memory; and conceptual frame structures that represent special types of network representations that embed descriptive information into high-level conceptual units.

Stratified models also have been developed in fields such as speech understanding (Ermann, 1977) and are similar in certain respects to stratificational and dependency syntax approaches in linguistics (Mel'cuk, 1979). The emphasis, however, in stratified models of comprehension is on semantic representations and the processing operations associated with them.

Representation of Linguistic Structures

We may identify three levels of representation of linguistic structure that are involved in providing input to the propositional-analysis component: *word and morpheme sequences* (which form the input to the syntactic parsing component), *syntactic parse trees* (which summarize syntactic information available to the semantic-analysis component), and *syntactic dependency relations* linking information across syntactic trees [e.g., anaphoric relations such as pronoun-referent ties (Halliday and Hasan, 1976) and topical patterns across sentences (Grimes, 1975)].

Convincing arguments for modular processing in sentence interpretation have been given based on experimental evidence (e.g., Ferreira and Clifton, 1986; Seidenberg and Tanenhaus, 1986). Properties of these various linguistic representations are known to exert independent effects on comprehension (Graesser,

Hoffman, and Clark, 1980) and to represent expressive alternatives in systems for text generation (McKeown, 1985).

Propositional Representation

In current theories, a proposition is regarded as an intermediate semantic representation that is specialized both for the representation of chunks of conceptual information in natural language and for logical reasoning. As a semantic base for natural language, propositions represent categories of semantic information that are distinguished in natural language sentences. As a basis for reasoning, propositions serve as truth-valued and quantified predicates for logical reasoning operations (Sowa, 1984), probably according to a fuzzy logic (Zadeh, 1974).

Current propositional models (such as that of Frederiksen, 1975, 1986) are capable of representing a great variety of semantic relations and structures found in natural and formal languages. These include the following types of information.

1. *Events.* A complex structure consisting of an action that causes a change in a state or process together with the agent or cause of that action plus other "resultive case relations" that specify the internal structure of the event and any "identifying relations" that specify properties of actions such as attributes, location, time, duration, and the like.
2. *Systems.* A complex structure composed of an object or objects and a "process" that characterizes the object or objects plus additional "processive case relations" that identify any related objects, states, actions, or processes that define the internal structure of the system, and any "identifying relations" that specify properties of the process (as for actions, previously).
3. *States.* Objects together with "identifying relations" that specify properties of the objects as well as their determination and quantification.
4. *Propositional relations.* Abstract concepts representing propositions (called "proposition identifiers") together with "identifying relations" that specify properties of abstract concepts.
5. *Identities.* Relations linking concepts or propositions into identity sets.
6. *Algebraic relations.* Transitive and intransitive "order" and "equivalence" relations applied to variables that may represent values identified in other propositions.
7. *Functions.* Operations defined on "operands" (variables identified in other propositions) that return "values" (e.g., distance, difference).
8. *Binary dependency relations.* Relations that make one proposition depend on another such as "causative relations," "conditional relations," and "logical implication" (material conditional and material biconditional).
9. *Conjoint dependency relations.* "And," "alternating or," and "exclusive or" relations.
10. *Tense, aspect and iterative components.* Components that specify temporal properties of propositions.

11. *Modality and truth value components.* Components that specify the asserted truth conditions for propositions.

Propositions are generated from syntactic trees and semantic markers in the lexicon. The only specifically linguistic information that occurs in propositions are lexical identifiers of concepts.

In addition to propositions that are encoded directly in natural language, propositions may be derived using local coherence inferences that bridge gaps or represent relations among a sequence of related propositions in discourse (Townsend, 1983; Tyler, 1983), or rules that summarize or extend the literal discourse meaning through the application of macro-structure and logical operators (van Dijk and Kintsch, 1983). Sowa (1984) has demonstrated how the operations of a first-order predicate calculus can be applied to predicates whose internal structure reflects the categories of semantic theories at the propositional level, and Emond (1989) has added this capability to our computer model and is currently working on rules for the resolution of problems of anaphora that operate on natural language or propositional representations. The general approach to inference is to write classes of rules that apply to propositional trees and that return new trees or modify the propositions on which they operate.

In stratified models of comprehension, the generation of propositions provides the semantic base information from which the construction of conceptual graph representations takes place.

Conceptual Graph Representations

Conceptual graph theory provides a bridge from the semantic representation of natural language as propositions to the structure of meaning in memory as conceptual frames. Conceptual graph representations (or, alternatively, "semantic networks") are connected network structures that are assumed to provide the means by which knowledge is represented in long-term memory. Unlike propositions, conceptual frames are not cut up into isolated chunks of information; they are networks of interconnected conceptual units.

Research in the field of knowledge integration (Hayes-Roth and Thorndyke, 1979) has shown that when relational links between concepts are expressed close together in a text (i.e., within propositions or neighboring propositions), subjects are likely to learn the relationships; but when they are expressed in widely separated parts of a text, subjects are less likely to remember the relationships. Furthermore, specific integrative operations are required to connect text information to information already in memory (Kubes, 1988). Such experiments suggest that there are distinct processes associated with linking conceptual information into a network that are required when information is not directly linked within propositions. This process is referred to as "semantic network generation" when it operates within a text and "integration" when it operates on existing semantic networks representing prior subject-matter knowledge in long-term memory. Integrative processes include a variety of retrieval, inferential, and reasoning processes that operate in using prior knowledge to understand or interpret new text-derived conceptual information.

In addition to such descriptive conceptual networks constructed from a propositional base and prior knowledge, research on the comprehension of particular types of texts such as stories, procedures, narratives, dialogue, and problems has demonstrated that text understanding involves in addition high-level knowledge about these structures (Frederiksen, 1985, 1989a). Both canonical frame and semantic frame grammar approaches have been proposed to characterize this knowledge of high-level conceptual frame structures.

Types of conceptual frames that have been studied include:

1. *Narrative/causal event frames* representing temporal and causally connected event structures (Frederiksen, Donin-Frederiksen, and Bracewell, 1986; Trabasso and Nichols, 1980).
2. *Procedural frames* representing declarative knowledge of procedures (Frederiksen and Breuleux, in press; Frederiksen, 1989b).
3. *Problem frames* representing the structure of problems and problem solving, a principal component of a "story grammar" (Newman and Bruce, 1986; Frederiksen, 1989a; Gick and Holyoak, 1983; Stein and Policastro, 1984).
4. *Descriptive frames* of various types (e.g., locative frames representing spatial-locative information, taxonomic systems representing classifications and definitions, logical frames representing proofs or derivations, part structures representing decompositions of complex objects, etc.).
5. *Dialogue frames* representing conversational structures composed of illocutionary events and relations (Frederiksen et al., 1986; Frederiksen, 1989a; Grosz, 1980; Sanford and Roach, 1987).

Frames define knowledge in various content areas and reflect conceptual structures of these types. For example, knowledge of procedures in chemistry is structured in terms of procedural frames together with descriptive frames, which represent the scientific knowledge underlying the procedure. Discourse comprehension can involve both the use of preexisting frame structures retrieved from memory to interpret new information or the generation of new frame representations when relevant prior knowledge is absent.

There is abundant evidence in the experimental literature to support the contention that frame-based processing is important to the comprehension of texts expressing information interpretable in terms of one or more types of conceptual frames, and that frame-level processing may be either "knowledge based" (i.e., involving the instantiation of frames previously stored in memory) or "rule based" (i.e., generated by means of the application of rules in a frame grammar).

The Semantic Representation of Discourse

In this section we discuss the problem of definition of a formal structure to model semantic representations of natural language discourse. We will discuss what is required for a definition of propositions and of particular types of conceptual frames. We will also discuss how these definitions, specified as "semantic grammars," are linked to procedures for generating them. The example and discussion are adapted from material previously presented (Frederiksen and Breuleux, in press). For a discussion of the computer implementation of the model, see Frederiksen, Décary, and Hoover (1988).

Canonical Frames and Semantic Grammars

Formally, a semantic network (or "conceptual graph") is a type of data structure composed of two kinds of entities: nodes and links (or arcs). The basic structural unit is a relational triple composed of two nodes that are connected by a link into a relational structure. Networks are data structures composed of sets of relational triples. Nodes are either simple or complex. Simple nodes, *S-nodes*, refer to: (1) lexical concepts, (2) primitive concepts defined by a particular semantic model, or (3) proposition identifiers; complex nodes, *C-nodes*, are nodes that are explicitly decomposed in a network into other nodes. *Links* are identified by names referring to the type of relation represented by the link.

To illustrate these ideas, consider the example in Figure 4.2, which contains a semantic network generated for the following sentence taken from a procedural text in chemical engineering.

Collect the samples in an air-tight bottle.

In the figure, nodes in the network are enclosed in rectangles and relational links are enclosed in ellipses. Examples of S-nodes are "samples," "DEF," and "7.2," and an example of a C-node is "OBJECT." Notice that an OBJECT node is decomposed into a S-node and another complex node (DETERMINER). Arrows in Figure 4.2 either connect nodes to links or connect C-nodes to other nodes that decompose them. In the theory of conceptual graphs, S-nodes contain "identifiers," entities that label semantic information. This information may be (1) a "primitive concept" (e.g., "TOK," token, a primitive determiner defined within the model), (2) a "lexicalized concept" represented by a word in the lexicon, or (3) a "proposition identifier," a numeric label for a proposition or word referring to one or more propositions.

A proposition is a particular type of network structure, specified by a model, that is composed of nodes and relations, has a truth value, and is a unit of semantic information that may be expressed in natural language. In Figure 4.2 there are three propositions: one event (proposition 7.1) and two states (propositions 7.2 and 7.3). When an arrow points from a relation to a proposition number (e.g., from RESULT.REL to "7.2"), the proposition labeled by the identifier is embedded in the node linked to the relation, that is, within another proposition. In the example, propositions 7.2 and 7.3 are embedded within 7.1 (i.e., in the "result node"). In Figure 4.2, positive truth value is implicit and is not marked explicitly.

To define a semantic network model requires (1) specification of the content of all nodes, (2) definition of all relational links and primitive concepts, and (3) specification of all patterns of relational structures and node decompositions that are permitted. Any model of semantic representation may be examined in terms

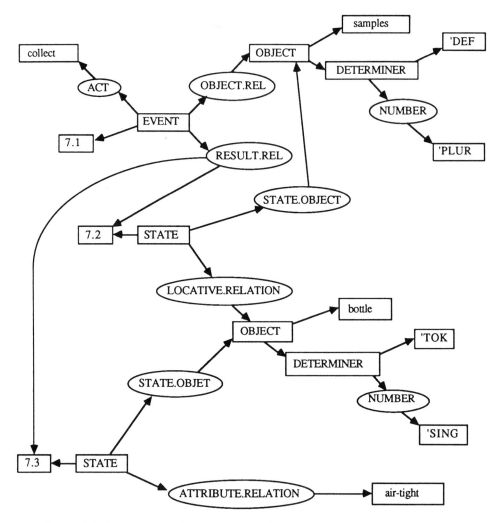

FIGURE 4.2. Conceptual graph representation of example sentence: "Collect the samples in an air-tight bottle." (Note. From "Monitoring cognitive processing in semantically complex domains" by C.H. Frederiksen and A. Breuleux (1989, in press), In N. Frederiksen, R. Glaser, A. Lesgold and M. Shafto (Eds.), *Diagnostic monitoring of skill and knowledge acquisition*. Hillsdale, N.J.: Erlbaum. Copyright 1989 by Lawrence Erlbaum Associates, Inc. Reprinted by permission.).

of how it accomplishes these specifications. Two approaches have been taken in the literature on semantic representations to defining a semantic representation model: definition by means of "canonical frames" (Schank, 1975; Sowa, 1984), or definition by means of "semantic grammars" (Frederiksen, 1986).

A "canonical representation" (or "frame") is a particular network structure or pattern that contains "variables." Variables are symbols in a pattern that can be replaced by specific values. For example, in proposition 7.1, all S-nodes might be replaced by variables.

```
(EVENT (7.1) (ACT(X)) (OBJECT.REL(OBJECT(Y) (DETERMINER
(P)(NUMBER (Q)) (RESULT.REL(Z) ('POS))*
```

which could be bound to (i.e., "assigned") the values given in proposition 7.1. Such a canonical frame could include "constraints" on values of variables; for example, X might be constrained to be a class of actions that includes "collect," Y might be an object, and Z might be constrained to be a stative proposition or propositions specifying a location. A canonical frame defined in this way thus is capable of representing a large number of structures, or "instantiations." The canonical frame approach to defining a propositional representation consists of defining an exhaustive set of such patterns, each of which represents a particular type of structural possibility. In computational semantic systems adopting this approach to propositional analysis, the set of such frames is stored in a dictionary. In linguistic terminology, this is an example of a "slot grammar." The power of a slot grammar depends on the number and kinds of canonical frames included in the dictionary.

A "semantic grammar" adopts a generative approach to definition, specifying a model by means of rules that generate all acceptable patterns within the grammar. It is well known within the theory of generative grammar that a relatively small set of recursive rules can be much more powerful than a large set of canonical frames. To illustrate, in Figure 4.3 we give the subset of rules from the semantic BNF grammar for propositions developed by Frederiksen (1986; Frederiksen, Décary, and Hoover, 1988) that are required to generate the conceptual graph in Figure 4.2. Rules are applied in order. Each rule specifies how a structure corresponding to the rule name may be formed by applying other rules (that are "called"). Eventually, the sequence of rules leads to lexical or proposition identifiers, or primitive concepts. The rules of this grammar are written so that rules whose names do not begin with the symbol # write their names into a parsing tree when they are applied. By this means, the application of rules directly generates a conceptual graph representation for each proposition.

Generating Propositions: Frame Instantiation and Parsing

These two approaches to defining a semantic representation have been associated with different computational approaches to generating propositions from natural language sentences (Ritchie, 1983). In the first approach, called "frame instantiation," propositions are generated by finding a canonical frame that can be matched to an input sentence. Frame matching normally involves matching semantic structures to syntactic patterns that instantiate them and assigning variables values derived from sentence information (e.g., lexical values). Canonical frames are often specific to particular entries in the lexicon (e.g., verbs), so that

---

*Here the graph structure is represented in terms of its list structure representation.

#PROPOSITION ::= EVENT I STATE I PROPOSITIONAL.RELATION I IDENTITY.RELATION
    ALGEBRAIC.RELATION I FUNCTION I BINARY.DEPENDENCY I
    CONJOINT.DEPENDENCY

EVENT ::= #PROP.NUMBER ACT #CASE.FRAME {#ACT.IDENTIFYING.RELATION}* {#TENSE}
    {#ASPECT}* {#ITERATIVE} {#MODALITY}* #TRUTH.VALUE*

ACT ::= #ACT.IDENTIFIER I 'EMPTY I 'WH-QUES

#CASE.FRAME ::= #PROCESSIVE.CF I #RESULTIVE.CF I 'EMPTY.CF

OBJECT.REL ::= #AFFECTED.OBJ* I 'EMPTY I 'WH-QUES

#AFFECTED.OBJ ::= OBJECT I #PROPOSITION.LABEL*

RESULT.REL ::= #RESULT* I 'EMPTY I 'WH-QUES

#RESULT ::= OBJECT I #PROPOSITION.LABEL*

STATE ::= #PROP.NUMBER STATE.OBJECT #STATE.IDENTIFYING.RELATION* {#TENSE}
    {#ASPECT}* {#ITERATIVE} {#MODALITY}* #TRUTH.VALUE*

STATE.OBJECT ::= OBJECT* I 'EMPTY I 'WH-QUES

OBJECT ::= #DETERMINED.OBJECT I #PRONOUN.IDENTIFIER I #PROPER.NOUN.IDENTIFIER

#DETERMINED.OBJECT ::= #OBJECT.IDENTIFIER DETERMINER I #PROPOSITION.LABEL
    DETERMINER

DETERMINER ::= #NON.GENERIC I #GENERIC

#NON.GENERIC ::= #NG.DETERMINER #NG.QUANTIFIER {DETERMINER}

#NG.DETERMINER ::= 'DEF I 'TOK

#NG.QUANTIFIER ::= NUMBER I DEGREE

#STATE.IDENTIFYING.RELATION ::= CATEGORY.RELATION.STATE I IS.A.RELATION.STATE I
    PART.RELATION.STATE I IS.PART.RELATION.STATE I ATTRIBUTE.RELATION I
    LOCATIVE.RELATION I TEMPORAL.RELATION I DURATIVE.RELATION I
    THEME.RELATION

ATTRIBUTE.RELATION ::= #ATTRIBUTE.IDENTIFIER {DEGREE}* {ATTRIBUTE.RELATION}* I
    'EMPTY I'WH-QUES

LOCATIVE.RELATION ::= #LOCATION* I 'EMPTY I 'WH-QUES

#LOCATION ::= #LOCATION.IDENTIFIER {DEGREE}* I OBJECT I #ACT.IDENTIFIER I
    #COORDINATES

NUMBER ::= #INTEGER I #NUMBER.IDENTIFIER {DEGREE}* I 'SING I 'PLUR I INTEGER.PAIR I
    'EMPTY I'WH-QUES

#TRUTH.VALUE ::= 'POS I 'NEG I 'INT

BNF Notation: Uppercase identifier = a rule name
                Quoted uppercase identifier = a primitive concept
                a # at the beginning of a rule name = a "hidden" rule
                ::= following a rulename = a rewrite rule
                I = or (choice among rule sequences separated by this symbol)
                { } enclose rules that are optional
                * following a rulename indicates that the rule is repeatable
                rules are applied in sequence given in the grammar

FIGURE 4.3. Subset of rules from the propositional grammar required to generate the example in Figure 4.2. (Note. From "Monitoring cognitive processing in semantically complex domains" by C.H. Frederiksen and A. Breuleux (1989, in press), In N. Frederiksen, R. Glaser, A. Lesgold and M. Shafto (Eds.), *Diagnostic monitoring of skill and knowledge acquisition*. Hillsdale, N.J.: Erlbaum. Copyright 1989 by Lawrence Erlbaum Associates, Inc. Reprinted by permission.).

much of the work that is done in building such a computational system involves building canonical frames into the lexicon.

In the second approach, "semantic parsing," rules in a semantic grammar have associated with them tests that are applied to lexical, morphological, and/or syntactic representations of the sentence being analyzed and to information (e.g., semantic markers) in the lexicon (Frederiksen, Décary, and Hoover, 1988). If the conditions associated with a test are satisfied, the rule is applied to generate a node in a parsing tree and transfer control to other rules (that are called by the rule). Most semantic parsing systems purport to carry out direct semantic parsing, that is, parsing in which there is no prior syntactic analysis of a sentence input to the system. However, Ritchie (1983) has observed that such systems inevitably incorporate syntactic categories into their semantic rules. Psycholinguistic evidence (Ferreira and Clifton, 1986; Morrow, 1986) and considerations involved in text generation systems (in which sentences are generated from semantic representations; McKeown, 1985) dictate a "mixed" approach to semantic parsing.

Generating Conceptual Frames

Conceptual frames also may be defined either by means of semantic grammars or canonical frames. While both approaches have been proposed, in theory and research on discourse comprehension the latter, referred to as "schema theory," has been the most popular in research on reading comprehension (Rumelhart, 1980). However, the considerations raised previously in relation to propositional models apply to frame representations as well. A rule-based model would seem to be required to account for the ability to construct new representations when existing frames are not appropriate to the interpretation of new information.

Conceptual frame representations may be illustrated using the example of Figure 4.2. This sentence was taken from a chemical (pulp and paper industry) text that describes a procedure for measuring the amount of solids in the liquor produced in the production of wood pulp. This text was analyzed by applying a procedure frame grammar that consists of rules specifying the components of a procedure and their relations to other procedure components. These procedure relations define the high-level structure of a complex (i.e., multicomponent) procedure. These rules are illustrated in the following listing, which gives semantic information required by the grammar to represent the component procedure (together with its relations to other components) in the example sentence.

```
(PROCEDURE.COMPONENT (PROC.NAME P7 collect liquor samples)
  (PROC.DESC
    (ACT(ACT.IDENTIFIER collect))
    (PROC.CASE.FRAME
      (PROC.SOURCE.REL EMPTY))
      (PROC.RESULT.REL (7.2) (7.3))
```

```
        (PROC.GOAL.REL EMPTY)
        (PROC.AGENT.REL EMPTY)
        (PROC.INSTRUMENT.REL EMPTY)
        (PROC.OBJECT.REL (OBJECT(samples) (DETERMINER(DEF)
            (NUMBER PLUR))))
      (TRUTH.VALUE POS))
   (PROC.SITUATION.DESC (7.3))
   (PROC.PRODUCTION.RULE (EMPTY))
   (PROC.RELATION
      (RELATION.ISPART(PROC.NAME P6))
      (REL.COND (PROC.NAME P19.1))
      (RELATION.CATEGORY (PROC.NAME P5.1))
      (RELATION.CATEGORY (PROC.NAME P5.8))))
```

The grammar defines a "procedure component," one node in a network representation of a procedure. A complex procedure is represented by a "procedure frame" consisting of a set of linked procedure components. For each procedure component, four types of information are required: (1) a "description" of the component (PROC.DESC) that includes information defined by the semantics of events and actions, (2) a "situation description" (PROC.SITUATION.DESC) that includes propositions specifying any states necessary to the procedure, (3) "production rules" (PROC.PRODUCTION.RULE), which are tests of conditions necessary for the enactment of the procedure, and (4) any "relations" linking the procedure to other procedures (PROC.RELATION). The relations for a set of procedure components define a procedural frame as a network in which nodes represent component procedures and links represent procedural relations connecting the nodes (see Figure 4.4). In the example the following relations link this procedure component to other procedure components: procedure component P7 is linked to procedure components P5.8 and P5.1 by "category relations," it is a *part* of procedure component P5.0, and it is *conditional* on procedure component P4.4. The "part relation" generally provides the basis for a hierarchical structure of a procedure in which general components are subdivided into more specific components.

Control of Processing during Comprehension

Research on discourse comprehension has dealt extensively with the problem of control of processing during comprehension. In any complex multilevel process,

▶

FIGURE 4.4. Graph of procedural frame representation for the text containing the example in Figure 4.2. (Note. From "Monitoring cognitive processing in semantically complex domains" by C.H. Frederiksen and A. Breuleux (1989, in press), In N. Frederiksen, R. Glaser, A. Lesgold and M. Shafto (Eds.), *Diagnostic monitoring of skill and knowledge acquisition*. Hillsdale, N.J.: Erlbaum. Copyright 1989 by Lawrence Erlbaum Associates, Inc. Reprinted by permission.).

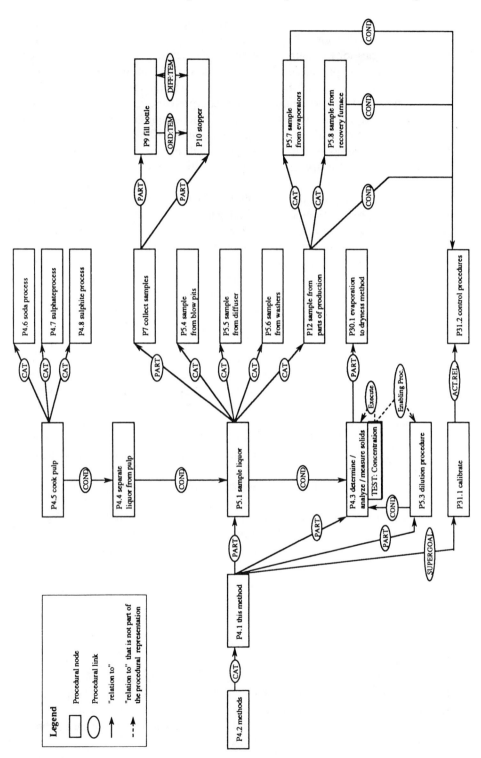

issues of control or management of processing occur. Researchers have given consideration to the normal flow of control in discourse understanding and explicit strategies for managing the processing of texts.

In the earliest comprehension models, the flow of control was assumed to be "bottom-up" or "text driven" (i.e., from the bottom to the top of Figure 4.1). In a bottom-up model, syntactic information is interpreted semantically, and propositions are constructed as component information becomes available. For example, when an "agent" is identified from a possible representation of "agency" in syntax, the agent component of a proposition would be generated. By this means, semantic forms are constructed from syntactic structures.

In a "top-down" model, the flow of control is the reverse. The reader is assumed to generate propositions (or other semantic representations) either by instantiating representations already existing in memory or by applying semantic rules. For example, in a rule-based system a procedure for generating propositions may look for evidence of an event in the currently available syntactic and lexical information, then, given such evidence, enter an event marker into a propositional data structure (i.e., a parse tree) and, finally, transfer control to the next rule that looks for an action, and so forth. In such a system the flow of control is reversed; lower levels of analysis serve the purpose of providing information pertinent to tests associated with high-level semantic rules.

In terms of the complete stratified model, control is assumed to flow from frame-level rules (e.g., if a procedural text is being read, the reader is assumed to be seeking information that completes a representation of the procedure). There is abundant evidence that top-down processes occur in comprehension, both from recall and on-line measures such as reading times and concurrent interpretations (Frederiksen and Renaud, 1987; Renaud and Frederiksen, 1988). In our computational model, the generation of propositions involves top-down application of rules, but there is also a bottom-up component that determines the likely number of propositions.

To supplant the normal flow of control, readers can employ specific control strategies that are based on their goals, the situation of text use, relevant prior knowledge (Frederiksen, 1989a; van Dijk and Kintsch, 1983), and monitoring of their own processing (Brown, 1980; Brown, Campione, and Day, 1981). While such high-level "meta-comprehension" strategies in reading comprehension have been demonstrated, they have not been identified in terms of how they relate precisely to the processing of discourse representations.

Discourse Production

In the production of discourse a process similar to that of comprehension takes place, but the problem is, in a certain sense, reversed. The production process may be thought of as proceeding from the specification of a conceptual representation to the generation of sentences in discourse. Unlike comprehension, the problem is gradually to constrain the production of semantic and language structures. In comprehension, there is a high degree of constraint on the generation of structures as one moves from text to conceptual representation, but in writing there frequently is very little specification of constraints on what is to be produced. Consequently, the writer must define strategies to guide the composing process as well as satisfy general "pragmatic" (e.g., coherence, relevance), "semantic" (e.g., to communicate particular knowledge), and "textual" constraints (e.g., topicalization, reference) that apply to her written product.

Levels of Processing in Text Generation

When text generation is viewed from the standpoint of the stratified model discussed in relation to comprehension, a number of distinct processes become apparent. In order to translate a conceptual representation into a text, a series of decisions must be made that successively constrain production until a unique linguistic structure is produced. Research on children's text production (Frederiksen et al., 1986) and on student writers' composing and revising operations (Bracewell, 1987; DeRemer and Bracewell, 1989) has demonstrated that writers do demonstrate an ability to manipulate both semantic and textual structures and to coordinate the two. However, experimental research on text generation is far less advanced than research on comprehension, and computer text generation systems have not yet provided truly comprehensive models (McKeown, 1985; Mann, 1984).

Nevertheless, it is possible to identify a series of modular component processes that enter into the generation process. These may be organized according to the type of structure they generate or operate on, (1) conceptual networks, (2) propositions, and (3) natural language structures. Each component process is necessary to establish constraints on the choice among alternative semantic and syntactic structures at the level of generation of sentence and textual structures.

While these processes will be described in terms of a sequence of operations in generation, it is by no means assumed that processing is necessarily sequential. An important goal for our research on production during the next few years is to construct and test computer models of these component processes and use them to study different strategies for controlling their application during text generation.

Processes Operating on Conceptual Networks

Frame Generation

If the goal of communication is to transmit an understanding of one or more conceptual frames (e.g., of a procedure, a narrative-causal event structure, a taxonomic system, or a problem) the generation of a discourse begins with the generation of one or more conceptual frames, or the retrieval of a frame structure from one's prior knowledge. The frames act as organizing principles for the discourse. If a writing task does not explicitly involve a particular type of conceptual frame structure (e.g., as in writing purely descriptive text on a topic), more general semantic network structures are involved. In such situations, it seems likely from research on planning in writing that writers implicitly organize their generation of descriptive semantic information in terms of a procedural frame (e.g., a plan or routine procedural strategy such as the production of an outline). A frame can be generated in two ways: by applying rules of a semantic frame grammar or by filling slots in a canonical frame that is already a part of memory structure.

Elaboration of Descriptive Networks

When a frame structure has been generated, descriptive semantic information is required to complete the specification of the frame. For example, a narrative-causal frame establishes event structures, but a detailed description of the internal structure of events, and states or situations surrounding them, is required to specify fully the events, their participants, and where and when they take place. The frame provides the superstructure that is "filled out" by networks of descriptive semantic information.

Integration of Semantic Information

As descriptive networks are generated, they may be linked to semantic networks already produced by means of integrative operations. The result of operations integrating semantic information is a more connected representation. Integrative operations also can lead to further elaboration of the network. These operations of elaboration and integration satisfy the pragmatic requirement of being complete.

Selection and Topicalization of Information

The translation of a fully specified conceptual structure (as produced by the preceding operations) would normally lead to extremely long and detailed discourse. In normal discourse communication, decisions are made as to what information to express explicitly and what to assume is already known to a reader or might be inferred on the basis of prior knowledge. Therefore, operations are required to select information for explicit communication to a reader. In addition, since topic structure is well known in studies of comprehension to (1) reflect the distinction between information that is assumed to be given and that which is new, and (2) signal priority of information to a reader, a writer must establish a prioritization of information for introduction as topics in discourse. Selection of topics is necessary to constrain order of introduction of information and selection of sentence structures to express information in text.

Processes Operating on Propositions

Sequential Generation of Propositions

To encode selected information in sentences, a complete specification of propositions is required. For example, sentences normally require a tense, aspect, modality, and truth value as well as specification of all information required by a given type of proposition. Since propositions represent discrete units of information, they are generated in a sequence that reflects the selection and topicalization of information from the descriptive network.

Local Inference and Selection of Propositions

A sequence of propositions must satisfy criteria of local coherence, that is, there must be inferential links from one propositional structure to the next. Propositions must be generated so that these links are either explicit or are likely to be inferred by a reader. A writer, therefore, makes local coherence inferences and decisions related to his assumptions about the likely inferences of a reader in the propositional context as well as the pragmatic situation of discourse communication (Morgan and Sellner, 1980).

Logical and Macro-Structure Inferences on Proposition Sequences

As local stretches of propositions are generated, criteria of logical development and summarization (e.g., through topic sentences) are frequently applied in writing. This entails a process of generating or evaluating logical and macro-structure inferences for the stretch of text.

Chunking of Propositions for Linguistic Encoding

One important property of text demonstrated in research on comprehension as having an important impact on a reader is "propositional density," the number of propositions encoded in a single clausal structure. Since natural language syntax theoretically places no limit on the number of propositions per clause, propositions must be chunked for encoding into a single linguistic structure. Chunking of information seems to be a mechanism for binding propositions together into units so that they are likely to be understood in terms of a connected semantic unit.

Processes Operating on Natural Language Units

Generation of Clauses to Reflect Chunking and Topicalization

The next step is the linguistic encoding of chunks of propositions. The generation of sentence structures reflects choice among alternative linguistic encodings to reflect the topicalization of information as well as the propositional content.

Specification of Lexical Information in Clauses Including Anaphoric Elements

Finally, all content words within sentences must be specified. Lexical specification may reflect common lexical identifiers for concepts already associated with propositions, modifications to common (default) lexical choices to improve style, and replacement of content words with anaphoric markers. The use of anaphoric markers enables the writer to produce shorter texts and to increase the likelihood that links will be made across semantic information expressed in different sentences.

Flow of Control in Structure Generation

The production of discourse results from the execution of a sequence of operations to build or retrieve an abstract conceptual network of information and to transform it, through a certain number of levels of representation, into a material, grammatical, and linear discourse structure. Processing within and among various levels of representation involves transformations that can be achieved through a top-down or bottom-up flow of control.

Through a top-down flow of control, a writer initially determines some conceptual structures and gradually instantiates these into discourse. This type of processing relies mainly on strategies for retrieving information from memory and emphasizes the rules responsible for the coherence of these information structures. The writer must also select from the frame structure a restricted quantity of information, eventually organizing it according to specific purposes, and specify the exact content of the propositions. At the level of surface structures, the task implies operations using the rules of syntax and lexical decisions to produce syntactic units in a language (clauses).

A bottom-up flow of control involves mainly linear coherence relations among units at lower levels of representation and establishing their relationship to conceptual representations. Thus, the writer generates sequences of propositions that make a coherent progression or development of a topic and then later edits them to make them adhere to an organizing conceptual frame. For example, in writing instructions, an initial draft may reflect a sequential production of steps of actions that are later edited to reflect their role in the procedural frame.

Normally both top-down and bottom-up processing would be expected to occur as mappings are established between conceptual/semantic structures and discourse structures. Studies of editing demonstrate writers' ability to operate in both ways (Bracewell, 1987; DeRemer and Bracewell, 1989).

Constraints on Structure

Representational structures at each level are defined by formation rules that can be considered as a set of constraints on the production process. These constraints also include earlier parts of the discourse that a speaker/writer produced. The usual task analysis for writing, for example, includes constraints that are internal to the writer and constraints that come from the external environment of the task. A first set of internal constraints is the availability of "declarative" information in memory, at the conceptual and lexical levels. Qualitative as well as quantitative characteristics of relevant prior knowledge affect the production of discourse (Voss, Vesonder, and Spilich, 1980). A second set of constraints is the availability of "procedures" for the construction and manipulation of both conceptual and linguistic structures. These include rules for expanding and modifying the conceptual information retrieved from memory and rules for generating language structures related to conceptual information. Discourse structures are produced according to two major levels of constraints: they must encode information that corresponds to propositions, and they must signal the higher-level structure of the frame in which the propositions take part. Recent studies show that even young writers are capable of exerting control over the construction of syntactic units in order to reflect the frame structure of the discourse (Bracewell, 1987). External constraints on writing or speaking involve mainly the characteristics of the hearer or audience, the genre, the situation of communication, and the purposes of the writer (Frederiksen and Dominic, 1981).

Writing tasks vary in the level of structure that they impose on the writer. For example, an extremely constrained writing exercise would be to produce a description of a simple sequence of events following its temporal order. In such cases, writing requires a detailed representation of the events in memory, and some skill in expressing that content in linguistic structures, but it involves few processing alternatives because the structure of the text to be produced is dictated by the structure of the events. Less constrained writing situations, in which the experimenter does not control the input to the task, usually involve more reorganization: the writer has some idea of the goal text, but no immediately available ways to achieve that goal. In these situations the writer must resort to more complex strategies.

Processing Strategies in the Production of Discourse

The multiple and simultaneous constraints imposed on the writer/speaker are sufficiently complex to warrant viewing the production process as a problem-solving task. Writers/speakers must operate on an initial situation—the information in memory—and transform it into another situation—discourse—that constitutes the goal of the problem. In terms of Greeno's (1978) typology of problems, the strong components of the problem are "arrangement" and "transformation." In contrast to well-defined problems, however, most of the information needed to attain a solution (selected information from memory and mapping rules from one representation to another) is not given as part of the problem. The production of discourse representations from knowledge structures implies the ability to generate and evaluate potential solutions at different levels; in this type of arrangement problem the search space is particularly vast and the discovery of a solution requires the availability of principles to avoid verifying all possible solutions randomly. In addition to these arrangement processes, once some content has been generated and/or selected, writing involves transformation processes to build language structures that correspond in specific ways to the semantic structure.

Planning as a Major Strategy in Writing

Planning is recognized as the strategy fundamental to attaining a solution in transformation problems. In writing, planning provides a useful strategy because it enables the exploration at an abstract level of the rich network of possible solutions, whereas the actual undertaking of these solutions would be time consuming and cognitively costly. By planning, a writer can delay much of the lower-level decisions, such as the specific ordering of goals and the elaboration of surface structures. The importance of planning in writing has been emphasized in research on writing (Breuleux, 1988a; Butterworth, 1980; Flower and Hayes, 1981; Matsuhashi, 1987). However, planning has not been tightly connected to these semantic and linguistic representations whose possibilities of arrangement and transformation define the boundaries of the problem space.

Planning is generally defined as the hierarchical and sequential organization of goals and subgoals representing a course of action (Newell and Simon, 1972). It consists in the "abstraction" of objects and operators of a problem to create a manageable representation in which a blueprint for the solution in the original problem space is produced. This process permits the exploration of a number of possible solutions by searching through a small and abstract problem space as opposed to working out a solution in the original, detailed problem space.

Planned writing involves setting up plans and executing them. The elaboration of a plan can be conceived of as the organization of goals that are associated with the communication of specific content, and the execution of the plan as the actual writing, that is, the realization of goals as sequences of propositions and linguistic structures in text. The execution phase consists essentially of producing grammatical sentences to form a text according to the goals in the plan that controls the actions. Plans, however, can appear at various levels along the hierarchy of processing described in this chapter. Initial content-related plans that encompass the whole text to be produced can be considered highest in the hierarchy, together with overall rhetorical plans (e.g., to convince or to trick the reader). More local plans are subordinated to goals that are set earlier, or do not involve new content but lower levels of the writing process (e.g., signaling or syntax). The objective of protocol analyses of writers' planning specifically concern the extent to which, in writing, the high-level decisions made during planning interact with decisions made at lower levels during the execution of plans. For example, detailed analyses of writers' think-aloud protocols show that subexpert writers produce shallow plans that are expanded, modified, or executed according to local properties resulting from earlier actions (see Breuleux, 1988a). Finally, plans can be routinized as procedures for particular registers or writing tasks such as generating an outline or following a script for an experimental article in psychology. In such cases, planning is largely superseded by a process of following a known generation procedure.

Methods for Studying Discourse Processing

The theory that we have elaborated provides a principled basis for the development of precise methods for assessing the processing operations underlying discourse comprehension and production. In this section we will review the three main methods for assessing discourse abilities: (1) discourse analysis of texts presented to or produced by an individual, (2) assessment of discourse comprehension, and (3) assessment of discourse production. For each method, we will consider the quality of the method in providing unambiguous information about both underlying representations and discourse-processing operations.

Discourse Analysis

The models of discourse representation discussed previously provide the basis for specific discourse-analysis procedures. Such analysis proceeds formally by applying the rules underlying either a particular representation (sentence parsing, a propositional grammar, etc.) or a type of operation on representations (e.g., a type of inferential rules) to a discourse. Assume that the rules underlying a particular representation are completely specified in the form of a grammar. Then the analysis can proceed in three ways: (1) by hand (requires complete knowledge or documentation of the rules), (2) with the assistance of a computer program that helps the analyst apply the rules, and (3) automatically by means of a computer program. In our laboratory we have developed computer software that assists in the application of rules to the analysis of discourse. This program, called CODA (for *Co*gnitive *D*iscourse *A*nalysis) interprets a grammar provided to it and generates dialogue questions to which the user responds. As rules are applied to a discourse, the program creates a list structure representation of the parse tree and displays it graphically on the screen. The program eliminates errors in analysis that are attributable to incorrect application of rules. It is currently used for propositional and frame analysis and can be used for syntactic parsing of sentences or application of other (e.g., inferential) rules. Syntactic analysis of sentences in a discourse is most efficiently carried out using an automatic parser.

Discourse analysis is normally carried out in steps, beginning with clausal analysis (if a complete syntactic analysis is desired), then propositional analysis to specify all propositions encoded in sentences, then construction of the semantic network from propositions (this step requires resolution of anaphoric reference) and, finally, frame analysis. We hope eventually to have enough rules in the proposition grammar implemented in our computer model to carry out automatic propositional analysis. For a more complete discussion of discourse analysis based on cognitive models, see Frederiksen (1986).

In assessing discourse abilities, three strategies can be used that apply discourse analysis methods.

1. *Development of a model of a discourse presented to subjects*. The strategy, most often adopted in experimental studies of text comprehension, is to carry out an analysis of the text presented to subjects and then to use this analysis to predict measures obtained during reading or post-hoc measures obtained using postinput tasks such as recall or question answering. By matching subjects' responses to units such as propositions from the text analysis, one can study information

acquired and inferences made on the basis of the text's propositional content. Selective recall and inference for information in frame structure provides strong evidence for frame-level processing of text. For example, Frederiksen and Renaud (1987) compared text measures reflecting a number of levels of text representation to predict recall, on-line interpretation protocols, and reading times and obtained evidence of processing at multiple levels during input and for parallel and top-down processing.

2. *Development of a reference model of expert knowledge.* A second method applicable to both comprehension and production applies discourse-analysis methods to protocols obtained from experts in a subject-matter domain to construct models of expert knowledge (Frederiksen and Breuleux, in press; Kubes, 1988). Segments from a subject's discourse or protocol are matched to nodes and links in the expert model to assess conceptual knowledge referred to in the protocol. For example, in studies of the writing of instructions, an expert model of a procedure is developed and used to analyze writers' strategies for incorporating conceptual information into their texts (Donin, Bracewell, Frederiksen, and Dillinger, in prep.). Inferences can be made about many of the component processes involved in writing in this manner.

3. *Discourse analysis of subjects' productions.* A third method is to apply discourse-analysis methods directly to the discourse produced by a subject. While this method is most costly, it can yield the most complete information about the discourse representations that are derivable from a subject's production. Machine analysis of discourse will be required to make this feasible as a routine research or assessment method. Breuleux (1988b) has successfully used machine analysis to analyze writers' plans from think-aloud protocols previously analyzed into propositions.

Assessment of Discourse Comprehension

In this section we will review methods used for the assessment of discourse comprehension and discuss the psychological assumptions they presuppose. "Product-oriented (post-hoc) methods" focus on assessing the memory representations that remain after a comprehension task has been completed. These include most conventional measures of comprehension such as recall, question answering, and the like. Increasingly, these methods are used in combination with "process-oriented (on-line) measures." These measures, such as reading times and on-line interpretations, are now widely used to study directly cognitive processes used during reading or other on-line performance based on text. When only post-hoc methods were used, processes had to be inferred from the occurrence of semantic information in recalls. The problem of post-hoc data is that they do not permit the direct study of processes as they occur during performance on the task. By combining post-hoc methods with on-line methods, semantic information and processing reflected in postinput memory structure can be traced to its locus of generation during input processing.

Product-Oriented (Post-Hoc) Methods

Recall and Probed Recall

The recall paradigm has been the most important method employed in testing and developing models of reading comprehension. Typically, characteristics of the comprehension process and representations are inferred from analyses of the match of semantic structures produced by a subject during recall, to semantic representations of the text. Analyses of products of comprehension yield data pertaining directly to the memory representation constructed by a reader. The processes that generated this representation are inferred from the mapping between a formal text representanatation and the information in the subject's recall protocol.

In this post-hoc method a free recall is obtained from a subject after some input task (e.g., reading a text). To assess the semantic representation acquired by the subject, propositions represented in a subject's recall protocol (at output) are compared to a detailed propositional analysis of an input text. One reason for the popularity of the recall method is that no new information is introduced into the assessment task that could lead the subject to modify her cognitive representation. However, a problem with free recall is that the subject's production during recall may not include information that is part of her memory representation. To overcome this problem, probes may be used to assess particular parts of the conceptual or propositional structure of the text. When probes are introduced, they must be carefully constructed to exert minimal biasing influence on the subject's representation.

Simple measures that have proven to be very useful in assessing processing at the propositional level are: number of propositions recalled, propositions recalled with inferential modifications (e.g., filling of empty slots), or propositions that served as a basis for generation of new inferred propositions. This coding, based on a systematic and reliable decision procedure, can be augmented by a coding of types of inferences and their locus of application to structural elements within a proposition. This categorization of inferences is based on a propositional model and requires, in addition to mastering the semantics of propositions, the development of a list of acceptable paraphrases and synonyms of terms and a set of inferential operators that are used to classify transformations of propositional information.

Recall protocols can also be evaluated to see how they reflect higher levels of conceptual representation and processing. Evaluation of frame structure can be carried out in two ways. First, selective recall and inference for propositions having particular roles in instantiating frame-level structure can be assessed by analyzing differential recall and inference for propositions classified in terms of the frame structure of the text. Second, information in a recall protocol can be matched directly to a "conceptual frame model" of the text (or to an "expert knowledge or task model" that includes text knowledge as a subset). In this case, the coding of a subject's protocol is against units (nodes and links) in the expert

model rather than to text propositions. The expert model is developed from protocols of experts elaborating the knowledge required to understand a text fully.
Coding against an expert model directly evaluates the subject's prior knowledge
in the domain or knowledge that the subject has acquired (regardless of whether
it was directly instantiated in text propositions or inferred). Thus, it provides a
means for studying semantic processing operations at the frame level (e.g.,
integration and frame generation). Of course, nodes and links in the expert model
that were instantiated explicitly in the text can be identified to keep track of the
subject's inferences.

To summarize, matching a subject's recall to text propositions enables an
assessment of how the subject operated on text information; matching to an
expert model enables assessment of how the subjected operated on knowledge
structures in memory.

Choice Response Tasks

A common method for assessing comprehension in standardized tests is to obtain
subjects' responses to yes-no questions based on a text. Multiple-choice questions
have also been widely used in which a subject has to select a sentence that is correct from among a set of alternatives. There are numerous advantages to this
approach: it is an objective measurement, it can be analyzed with standard
statistical tools, and it is an easy task to build quantitative models for the data.
However, there is often an inadequate theoretical specification of how these
questions were constructed. In the absence of such specification in terms of text
information and operations required to answer the question, it is not clear what
a test composed of such items measures. Moreover, frequently such items can be
answered simply by locating factual information in a text presented together with
the items. Pourafzal (1984) demonstrated that answering questions with a text
present is not a good measure of comprehension (as assessed by recall), even
when the questions require free verbal responses. However, when the text was
not made available to subjects while they answered the questions, question
answering provided a much better assessment of comprehension.

Choice-response questions could be improved if questions were constructed on
the basis of a semantic model of the text, an expert model, and an analysis of the
operations required by a subject to answer questions, and if the task required that
questions be answered on the basis of a subject's memory representation and
without access to the text. However, the possibility would remain that the answer
was based on inferences made during response to the question rather than on
processes occuring during comprehension.

Question Answering Requiring Natural Language Response

Most natural questions are not simple yes-no questions but, instead, invite complex verbal responses. Therefore, a more open-ended type of question requiring
answers in the form of verbal protocols is necessary to assess more fully question
answering based on text-derived or prior knowledge. The two major areas of

research on questions in cognitive science are "question construction" and "question answering" (Graesser and Black, 1985). Answering a question requires that there is compatibility between the information required for answering and a person's knowledge representation of this information, in addition to knowing why the question is being asked. This requires an identification of both processes and knowledge structures underlying questions. Constructing questions requires that we relate the information to be processed for answering to a reference model. Frederiksen and Breuleux (in press) have presented a general approach for monitoring and evaluating knowledge. This approach is based on the detailed analysis of semantic information at various levels, from the propositional information to high-level frames.

Process-Oriented (on-line) Methods

The on-line study of comprehension tries to identify the temporal organization of the various component processes involved in processing text and the manner in which they interact. Real-time measures that are typically used are eye movements and reading times for various units of text (Rayner and Carroll, 1984; Haberlandt and Graesser, 1985; Renaud and Frederiksen, 1988). The underlying assumption is that the time spent reading each of these units is an indication of the amount of processing each requires. The assessment of correlations between real-time measures and theory-based components of a psychological process are taken as indicators of their contribution. One difficulty underlying this research is in specifying how temporal measures relate to specific discourse processes. Identifying theoretically based variables requires a detailed model. However, such a model often has been lacking in research applying this approach (Danks, 1986).

Segment Reading Times

This method measures reading times for segments of text such as phrases, clauses, or sentences that are presented one at a time on a computer screen. Reading times for segments such as clauses or sentences allow for all levels of processing to take place in parallel and avoid a major criticism addressed to the use of smaller units (e.g., words) that assume immediacy of processing (Mitchell, 1984; Aaronson and Ferres, 1984). Segments of various sizes have been used in studies of reading time, including phrases (Wisher, 1976), clauses (Carver, 1970), sentences (Graesser et al., 1980), and longer stretches of discourse (Coke, 1974; Kintsch and Keenan, 1973).

Eye Fixation Data

Eye movement data have been widely used in the study of reading, since it is a naturally occurring phenomenon that can be measured. It is reasonable to suppose that they indicate what might be going on during reading (Rayner, 1977; McConkie, Hogoboam, Wolverton, Zola, and Lucas, 1979). However, there has been considerable debate concerning the extent to which eye movements reflect the cognitive processing of text. Eye movement records do not directly provide a measure of processing time. They only indicate that the eyes fixated certain locations, in a particular sequence, and for a certain period of time. Processing-time profiles must then be constructed on the basis of assumptions concerning what the eye movements reflect. If more were known about specific relationships between cognitive processes and eye guidance mechanisms, more accurate profiles could be constructed but, until then, great care must be taken in interpreting these measures. Particular positions on these issues cannot be taken strongly, since there is little evidence on which to base them (Hogoboam and McConkie, 1981). In fact, the vast amount and high degree of precision of eye movement data stand in the way of a theory of reading (Rayner and Carroll, 1984). Researchers using them are still testing specific as opposed to more global hypotheses about cognitive processing in reading.

Think-Aloud and On-Line Interpretation Protocols

A major difficulty with reading time measures used alone is that time measurements do not provide direct evidence of the representation that is being generated or the operations that are being applied during reading. A possible solution to this problem is the collection of on-line interpretation or think-aloud protocols. This approach has been modeled on the use of think-aloud methods in the study of problem solving (Collins, Brown and Larkin, 1980; Ericsson and Simon, 1984). While the rigorous analysis of verbal protocols presents its own problems, the think-aloud method seems promising, especially if well-developed models of semantic processing and representation are applied to their analysis and interpretation (Olson, Duffy, and Mack, 1984).

A typical instruction to subjects for such a task is to express orally all ideas, associations, or thoughts that occur to them while reading (Ericsson and Simon, 1984). It is assumed that these processes are not unconscious, they occur slowly enough to be described by the reader, samples of them are sufficient for the experimenter to infer what went on, and the use of the think-aloud task does not itself influence text processing. Frederiksen and Renaud (1987) obtained evidence that an on-line interpretation task does not influence the normal processing of text. The use of the think-aloud method during comprehension can reveal the strategies used by a reader, the sources of knowledge employed, and the representations constructed.

Olson, Duffy, and Mack (1984) identify three major types of think-aloud tasks in reading comprehension research in which talking takes place after each sentence, selectively or retrospectively. In a "sentence-by-sentence" talking condition the subject is asked to talk after each sentence of the text, without being able to look at the next sentence. What is often varied is the extent to which the reader can look back at previous text. "Selective talking" implies that a subject will talk only at particular points in the text. One may have a process theory that pinpoints certain places in the text as crucial tests for an aspect of the theory, or there may be certain features of interest that occur at particular points in the text. In the last type of task, "after the fact talking," the subject gives an account of his cognitive processes only after a certain criterion is attained, a type of retrospective protocol. Ericsson and Simon (1984) point out that memory is too fallible to allow for accurate reporting of earlier mental states. This procedure should only be used with short texts or after a few sentences have been read.

An advantage of this method is that is provides rich material and is useful in helping to generate hypotheses. The types of elaborations that might help the reader remember a text can be directly observed. In addition, this method allows the use of ecologically valid texts that were not necessarily designed by experimenters for the purpose of controlling the experimental material. Other advantages of this method are that it provides a way of studying individual differences in higher-level processes and it correlates with other forms of reading behavior, such as sentence reading times.

Some problems of this method are that it is sensitive to instructional variables that have to be clear; it works better for certain kinds of texts than for others; data obtained are difficult to analyze; there are "good" and "bad" subjects for a think-aloud task—while training is possible, it is sometimes long; and, finally, the think-aloud method itself may influence the nature of the comprehension process. However, the greatest problem with verbal protocols has been in specifying the type of information that is of interest and in analyzing it. This problem is not so much inherent to the method but has been a result of the lack of a detailed model on which to base the analysis of verbal protocols (Breuleux, 1988b).

Identification of Comprehension Measures with Representations and Processes Specified in the Model

The most important criterion in selecting or evaluating measures of comprehension is the ability to identify unambiguously a measure with particular representations or processing operations. The previous discussion of individual measures noted the variability across methods in the quality of this identification. In general, we advocate the use of both post-hoc and on-line measures that are closely identified with units of information in a text or expert model and that reflect particular processing operations applied to these units of information. While it is desirable under certain circumstances to manipulate structures in texts presented to readers, we prefer the use of natural texts. High-level cognitive processes such as comprehension are so embedded in the knowledge people have that it is necessary to study them in a way that takes that knowledge into account. Kubes (1988) has shown that by using an expert model of knowledge in a domain as a reference model, it is possible to evaluate precisely prior knowledge and its use in comprehension and knowledge integration tasks. Expertise in comprehension in particular knowledge domains (such as chemistry) is heavily knowledge dependent. Therefore, methods for assessing comprehension should be capable of assessing a subject's knowledge, whether it is acquired from a text, already known, or inferred. By using well-identified post-hoc and on-line measures, it is possible to assess unambiguously specific representations and processes in comprehension.

Assessment of Discourse Production

Methods to assess subjects' ability and skill in producing discourse can be divided into two major approaches: product-oriented methods that are based on analysis of the structure of discourse that has been produced, and process-oriented methods that are based on information collected during the discourse and text production.

Product-Oriented Methods

Methods of assessment that are based on an analysis of the product can themselves be divided into two major approaches: subjective evaluations and analyses of text structure.

"Subjective evaluations" are methods that rate the overall quality of a text as a whole, or the quality of major characteristics of a text. In "holistic evaluation" the entire text serves as a unit to be rated; the measurement procedure itself can be either placement of a text on a scale or establishment of a ranking across different texts. In the simplest form of this type of assessment a text is evaluated on a single general criterion of quality. More complex holistic assessments, sometimes called "analytic evaluation," require ratings for a number of criteria, with organization, interestingness, and mechanics being the most common.

"Trait analysis" is a subjective method that is applied to major characteristics of a text. These characteristics, or traits, are defined through a rhetorical analysis that is applied to a text to determine salient themes and the manner of their presentation. For example, a text that advocates one side of a an argument might present counterarguments and then show why they are not valid. The presentation and refutation of counterarguments would constitute a primary trait of the text. A rater assesses the extent to which one or more of these traits are elaborated in a text, usually assigning a score from a scale for each trait.

In both types of subjective evaluation methods, the reliability of scoring is a major concern. To increase reliability, raters are usually trained on a subset of the texts to be scored, and benchmark texts that present salient features of the rating system are established and used as references throughout the scoring procedure.

Analyses of text structure are more objective methods that provide data on the representations that make up a text. According to the stratified theory of text generation, a text's representations occur at a number of levels and, consequently, analyses of text structures can be categorized on the basis of which level is being analyzed. The major division in structural analyses occurs between analysis of linguistic representations and analysis of conceptual (or semantic) representations. Within each of these general categories, structural analysis of further levels of representation can be undertaken.

Analyses of the linguistic structure of a text are made at three levels: lexical, syntactic, and suprasentential. "Lexical analyses" take a number of forms, depending on what the unit of lexical analysis is. If the unit is the individual word, dependent measures based on counts (fluency) are obtained. If the unit is occurrence of a word in the text, then measures of type/token ratios are obtained. Specific features of words can also be scored in reference to norms, yielding dependent measures for concreteness of vocabulary and frequency of use. These last measures are often combined to yield a readability index.

"Syntactic analyses" also take a number of forms. Simpler analyses are based on a parts-of-speech unit (e.g., noun, verb, or participle) and result in general indices of syntactic complexity. More complex syntactic analyses are based on parse trees for clauses as a unit. Such analyses provide more detailed data on syntactic complexity and on the types and range of syntactic structures used in a text. When combined with lexical counts (e.g., number of words per clause) or used to define syntactical "errors" and incomplete structures (false starts), indices are obtained that have been demonstrated to reflect the development of writing ability (Hunt, 1970; Loban, 1976).

Analyses of "syntactic dependency relations" reveal the structure of text across sentences. Cohesion analysis (Halliday and Hasan, 1976) takes as its unit the relationships between lexical items in a text (e.g., word repetition, anaphoric reference denoted by pro-forms, and conjunctions). Topical structure analysis is based on the constituent structure of clauses, taking as its unit the semantic information that appears in major constituent structures (e.g., subject position). Dependent measures for both types of analysis include: (1) frequency and variety of structure types in a text, and (2) relational measures that are combined with clause structure (e.g., number of clauses between a pronoun and its reference, and number of clauses in which the same information is maintained in topic position). Both types of measure have been found to index writing ability (Witte and Faigley, 1981; Witte, 1983; Bracewell, 1987).

Analyses of the conceptual, or semantic, structure of a text are made at two levels: the propositional and the frame level. The unit of the "propositional analysis" consists of a concept-relation-concept triple. Both concepts and relations are defined so that propositions can represent the detailed semantic and logical relations of the information that is presented in a text. A propositional analysis of a text yields a data base from which dependent measures can be derived. These include frequency and variety of structures and also relational measures such as the number of propositions per clause, referred to as propositional density.

A "frame analysis" of a text is conducted to represent the text's higher levels of semantic structure. Frame structures differ in type, each type being defined by a semantic grammar that specifies the constituents of the frame and the relations among constituents. As with a propositional analysis, a frame analysis of a text yields a data base from which dependent measures can be taken. These include frequency and variety of frame constituents and measures of the proportion of different frame structures in a text. In addition, in situations in which a semantic domain can be defined independently (e.g., a sequence of procedures for accomplishing a task), a comparison can be made between a frame representation of the situation and frame structures that subjects are able to produce in text (e.g., written instructions for carrying out the task).

One of the most promising areas of assessment concerns the development of methods that index the *relationship between linguistic and conceptual structure*. Global measures that relate these types of structures (e.g., propositional density) have been referred to previously. More sensitive measures are based on specific relationships between types of representation at the conceptual and linguistic levels. For example, it has been found in stories produced by children that whether information remains in topical position across clauses at the linguistic level depends on the narrative frame constituents at the conceptual level (Bracewell, 1986). Such findings revise the perspective on linguistic structure in assessment. Linguistic structures should not be evaluated in themselves, but rather for the role that they play in marking or signaling the conceptual structure of a text.

Process-Oriented Methods

Methods of assessment that are based on an analysis of the process of production consist of two major approaches: think-aloud protocols and timing measures of production.

"Think-aloud protocols" are records of verbalizations made by a subject as she is composing (see the previous discussion). The principal problem in using think-aloud protocols as an assessment device lies in the encoding of the verbalizations. That is, how can a coder recognize an instance of the use of an operation to elaborate a frame structure, for example? Breuleux (1988) has shown that the resolution of this problem lies in treating the think-aloud protocol itself as a discourse in order to apply discourse-analysis techniques that reveal the procedures that the subject is using to guide composing.

"Timing measures of production" are temporal records of the acts carried out by subjects in writing a text. The resolution of the unit of measurement can vary from the micro-level (e.g., keystrokes) to the macro-level (e.g., time to prepare a draft). Although the principal problem with such measures lies in inferring the production processes that they index, reference to the local text structure can be used to constrain the identification of processes. Such studies have revealed temporal features of planning when writing (Mastuhashi, 1981).

As is the case with reading-time measurements in assessments of comprehension, the true potential of these process-oriented measures would seem to lie in their integration with measures based on the analyses of text structure. Think-aloud protocols can provide data on at least part of the control structure and processes that are guiding text production; timing measures can provide an index of transfer of control between processes and the application of processes; and discourse analysis can specify the representations that are being constructed and modified. This combined approach would yield a record of operations made in real time of the production or revision of a text.

Identification of Production Measures with Representations and Processes Specified in the Model

A considerable variation in quality exists in the potential of the prior assessment methods for identifying characteristics of levels of representation and component processes in the production of a text. In general, the subjective measures are of little utility in focusing on either representations or processes.

Evaluation that is based on models of representation is more precise; however, the utility of such evaluation is likely to depend on the sophistication used in constructing dependent measures. This is perhaps best illustrated with a reference to specific studies. Loban (1976) conducted a longitudinal study that measured (among other things) the increase of syntactic complexity in writing for children from ages 5 to 17 years. Although the measures of syntactic representation used were both objective and precise, the semiinterquartile range of ability found for any one age tended to span plus or minus 3 years. That is, knowledge of the syntactic complexity of a child's writing provided only a very rough index of the degree of development. More significantly, this type of knowledge provides little direction about what should be done to improve or remediate writing. (One certainly would not want simply to advocate the writing of more complex sentences.) Contrasting data can be found in Bracewell (1987) from a cross-sectional study of children's text production at ages 7 and 9 years. This study also examined syntactic complexity, but the focus was on the use of sentence constituents as topical markers and their relationship to constituents of the narrative frame at the conceptual level. For certain types of marking, very consistent differences were found between the grades. For example, narrative frame constituents that signaled a change in time (e.g., "later that night") were almost always topicalized by the older students, whereas younger students showed no preference. Thus, for this particular measure, an age span of only 2 years shows a very strong developmental trend. In addition, the trend can be accounted for in principle by the communicative function of such a relationship between linguistic and semantic structure, and methods of instruction for promoting the relationship follow directly from the representations that have been identified.

A more adequate method for the identification and evaluation of production abilities will require the concurrent use of process-oriented methods. The semantic and linguistic structures (and their integration) that writers achieve in their texts are the products of specific processes. For example, writers must decide which components of a conceptual frame to elaborate and then implement a process (e.g., memory search) to achieve the elaboration. The characteristics of such decisions and procedures can only be determined through the use of process methods such as think-aloud procedures and timing measures.

Applications in Research on Brain Damage

The application of models of cognitive representation and processing of discourse in research on and assessment of brain-damaged subjects is important both for cognitive science and for medical research in brain science. As indicated in the introduction to this chapter, for cognitive science the dysfunctions associated with brain damage constitute an important domain for testing assumptions and examining adaptive properties of the cognitive system. For medical brain science, cognitive discourse models provide the basis for more specific assessment and diagnosis of brain dysfunction and for theoretically derived treatment methods that lead either to the recovery of function or the development of compensatory processes.

It is beyond the scope of this chapter to present a comprehensive review of literature on discourse-related deficits in brain-damaged subjects from the perspective of cognitive discourse models; however, something of the promise of this approach can be illustrated by discussing a specific study by Joanette, Goulet, Ska, and Nespoulous (1986) on discourse production in the brain damaged. This study is an exemplary one that employed both linguistic and semantic analyses of discourse and provided evidence that implied specific deficits in the cognitive processing of discourse. Because of the sophistication of the design and treatment of the data, the results of the study raise theoretical issues that can be addressed using the discourse-analysis methods previously summarized.

Joanette et al. studied the ability of right-brain-damaged subjects to produce a simple story orally from a short picture sequence. Story productions were analyzed at a number of levels of representation, including lexical (word count), syntactic (T-unit count), and propositional (number of propositions). Extensive exploratory analyses of the propositional data were carried out using cluster-analysis techniques to investigate empirically the semantic structure of the stories produced. Results revealed that (compared to hospitalized control subjects) brain-damaged subjects included fewer informative propositions in their stories despite producing as much language as the controls. Examination of the conceptual structures of the stories indicated that the brain damaged tended to include setting and resolution information rather than information that presented the complication in the story. Substantial overlap, however, in this pattern of structure existed between the brain-damaged and control groups. These results suggested that the brain-damaged subjects had a problem specifically with the organization of a specific type of conceptual representation in narrative discourse production.

The outcomes of the Joanette et al. study highlight research questions in the study of deficits in discourse processing that range from the processing of linguistic structures to the pragmatic context of text processing. These include the following.

How can deficits in linguistic as opposed to semantic functions be separated in the processing of natural-language discourse? Phrased more generally, the issue is how to isolate either a specific level for effects of processing or representation, or a particular process that mediates two specific levels. For example, is a deficit in propositional interpretation due to a breakdown in syntactic processing, rules for generating propositions, or the tests for syntactic instantiations of semantic rules? The first is purely linguistic processing, the second is knowledge of semantic structures, and the third mediates between the two.

The general solution for comprehension is to test with discourse in which syntactic and semantic structures are independently manipulated (e.g., syntactic structure, semantic structure, or the type of instantiation of propositional information in sentence syntax). A deficit in performance may be found to correlate with a particular manipulated structure. The difficulty in implementing this solution lies in the potentially large variety of texts and situations available and the constraints one level of structure imposes on another. For example, in one comprehension study it was found that when level in the hierarchy of topicalization of information in text (text level) was varied independently of level in a procedural hierarchy (conceptual level), both predicted recall and inferences based on text propositions and their interaction had only a minor effect (Frederiksen, 1989a). The stratified theory of discourse processing just presented provides a model of the structures that can be independently manipulated and of the constraints the one type of structure has on another.

In studies of production, the only way to eliminate this ambiguity is to look for or elicit productions in which one structure is manipulated independently of the other. For example, production tasks might require the production of different syntactic forms to express propositions or different propositional meanings, or they might exhibit or require independent manipulation of topicalization or conceptual hierarchies. This problem of ambiguity is illustrated by the Joanette, et al. finding that brain-damaged subjects produced relatively fewer complex propositions. This result may indicate dysfunction at the propositional level, or it may reflect a dysfunction at a frame level that has consequences for productions at the proposition level. If the effect were specific to the propositional level, however, it would be expected to appear independently of frame structure within a text; if the effect operates at a conceptual level it would be specific to particular frame-level conceptual structures.

Can deficits be demonstrated in comprehension or production that involve purely conceptual representations and functions and not linguistic processing? This issue is related to the issue of how to characterize effects as linguistic or conceptual. Specific conceptual deficits in discourse processing should reveal themselves in testing procedures that are nonlinguistic as well as linguistic. From the point of view of the stratified discourse model, semantic processing levels would be expected to function in the comprehension or verbal description of scenes, events, procedures, and so on. One way to assess deficits in nonlinguistic conceptual functions, therefore, is to use text materials in comprehension studies in which comprehension can be assessed nonverbally (such as the performance of textually presented instructions), or discourse produced on the basis of comprehension of natural activities (such as the demonstration of a procedure). A subset of the Joanette, et al. subjects seemed to have a deficit in organizing the "complication" content of their stories. In the stratified model, this content would be analyzed as a problem representation based on a procedural frame. If this deficit is truly conceptual, it should be observed also in subjects' comprehension of procedural demonstrations and performance of textually presented procedures.

To what extent are deficits in comprehension related to (or independent of) deficits in production? There are no "pure" tasks calling only for comprehension or production processes; instead, tasks can be arranged on a continuum of varying demand for comprehension as opposed to production processes (Bracewell, Frederiksen, and Frederiksen, 1982). The Joanette et al. task calls for comprehension of stimulus pictures as well as story production, and a careful concern of the authors for this comprehension component can be seen both in the attention paid to possible perceptual deficits and in the categorization of output as either "referential" or "modalized." (Referential content contains specific information on the persons, objects, and ideas of the story; modalized content has to do with the speaker's attitude toward what she is saying.) The propositional-analysis theory and methods outlined previously allow the direct analysis of the information that is presented in the picture sequences (Donin-Frederiksen, 1984) and can form the basis of a procedure (using questions for example) that would more directly test for comprehension of the picture stimuli. When paired with discourse-analysis techniques for text productions, such an approach would lead to the differentiation of comprehension and production processes.

How can texts be analyzed to provide unambiguous information about particular deficits in discourse representations? In their study, Joanette et al. adopted an exploratory-empirical approach to the examination of semantic structure of texts, using frequency data to establish important (or "core") propositions and cluster analyses to investigate patterns of propositional production. These techniques allowed them to observe a specific conceptual deficit in the story production of the majority of their brain-damaged subjects. Given the heterogeneity of the Joanette et al. findings, however, the further investigation of these effects is likely to require more powerful methods such as those deriving from the stratified discourse-processing model. This model provides a comprehensive and precise definition of representations and processes at the suprapropositional level in terms of conceptual frames. It specifies what is reflected in the propositions as opposed to using the co-occurrence of propositions to specify the semantic structure. Such models, when used with a variety of testing situations and subject populations, should provide unambiguous comparative data on specific dysfunctions in brain-damaged subjects.

How can textual or semantic structure differences be related to deficits in discourse-processing functions? The specific deficit in the Joanette et al. data was a reduced amount of information for the "complication" component of the story. This effect was not a simple problem of inferencing or organization, however, since deficit subjects tended to include a general proposition (that one protagonist had tricked another) that expressed the gist of the complication more frequently in their stories than nondeficit subjects. The constituents specified by the procedural frame grammar (which would apply to the complication content) of our discourse model provide a basis for testing the nature of this deficit. The presence or absence of particular constituents and the relations among them could be tested by means, for example, of probe questions motivated by the procedural frame model. Data from such a procedure would provide more convincing evidence related to the subjects' ability to elaborate and integrate the complication component of a story. In general, the types of discourse frames (dialogue, procedural, narrative, and descriptive) specified by the model provide a principled basis for the assessment of conceptual structure deficits in discourse processing.

Can specific deficits be found that affect the pragmatic aspects of discourse processing? As Joanette, et al. discuss, it is not clear from their data whether the semantic structure deficits were the result of a specific deficit in discourse processing or the result of a different pragmatic approach to the task. This is, of course, a problem in the interpretation of any effects for tasks in which the task definition itself is complex or must be constructed in large part by the subject. A precise discourse model can be used to examine the subject's comprehension or definition of the task situation and thus help establish whether an effect is attributable to a dysfunction or to a specific approach to the task, or it can be used as a basis for manipulating aspects of the pragmatic context (by providing different goals of communication, assumptions about the reader's or listener's knowledge, etc.; Frederiksen, 1988). Investigation of how the subject understands the task and uses pragmatic considerations to control production would be accomplished through analysis of discourse produced and of think-aloud protocols (Breuleux, 1988). It would seem, in fact, that verbalizations relevant to task definition appeared in the stories in the form of the modalized content that was produced. This type of verbalization can be an important source of data on discourse processing. It constitutes a type of think-aloud protocol in that it gives information about the author's stance toward the referential content as the story is being produced. The procedural frame models and coding procedures presented earlier and, in particular, Breuleux's research on planning, provide a method for analyzing such modalized content and determining in part how a subject defines a task.

There are two additional problems, not specifically raised in the Joanette et al. study, that also should be mentioned as potential sources of deficiency in discourse processing.

Is there any evidence that brain damage can produce deficits in the control of processing, that is, of disruption in either the normal flow of control of component processes, or plans or strategies that are used to organize the processing of discourse? Deficits may occur in the management of processing, both through a disruption of the normal flow of control or through a reduction in planning or the use of preestablished management methods (e.g., the ability to use an outline). For example, a disruption of the flow of processing in comprehension might involve the loss of top-down methods that are replaced by a bottom-up flow. This would be reflected in reading-time data as well as the locus of inferences related to propositional coherence and conceptual structure. Disruptions in plans or use of preestablished heuristic methods would be reflected in subjects' think-aloud protocols.

To what extent can deficits in discourse processing be traced to the loss of declarative knowledge, and what is the role of such memory loss in comprehension and discourse production? Research on both discourse comprehension and production has clearly established that discourse processing involves the use of prior declarative knowledge relevant to the content of text being understood or produced. Since brain damage can produce loss of information from memory as well as loss of functions, it is particularly important to determine the role loss of knowledge plays in a given patient. This would require an independent assessment of domain knowledge pertaining to a given discourse-processing task. Frederiksen and Breuleux (in press) have described methods for assessment of knowledge based on the use of semantic models, and these models could be used in studies with brain-damaged patients. Furthermore, if specific loss of knowledge is involved, the deficits observed should be found only in discourse processing involving that knowledge domain.

In summary, the research issues considered here constitute a "first pass" at a research agenda that would both test the models of discourse processing and representation developed in cognitive science and contribute to the understanding and assessment of discourse dysfunction associated with brain damage. Other issues could, of course, be added to the agenda. We feel confident, however, that cognitive discourse models such as that presented here can contribute in a major way to discourse-processing research in medical brain science, and that such studies would be a significant contribution to the cognitive science of discourse.

Acknowledgment. The research reported here was supported by grants from the Natural Sciences and Engineering Research Council of Canada; an Actions Structurantes grant from the Ministère de l'Enseignement Superieur et de la Science, gouvernement de Québec; the Social Sciences and Humanities Research Council of Canada, and the Fonds FCAR, Gouvernement de Québec.

References

Aaronson, D., & Ferres, S. (1984). Reading strategies for children and adults: Some empirical evidence. *Journal of Verbal Learning and Verbal Behavior, 23*, 189–220.

Bracewell, R.J. (1986). *Signalling semantic representation: The role of topical patterning in text.* Paper presented at the Fourth Annual International Conference on the Teaching of English, Ottawa.

Bracewell, R.J. (1987). *Semantic and textual constraints students use in revising their writing.* Paper presented at the annual meeting of the American Educational Research Association, Washington, D.C.

Bracewell, R.J., Frederiksen, C.H., & Frederiksen, J.D. (1982). Cognitive processes in composing and comprehending discourse. *Educational Psychologist, 17*(3), 146–164.

Breuleux, A. (1988a). *L'élaboration et l'exécution de plans dans une tâche de rédaction.* Unpublished doctoral thesis, Université de Montréal.

Breuleux, A. (1988b). The analysis of writer's think aloud protocols: Developing a principled coding scheme for ill-structured tasks. In G. Denhière & J.-P. Rossi (Eds.), *Texts and text processing*. Amsterdam: North-Holland.

Brown, A.L. (1980). Metacognitive development and reading. In R.J. Spiro, B.C. Bruce, & W.F. Brewer (Eds.), *Theoretical issues in reading comprehension*. Hillsdale, NJ.: Erlbaum.

Brown, A.L., Campione, J.C., & Day, J.D. (1981). Learning to learn: On training students to learn from texts. *Educational Researcher, 10*(2), 14–21.

Butterworth, B. (1980). Evidence from pauses in speech. In B. Butterworth (Ed.), *Language production, Vol. 1: Speech and talk*. New York: Academic Press.

Carver, R.P. (1970). Effect of a "chunked" typography on reading rate and comprehension. *Journal of Applied Psychology, 54*, 288–296.

Coke, E.U. (1974). The effects of readability on oral and silent reading rates. *Journal of Educational Psychology, 66*, 406–409.

Collins, A., Brown, J.S., & Larkin, K.M. (1980). Inference in text understanding. In R.J. Spiro, B.C. Bruce, & W.F. Brewer (Eds.), *Theoretical issues in reading comprehension* (pp. 385–407). Hillsdale, N.J.: Erlbaum.

Danks, J.H. (1986). Identifying component processes in text comprehension: Comment on Haberlandt and Graesser. *Journal of Experimental Psychology: General, 113*(2), 193–197.

DeRemer, M., & Bracewell, R.J. (1989). *Students' use of semantic structure in revising their writing*. Paper presented at the annual meeting of the American Educational Research Association, San Francisco.

Donin, J., Bracewell, R.J., Frederiksen, C.H., & Dillinger, M. (1989). *Students' strategies for writing instructions: Organizing semantic information in text*. Manuscript submitted for publication.

Frederiksen, C.H., Bracewell, R.J., & Donin-Frederiksen, J. (1984). *Toward a psychology of rhetoric*. Paper presented at the annual meeting of the American Educational Research Association, New Orleans.

Emond, B. (1989). *Charles S. Peirce system of existential graphs and automated reasoning*. Manuscript submitted for publication.

Ericsson, K.A., & Simon, H.A. (1984). *Protocol analysis: Verbal reports as data*. Cambridge, Mass.: MIT Press.

Ermann, L.D. (1977). A functional description of the Hearsay II speech understanding system. *Proceedings of IEEE-ICASSP*, Hartford, Conn., pp. 799–802.

Ferreira, F., & Clifton, C. (1986). The independence of syntactic processing. *Journal of Memory and Language, 25*, 348–368.

Flower, L., & Hayes, J.R. (1981). Plans that guide the composing process. In C.H. Frederiksen & J.F. Dominic (Eds.), *Writing: Process, development, and communication, Vol. 2*. Hillsdale, N.J.: Erlbaum

Frederiksen, C.H. (1975). Representing logical and semantic structure of knowledge acquired from discourse. *Cognitive Psychology, 7*, 371–458.

Frederiksen, C.H. (1986). Cognitive models and discourse analysis. In C.R. Cooper & S. Greenbaum (Eds.), *Written communication annual: An international survey of research and theory, Vol. 1: Studying writing: Linguistic approaches*. Beverly Hills, Calif.: Sage.

Frederiksen, C.H. (1989a). Text comprehension in functional task domains. In D. Bloom (Ed.), *Learning to use literacy in educational settings*. Norwood, N.J.: Ablex.

Frederiksen, C.H., & Breuleux, A. (in press). Monitoring cognitive processing in semantically complex domains. In N. Frederiksen, R. Glaser, A. Lesgold, & M. Shafto (Eds.), *Diagnostic monitoring of skill and knowledge acquisition*. Hillsdale, N.J.: Erlbaum.

Frederiksen, C.H., Décary, M., & Hoover, M.L. (1988). The semantic representation and processing of natural language discourse: Development of a computational model. *Proceedings of the International Colloquium on "Informatique et langue naturelle,"* Nantes, France.

Frederiksen, C.H., & Dominic, J.F. (1981). Introduction: Perspectives on the activity of writing. In C.H. Frederiksen & J.F. Dominic (Eds.), *Writing: The nature, development, and teaching of written communication*, Hillsdale, N.J.: Erlbaum.

Frederiksen, C.H., Donin-Frederiksen, J., & Bracewell, R.J. (1986). Discourse analysis of children's text production. In A. Matsuhashi (Ed.), *Writing in real time*. Norwood, N.J.: Ablex.

Frederiksen, C.H., & Renaud, A. (1987). *On-line processing of text propositions: Linking reading time, on-line interpretation and recall*. Paper presented at the joint meeting of the Canadian Psychological Association and the British Psychological Society, Oxford University.

Gidk, M.L., & Holyoak, K.J. (1983). Schema induction and analogical transfer. *Cognitive Psychology, 15*, 1–38.

Graesser, A.C., & Black, J.B. (Eds.). (1985). *The psychology of questions*. Hillsdale, N.J.: Erlbaum.

Graesser, A.C., Hoffman, N.L., & Clark, L.F. (1980). Structural components of reading time. *Journal of Verbal Learning and Verbal Behavior, 19*, 135–151.

Greeno, J.G. (1978). Nature of problem-solving abilities. In W.K. Estes (Ed.), *Handbook of learning and cognitive processes, Vol. 5: Human information processing*. Hillsdale, N.J.: Erlbaum.

Grimes, J. (1975). *The thread of discourse*. The Hague: Mouton.

Grosz, B.J. (1980). Utterance and objective: Issues in natural language communication. *AI Magazine, 1*, 11–20.

Haberlandt, K.F., & Graesser, A.C. (1985). Component processes in text comprehension and some of their interactions. *Journal of Experimental Psychology: General, 114*, 357–374.

Halliday, M.A.K., & Hasan, R. (1976). *Cohesion in English*. London: Longman.

Hayes-Roth, B., & Thorndyke, B.W. (1979). Integration of knowledge from text. *Journal of Verbal Learning and Verbal Behavior, 18*, 91–108.

Hogoboam, T.W., & McConkie, G.W. (1981). *The rocky road from eye fixations to comprehension*. Technical Report No. 207, Center for the Study of Reading, University of Illinois at Urbana-Champaign.

Hunt, K.W. (1970). Syntactic maturity in schoolchildren and adults. *Monographs of the Society for Research in Child Development, 35*.

Joanette, Y., Goulet, P., Ska, B., & Nespoulous, J.-L. (1986). Informative content of narrative discourse in right-brain-damaged right-handers. *Brain & Language, 29*, 81–105.

Kintsch, W., & Keenan, J.M. (1973). Reading rate as a function of the number of propositions in the base structure of sentences. *Cognitive Psychology, 5*, 257–274.

Kubes, M. (1988). *The use of prior knowledge in integration of information from technical materials*. McGill University, unpublished Ph.D. thesis.

Loban, W. (1976). *Language development: Kindergarten through grade twelve (Research Report No. 18)*. Urbana, Ill.: National Council of Teachers of English.

Mann, W.C. (1983). An overview of the Penman text generation system, Information Sciences Institute Report 83-114. Los Angeles, Calif.: University of Southern California.

Matsuhashi, A. (1981). Pausing and planning: The tempo of written discourse production. *Research in the teaching of English, 15*, 113–134.

McConkie, G.W., Hogoboam, T.W., Wolverton, G.S., Zola, D., & Lucas, P.A. (1979). *Toward the use of eye movements in the study of language processing.* Technical Report No. 134, University of Illinois, Center for the Study of Reading.

McKeown, K.R. (1985). *Text generation.* Cambridge: Cambridge University Press.

Mel'cuk, I.A. (1979). Studies in dependency syntax. Ann Arbor: Karoma Publishers.

Mitchell, D.C. (1984). An evaluation of subject-paced reading tasks and other methods for investigating immediate processes in reading. In D.E. Kieras & M.A. Just (Eds.), *New methods in reading comprehension research.* Hillsdale, N.J.: Erlbaum.

Morgan, J.L., & Sellner, M.B. (1980). Discourse and linguistic theory. In R.J. Spiro, B.C. Bruce, and W.F. Brewer (Eds.), *Theoretical issues in reading comprehension.* Hillsdale, N.J.: Erlbaum.

Morrow, D.G. (1986). Grammatical morphemes and conceptual structure in discourse processing. *Cognitive Science, 10,* 423–455.

Newell, A., & Simon, H.A. (1972). *Human problem solving.* Englewood Cliffs, N.J.: Prentice-Hall.

Newman, D., & Bruce, B.C. (1986). Interpretation and manipulation of human plans. *Discourse Processes, 9,* 167–195.

Olson, G.M., Duffy, S.A., & Mack, R.L. (1984). Thinking-out-loud as a method for studying real-time comprehension processes. In D.E. Kieras and M.A. Just (Eds.), *New methods in reading comprehension research.* Hillsdale, N.J.: Erlbaum.

Pourafzal, F.K. (1984). *Comprehension and question answering: A comparative study.* Unpublished master's thesis, McGill University, Montréal.

Rayner, K. (1977). Visual attention in reading: Eye movements reflect cognitive processes. *Memory and Cognition, 4,* 443–448.

Rayner, K., & Carroll, P.J. (1984). Eye movements and reading comprehension. In D.E. Kieras & M.A. Just (Eds.) *New methods in reading comprehension research.* Hillsdale, N.J.: Erlbaum.

Renaud, A. & Frederiksen, C.H. (1988). On-line processing of a procedural text. *Proceedings of the Cognitive Science Society,* Montréal.

Ritchie, G. (1983). Semantics in parsing. In M. King (Ed.) *Parsing natural language.* New York: Academic Press.

Rumelhart, D.E. (1980). Schemata: The building blocks of cognition. In R.J. Spiro, B.C. Bruce, & W.F. Brewer (Eds.), *Theoretical issues in reading comprehension.* Hillsdale, N.J.: Erlbaum.

Sanford, D.L., & Roach, J.W. (1987). Parsing and generating the pragmatics of natural language utterances using metacommunication. *Proceedings of the Ninth Annual Conference of the Cognitive Science Society,* Seattle.

Schank, R.C. (1975). *Conceptual information processing.* New York: American Elsevier.

Seidenberg, M., & Tanenhaus, M. (1986). Modularity and lexical access. In I. Gopnik (Ed.) *McGill studies in cognitive science.* Norwood, N.J.: Ablex.

Sowa, J.F. (1984). *Conceptual structures: Information processes in mind and machine.* Reading, Mass.: Addison-Wesley.

Stein, N., & Policastro, M. (1984). The concept of a story: A comparison between children's and teachers' viewpoints. In H. Mandl, N.L. Stein, & T. Trabasso (Eds.), *Learning and comprehension of text.* Hillsdale, N.J.: Erlbaum.

Townsend, D.J. (1983). Thematic processing in sentences and texts. *Cognition, 13,* 223–261.

Trabasso, T., and Nichols, D.W. (1980). Memory and inferences in comprehending narratives. In J. Becker and F. Wilkins (Eds.), *Information integration by children.* Hillsdale, N.J.: Erlbaum.

Tyler, L.K. (1983). The development of discourse mapping processes: The on-line interpretation of anaphoric expressions. *Cognition, 13*(3), 309–341.

van Dijk, T., & Kintsch, W. (1983). *Strategies of discourse comprehension*. New York: Academic.

Voss, J.F., Vesonder, G.T., & Spilich, G.J. (1980). Text generation and recall by high-knowledge and low-knowledge individuals. *Journal of Verbal Learning and Verbal Behavior, 19*, 651–666.

Wisher, R.A. (1976). The effects of syntactic expectation during reading. *Journal of Educational Psychology, 68*, 597–602.

Witte, S.P. (1983). Topical structure and recision: An exploratory study. *College Composition and Communication, 34*, 313–341.

Witte, S.P., & Faigley, L. (1981). Coherence, cohesion, and writing quality. *College Composition and Communication, 32*, 189–204.

Zadeh, L.A. (1974). Fuzzy logic and its application to approximate reasoning. *Information Processing, 74*, 591–594.

Section 2
Empirical Perspectives

5
Discourse Comprehension by Right-Hemisphere Stroke Patients: Deficits of Prediction and Revision

Raymond Molloy, Hiram H. Brownell, and Howard Gardner

Discourse: n. [L. *discursus*, a running to and fro] 1. A communication of thoughts by words; expression of ideas; conversation. (Webster's Unabridged Dictionary, Second Edition)

This etymological definition can serve as a useful reminder of some facts that will concern us. The first of these is that the meaning of a conversation does not follow simply from the meanings of the individual sentences that compose it—at least not in the way that the conclusion of a syllogism can be inferred directly from its premises. Instead, it is part of the nature of discourse that it requires a listener who must work to understand how different sentences or utterances are related. (See Chapter 2 for a discussion of the kinds of rules that govern conversations.) To be successful at this kind of understanding entails much more than a knowledge of what individual sentences mean. One must also know when words and sentences depart from their usual functions and how this discrepancy may relate to the speaker's own purposes or to the subject at hand. Both words and speech acts—declarations, commands, and questions—are like tools in this respect. One can, if one chooses, stir a cup of coffee with a knife; it is also possible to make a joke with a deadpan statement (Millikan, 1984, p. 1).

In this chapter, we describe how the ability to understand discourse can be impaired by damage to the right cerebral hemisphere. The discussion begins with a general introduction to deficits that result from right-hemisphere damage and a comparison of these with the better-known deficits that result from left-hemisphere damage. We then discuss two kinds of discourse impairment we have observed in right-hemisphere-damaged (RHD) patients. We conclude by placing these results in the context of recent work in related fields.

Stroke and Its Aftermath

The patients whom we test have each suffered unilateral brain damage as a result of stroke. A stroke, or cerebrovascular accident, is a disruption of the flow of blood to an area of the brain. Such disruptions can ensue from the buildup of artherosclerotic plaque on the walls of the cerebral arteries, and it is the subsequent oxygen deprivation that leads to the death of the starved tissue. Blockages of this kind occur most frequently in particular blood vessels (i.e., the middle cerebral arteries) and, as a result, certain areas of a stroke victim's brain are more likely than others to be damaged. In addition, there is sometimes considerable variation in the effects of damage to a particular neural area. The deficits described next, therefore, are usual, not universal, effects.

Patients who have suffered strokes in the right hemisphere do not usually exhibit the kinds of obvious language impairments that are common among left-hemisphere-damaged (LHD) patients. For example, RHD patients do not usually have difficulty naming objects or understanding most syntactically complex sentences. They may, however, have other language-related disabilities. Right-hemisphere-damaged patients have been shown to have difficulty understanding the significance of idiomatic and metaphoric statements (Myers and Linebaugh, 1981; Van Lancker and Kempler, 1987; Winner and Gardner, 1977) and to have difficulty interpreting and organizing paragraphs, conversations, and stories (Delis, Wapner, Gardner, and Moses, 1983; Gardner, Brownell, Wapner, and Michelow, 1983; Huber and Gleber, 1982; Joanette, Goulet, Ska, and Nespoulous, 1986; Moya, Benowitz, Levine, and Finklestein, 1986; Tompkins and Mateer, 1985; Stachowiak, Huber, Poeck, and Kerchensteiner, 1977; Wecshler, 1973). In addition, RHD patients can exhibit a variety of attentional, visuospatial, and prosodic disorders (e.g., Heilman, Bowers, Speedie, and Coslett, 1984; Heilman, Watson, and Valenstein, 1985; Hughes, Chan, and Su, 1983; Ross, 1981).

In contrast, the most striking impairment of patients who have suffered unilateral left-hemisphere brain damage is usually aphasia: a related set of language impairments that may impoverish the stroke victim's ability to speak, to understand syntactically complex sentences, or to understand the meanings of single words. The pattern of linguistic deficits varies with the site of lesion within the left hemisphere (Benson and Geschwind, 1985). Surprisingly, LHD patients often demonstrate a pragmatic understanding of discourse. (See, e.g., Chapter 8.) In particular, LHD aphasics can often make use of a speaker's gestures, facial expression, and tone of voice in addition to such language as they may understand in order to determine the main point of a story (Stachowiak et al., 1977).

Affective changes also differ with side of lesion, with the right hemisphere often described as dominant for many types of emotional processing (see Tucker, 1981; Tucker and Frederick, 1988, for reviews). In particular, RHD patients are more likely to become inappropriately jovial, disinhibited, or apathetic (Heilman, Bowers, and Valenstein, 1985; Tucker and Frederick, 1988; Weinstein and Kahn, 1955). It has long been noted that LHD patients are more likely to become depressed after their illness (Gainotti, 1972; Robinson and Benson, 1981). This asymmetry has been associated with left versus right frontal lesions. Recently, Robinson and his colleagues (Robinson, Kubos, Starr, Rao, and Price, 1985; see also Tucker and Frederick, 1988) have shown that the likelihood of depression is related to the anterior extension of left-hemisphere lesions. In contrast, the closer a right-hemisphere lesion is to the frontal pole, the less likely the patient will become depressed.

Despite an ability to understand single sentences, then, RHD patients are often decidedly impaired in their ability to communicate. Indeed, the right hemisphere may play an essential role in processing the inferences that are necessary to comprehend the uneven logic of discourse. To examine this possibility in detail, we have studied how well RHD patients comprehend four kinds of discourse: indirect requests, verbal irony, jokes, and simple inferences.

These four genres of discourse can be divided into two classes on the basis of what kind of inferences a listener must make to understand them. Both indirect requests and verbal irony, for example, require a listener to note the difference between the literal meaning of what a speaker says and what he or she means. They are thus examples of figurative language. When considered in isolation, such statements are ambiguous, and a listener must make use of contextual information to understand a speaker's intended meaning. Hence the flow of meaning is from context to sentence, and this kind of comprehension may be said to move from the top down as one's knowledge exerts its influence on one's interpretation of the figurative sentence. To understand this kind of language, then, a listener must use contextual knowledge to make assumptions or predictions about what a speaker means.

Both the jokes and the bridging inferences that we describe in a later section also turn on the interpretation of a single sentence. In this second group, however, the relationship between sentence and context is reversed. That is, the critical sentence—in the case of a joke, the punch line—alters one's initial assumptions instead of being altered by them. They are thus examples of comprehension that moves from the bottom up as one's understanding of the context changes in order to accommodate new information. This class of discourse, then, entails a major revision or repair component.

The studies described next focus on these two discourse processes separately; insofar as possible, the processing examined in each study is restricted to either revision or prediction, and the other processing requirements are reduced to a minimum. In addition, other channels of information relevant to discourse comprehension have been eliminated or controlled across studies. The verbal nature of most stimulus items used avoids visuospatial problems in the perception of facial expression, or the need to make sense of other visual cues. Care has also been taken to remove obvious prosodic cues to speaker meaning through the use of stimulus items that are spoken in a natural-sounding but neutral tone of voice (Heilman, Watson, and Valenstein, 1985; Ross, 1981).

Indirect Requests and Verbal Irony

An indirect request is a question that is meant as a request for action but that takes the form of an inquiry about a fact (e.g., "Can you fix the typewriter?"). Although such requests often employ conventional forms (see examples), it is not possible to know for sure how one should interpret them without knowing the context in which they occur. For this reason, they are a good example of the kind of discrepancy between sentence meaning and speaker meaning that can occur in conversation. Consider, for example, the question "Can you see the house number?" in the following two contexts: (1) spoken by a husband to his wife immediately after he has affixed a new number to their home; and (2) spoken by husband to wife as they drive down an unfamiliar road in search of a friend's new home. In the first context, one answers the question directly ("Yes, it's quite clear"); in the second, one responds to the indirect request ("Yes, it's 259"). In both cases context drives the interpretation.

Some authors argue that, when it is appropriate to do so, normal listeners are able to comprehend the nonliteral meaning of such utterances directly without a prior understanding of the literal meaning (e.g., Gibbs, 1986; but see Clark and Lucy, 1975, for an alternative view). Presumably, this direct access to the nonliteral meaning of an indirect request rests in part on the comprehension of prior context as a guide to interpretation. The focus of the research we present here, however, is on how indirect interpretations can be disrupted.

It is important to realize that even when a listener successfully infers that a speaker is making an indirect request, it is not simply the case that the literal alternative interpretation is suppressed. As the philosopher Ruth Millikan has pointed out, the situation here is similar to the way that declaratory statements are sometimes used as commands (e.g., "You will hike 50 miles with a pack before breakfast. You will proceed to the top of Mt. McKinley."). She writes, "The suggestion in using an indicative form for giving orders is that the one who receives the order is being presented with a *fait accompli* rather than with a choice. He is being told the *facts* about his future" (1984, p. 77).

Indirect requests make comparable use of the sentence form/speaker meaning discrepancy but for different ends. They are a polite form of expression because they concisely signal the speaker's assumption of goodwill between speaker and listener; they assume that if the listener *can* do X, he will. At the same time, such requests also place the options in the hands of the listener. As explained by Murphy (Chapter 2), the listener is given the option of not complying with the implied request for action because he or she may simply ignore this aspect of the utterance's meaning. To respond appropriately to the indirect request, the listener must use preceding context as a guide to the speaker's intended meaning (i.e., a request for performing some action). This kind of ambiguity is useful because it allows a single sentence to convey more meaning than a simple literal utterance.

Work by Hirst, LeDoux, and Stein (1984) and by Foldi (1987) has demonstrated that both LHD, aphasic patients and RHD, nonaphasic patients are impaired in their ability to use context to interpret indirect requests. (In some respects, the RHD patients in the Foldi study performed more aberrantly than the LHD patients.) However, both studies used stimuli that were in part pictorial (videotapes with dialogue on the one hand and still slides with taped dialogue on the other). In light of the visuospatial and paralinguistic deficits RHD patients typically exhibit, it was unclear whether their relative deficit would still be present when the stimuli were entirely verbal.

In order to answer this question, a group from our laboratory constructed a verbal test of indirect request comprehension (Weylman, Brownell, Roman, and Gardner, 1989). This test consisted of a set of short vignettes that described two characters engaged in some activity. Each vignette ended with a question that could be interpreted as either an indirect request or as a fact question. Half of the vignettes were designed to encourage the first interpretation, and half the second. After hearing a vignette, subjects were asked to choose the most appropriate response from a set of four choices: (1) an appropriate response to the question as indirect request; (2) an appropriate response to the question as literal inquiry; and (3 and 4) two distractor responses syntactically similar to, but different in content from, the first two responses. These last two responses were included to insure that patients were responding specifically on the basis of the information contained in the stimulus vignette.

In addition, the form of the question itself was also varied. Half of the critical utterances in each context condition were of a form conventionally associated with indirect requests (i.e., "Can you ...?" or "Could you ...?"); the remaining questions were of a form not canonically used in this way (i.e., "Are you able to ...?" or "Is it possible for you to ...?", cf. Clark, 1979). Together, the different wordings provided a test of whether the good or bad performance of different patient groups would be better attributed to use of context or to a focus on the superficial, surface form of an utterance.

Initially, the vignettes were presented (using a tape recorder) to RHD, LHD, and normal control subjects. LHD patients, however, found the task too difficult, and testing with this group was discontinued. The fourteen RHD patients and fourteen normal control subjects tested completed the task. Since most patients were recruited from a Veterans Administration Medical Center, the subject groups used in both this and the other studies from our laboratory were composed primarily of men. After the stimulus vignette was presented, a written set of four possible responses was given to subjects, which the examiner also read aloud. A subject then selected the most appropriate response.

Subsequently, a modified version of the same task was administered to twelve of the RHD patients who had participated earlier, and also to a group of twelve LHD, aphasic patients. In the modified procedure, subjects were allowed to read a typescript of the vignettes as they listened to them. After each vignette was presented in this way, the transcript was removed from view and the candidate responses were presented.

The results from this study indicate that RHD patients are not completely insensitive to the role of context in making sense of ambiguous questions; they were more likely to choose indirect responses in the indirect context, and they were more likely to choose direct responses in the direct condition. But they were shown to be significantly impaired in making this distinction when their performance was compared to that of normal controls. This basic finding successfully replicates those of earlier studies (Foldi, 1987; Hirst et al., 1984) and extends the domain of this deficit to a purely verbal task. When the performances of the RHD patients were compared to those of the LHD patients, no reliable statistical difference was found between the two groups' sensitivity to verbal context, although the pattern of means indicated that the LHD patients performed slightly less well than the RHD patients.

The data on the role that conventionality of wording plays in cuing subjects' interpretations are less clear but do not qualify the interpretation of the effects of context outlined previously. In fact, in the initial study, neither the RHD nor the control subjects were significantly affected by the conventionality of wording. This result is surprising. Clark (1979), for example, has reported that normal speakers are sensitive to such conventions. In the Weylman et al. study, however, the different contexts used were designed to be clear cases: examples that strongly encouraged or discouraged the indirect request interpretation. It is possible that for normal subjects conventionality of wording is of most use in ambiguous contexts — contexts where an indirect interpretation is possible but not clearly required. In the Weylman et al. stimuli, the difference between the direct and indirect conditions was, in general, quite clear. This finding suggests that the two variables (context and conventionality of wording) are, in fact, separate factors in comprehension.

On the retest that included LHD patients, both the LHD and the retested RHD patients demonstrated a small but statistically significant sensitivity to the conventionality of wording. The data on the sensitivity of RHD patients to conventionality of form are thus equivocal. In the absence of further evidence, there is not sufficient evidence for conclusions about this point. In either case, these patients' use of context to direct interpretation of the critical utterance was deficient, apart from whatever attention they paid to the surface form of the critical utterance.

One other general interpretation of RHD patients' impairment in this task needs to be considered. Several studies have documented that RHD patients tend to be literal in their interpretations of, for example, phrasal metaphors and idioms (Van Lancker and Kempler, 1987). However, the abnormal interpretation of indirect requests is not simply another example of pervasive literalness — by which we mean inability to understand anything other than the denotational meaning of a sentence. It was not the case that the RHD patients tested were uniformly more literal in their responses; instead, the major finding was that they did not *vary* their interpretations (as much as the control subjects) as a function of the preceding context. That is, the RHD patients were neither as literal as the control subjects in the direct interpretation (literal) condition, nor were they as nonliteral as the controls in the indirect condition. And, when compared to the LHD patients (in the modified version of the task), the RHD patients were, on average, reliably less likely to pick a literal interpretation than were the LHD patients. (There was no such main effect of subject group separating the RHD patients from the normal control subjects.) In sum, the impaired performances of the RHD patients reflect, to a large degree, a reduction in their use of prior discourse in a top-down manner.

Verbal Irony

Other kinds of figurative speech also capitalize on a listener's ability to negotiate the difference between sentence and speaker meaning. One may say the opposite of what one means to tease or to be sarcastic. Both are uses of verbal irony (Perrine, 1977). As with indirect requests, one uses contextual information as well as other cues to understand the intent of ironic statements. Here, too, context drives the interpretation.

One way in which the two forms of discourse differ, however, is in affective content. Ironic statements are usually made to be funny and/or to be sarcastic. Given the affective changes RHD patients sometimes experience, it is possible that they might demonstrate a selective impairment in the kinds of irony they comprehend.

Recently, researchers from our laboratory looked at the ability of RHD patients to understand verbal irony (Kaplan, Brownell, Jacobs, and Gardner, in press). Right-hemisphere-damaged and normal control subjects were again asked to listen to paragraph-length vignettes that ended in a critical sentence. Here, too, each vignette described a pair of characters engaged in some activity. One character's performance was always further described as good or bad, and each story ended with the second character's positive or negative comment about how the first had done. Together, the performance description and the comment were varied to create four possible performance-statement contexts. In two congruent contexts, the performance and the comment were either both positive or both negative; that is, the comment was literally true. In two discrepant contexts, the performance and the comment differed, and thus allowed the critical statement to be interpreted figuratively.

In order to know whether an ironic statement is meant to be supportive or wounding, one must know about the relationship between the participants in a conversation. Thus, to evaluate how well subjects would be able to use speaker motivation to interpret a critical sentence, a final variable was also included. The speaker of the final utterance in each vignette was always explicitly described as liking or disliking the performer. The following examples taken from the Kaplan et al. study illustrate a *poor performance—positive utterance* vignette presented first with a *friendly* and then with a *hostile* speaker-performer relationship.

Friendly:
Hal and Mark were both amateur golfers. Hal had played golf with Mark for years and liked him very much. Mark was entered in a tournament where he played very badly and kept missing easy shots. Hal watched the tournament, and afterwards he said to Mark, "You sure are a good golfer."

Hostile:

Hal and Mark were both amateur golfers. Hal hated Mark because Mark was not courteous to the other golfers and sometimes cheated. Mark was entered in a tournament where he played very badly and kept missing shots. Hal watched the tournament, and afterwards he said to Mark, "You sure are a good golfer."

As in the study by Weylman et al. described previously, subjects were given a typescript of each vignette to read as a tape of the vignette was being played. Again, the vignettes and final utterance were recorded in a natural, neutral-sounding tone of voice to remove obvious prosodic cues to sarcastic intent. A group of twelve RHD patients and a second group of twelve normal control subjects were tested.

After hearing each vignette, a subject was questioned first about the quality of the performance and about the speaker-performer relationship described. If the subject erred on either of these factual questions, he or she was asked to point out "where it says that in the story." Once it was assured that the subject knew how the speaker felt about the performer and knew too how the performer had done, he or she was given a multiple-choice question concerning the pragmatic intent of the utterance, that is, whether the speaker was (1) telling the truth; (2) joking or making fun; (3) trying to be sarcastic and nasty; (4) saying something wrong by mistake; or (5) telling a lie on purpose. (These functional descriptions, which had been refined on the basis of pilot work, were used instead of linguistic labels because they were easier to understand.)

The RHD patients and normal control subjects performed similarly in the congruent conditions. In these conditions both groups almost invariably described the speaker's statement as "telling the truth." This was true no matter how the characters' relationship or the performance description varied. In the discrepant conditions, RHD patients were significantly less consistent that the controls in their use of a speaker-performer relationship to interpret the intent of the final utterance. RHD patients were impaired in their ability to assign pragmatic motives accurately and to interpret a speaker's utterances on that basis.

As an illustration, consider how the RHD patients responded to the type of vignette just shown. For this combination of performance and utterance, the two most relevant interpretations were "telling a lie on purpose" and "trying to be sarcastic and nasty." When there was a friendly speaker-performer relationship, the control subjects most often opted for a lie interpretation (78 percent of their responses to vignettes with this relationship), that is, that the speaker was telling a lie to make the performer feel better. They rarely thought the speaker was trying to be sarcastic (11 percent), even though a literally positive utterance in the context of a poor performance could be considered the canonical situation for eliciting sarcasm (Clark and Gerrig, 1984; Gibbs, 1986; Jorgenson, Miller, and Sperber, 1984). With an opposite, hostile speaker motivation, the control subjects exhibited a very different view of the conversation and most often characterized the speaker as trying to be sarcastic (71 percent) and less often as telling a lie (22 percent). While the RHD patients showed a similar pattern, they were significantly less swayed by variation in speaker motivation. When provided a friendly speaker-performer relationship, the RHD patients chose the lie interpretation less often than the controls (36 percent versus 78 percent) and also chose the sarcasm interpretation more often (21 percent versus 11 percent). With a hostile relationship, the RHD patients were not as consistent as the control subjects in favoring sarcasm (51 percent versus 71 percent), often choosing instead "telling a lie on purpose" (24 percent versus 22 percent for the controls).

Together with previous work on indirect request comprehension, these results illustrate an impairment in interpretation of utterances in context, specifically when that context consists of a speaker's motivation to be supportive or hurtful. The utterances of most interest were all literally false and could be normally understood only in light of the preceding context. The RHD patients tested were not totally insensitive to this information, but they evidenced a decreased flexibility in its use. In addition, their explanations for their responses reflected a reduced capacity to reason on the basis of a speaker's motivations in conversation.

Jokes and Inference Revision

Both verbal irony and indirect requests are examples of discourse where context is used to give determinate meaning to ambiguous sentences. Our predictions are sometimes imperfect, however, and an attentive listener must also be able to revise the assumptions he or she makes in the course of understanding a story or conversation. An inability to engage in such revision can quickly lead to confusion. Without repair and updating, the mutual knowledge shared by participants in a conversation (a basis for effective communication) may rapidly diminish to the point where those involved are talking about very different topics and will misunderstand each other (Clark and Marshall, 1981).

In the studies we describe next, subjects were again asked to interpret stories that contained a critical final utterance. Here, however, the critical utterance was not an ambiguous statement, but one meant to alter the listener's understanding of what had been described previously in the discourse. The results are evidence for an impairment in the ability of RHD patients to use new information to revise their initial assessment of the context.

Jokes

Jokes are funny in part because they are misleading. Suls (1983), for example, describes two properties of narrative jokes that we have named *surprise* and *coherence* (Brownell, Michel, Powelson, and Gardner, 1983; Brownell and Gardner, 1988). When a joke begins, the listener must make initial assumptions about what is and will be occurring; the punch line is surprising because it disconfirms these assumptions. Thus, once the listener has been surprised, he or she must revise the initial assumptions in order to establish how the punch line can follow coherently from the opening. The following joke provides an apt example (Brownell et al., 1983).

The quack was selling a potion which he claimed would make men live to a great age. He claimed he himself was hale and hearty and over 300 years old.
  "Is he really as old as that," asked a listener of the youthful assistant.
  "I can't say," replied the assistant, "I've only worked for him 100 years."

At first, one assumes that the assistant's response will be an honest one. But the rest of his demurral—that he has worked for a century—is surprising, and a listener must reevaluate the significance of the utterance and its relationship to the opening in order to arrive at a coherent understanding of the joke. Thus one realizes that far from answering honestly, the assistant is simply performing his part of the ruse.

To assess the sensitivity of RHD patients to the roles that surprise and coherence play in narrative jokes, a group of twelve RHD patients and a second group of twelve normal control subjects were asked to choose the punch lines of jokes whose opening lines they had just heard. Subjects were tested individually and the jokes presented in succession. On each trial of a testing session, each subject listened to the opening of a narrative joke and subsequently decided which of a set of candidate statements was the best punch line. In addition to being read out loud, written versions of the candidate punch lines for each joke were also provided.

The most relevant alternative endings for the patent medicine joke are shown here.

Correct punch line. "I've only worked for him 100 years."
Non sequitur. "There are over 300 days in a year."
Straightforward ending. "I don't know how old he is."

The non sequitur and straightforward endings were included to test whether RHD patients exhibited deficits specific to either the surprise or coherence requirements of the narrative jokes. The non sequitur ending for the preceding patent medicine joke, for example, satisfies the first of these requirements since it is incongruent with what has come before, but not the second, since it cannot be reinterpreted to cohere with the opening. The straightforward ending is not surprising but is coherent in that it follows naturally from the opening. The premises of the experiment were that a consistent preference for the non sequiturs by RHD patients would be indicative of insensitivity to the coherence requirement, while a consistent preference for the straightforward endings would be indicative of insensitivity to the surprise requirement of narrative jokes.

Error analyses revealed that, in addition to making more errors than normal controls, RHD patients did show a selective impairment in their comprehension of the jokes. While the groups did not differ in the proportion of straightforward out-of-total errors, RHD patients were significantly more likely than normal controls to choose non sequitur endings. That is, although they realized that the ending of a joke should be surprising, RHD patients were not sensitive to the narrative requirement that the incongruity be resolvable when considered in light of the opening. This finding suggests that RHD patients are impaired in their ability to use new information to arrive at a coherent reinterpretation of an utterance or a unit of discourse.

Since the stimuli for this study were entirely verbal, aphasic LHD patients were not included. As a result, it was not possible to determine if the impairments the RHD patients demonstrated were specific to right-hemisphere pathology. Both LHD and RHD patients were tested, however, in one section of a second study of humor comprehension conducted in our laboratory (Bihrle, Brownell, Powelson, and Gardner, 1986). Stimuli for this second humor study included both verbal narrative jokes and captionless, four-frame cartoons. Both the jokes and cartoons conformed to the incongruity resolution model proposed by Suls in that the correct conclusions were surprising on one interpretation and coherent with the opening on another.

As before, this study also made use of alternative endings — or, in the cartoon section, alternative final frames — that were varied to test for a selective deficit in the surprise or the coherence requirements of the jokes. The following is an example from the verbal task along with examples of the alternative endings. Comparable endings were designed for the cartoon stimuli.

A man walked up to a lady in a crowded square.
  "Excuse me," he said,
  "Do you happen to have seen a policeman anywhere around here?"
  "I'm sorry," the woman answered, "but I haven't seen a sign of one."
Then the man said, ...

Correct punch line. All right, hurry up and give me your watch and pocketbook then.
Straightforward ending. Damn, I've been looking for a half hour and can't find one.
Neutral non sequitur. Baseball is my favorite sport.
Humorous non sequitur. All of the wheels fell off my car.

The important difference between the alternative responses in this study and those used in the earlier humor study was the inclusion of a humorous non sequitur ending. As before, these non sequiturs were designed to be surprising, but were also meant to contain an element of slapstick that was not dependent on the opening of the joke for its humor. Comprehension of the humor in these statements, then, demanded only a response to the non sequitur as an isolated statement. Ten LHD, aphasic patients, ten RHD patients, and ten normal control subjects were tested for this second study of joke comprehension.

The data from both sections of the second humor study confirmed and extended those of the first. As above, RHD patients demonstrated a selective impairment in the coherence requirement of jokes by demonstrating a preference for the non sequitur endings, and the humorous non sequiturs in particular. LHD aphasics, in contrast, were consistently more likely to choose the straightforward endings, but showed little preference for non sequiturs. That is, they realized that the ending of a cartoon should be consistent with the opening but failed to satisfy the surprise requirement. This dissociation indicates that the impairment in the ability of RHD patients to revise their assumptions as they integrate new information with old is not a result of brain damage in general but of right-hemisphere damage in particular.

Inference

A similar deficit among RHD patients in the ability to revise assumptions has also been demonstrated with nonaffective and less formulaic stimuli. Consider the following two-sentence story taken from a recent study (Brownell, Potter, Bihrle, and Gardner, 1986).

Jane hurried into the dentist's office.
She saw her purse on the table in the waiting room.

When the first sentence is presented, a normal listener usually infers that Jane is late for an appointment with the dentist. However, once the second sentence has been presented, a listener must revise his or her assumptions and make a new inference based on the two sentences together—that is, that Jane had forgotten her purse when she left the office.

Two-sentence vignettes such as this one were read to a group of eight RHD patients and to a group of eight normal control subjects in order to see how well subjects in each group could revise their assumptions. Subjects were tested individually and told to treat each pair of sentences as a single story or event. As before, subjects were shown written versions of the vignettes to read to themselves as the stories were read aloud. Once a subject indicated that he understood a particular vignette, the two-sentence typescript was covered with an index card and four test statements were presented in succession. Subjects were asked to state whether each test statement was true or false.

One statement always expressed the "incorrect inference" that could be generated from the misleading information contained in the first sentence of the story—for example, that Jane was late for her dental appointment. Another statement always expressed the "correct inference" that would be generated on consideration of both story sentences as a unit. To respond correctly to this statement, a subject was required to revise his initial assumptions and create a new inference formed with the help of the additional information in the second story sentence (e.g., "She had forgotten her purse when she left the office.").

In addition, two statements for each vignette assessed subjects' knowledge of facts mentioned in the story sentences. By including these questions, it was possible to control for any failures by the subjects to encode or remember the information that the story sentences presented. These control questions were added, then, to insure that errors on the inference questions were, in fact, the result of an inference deficit.

One-half of the vignettes, as in the preceding example, presented misleading information in the first sentence of the pair. The other vignettes used in the study also contained ambiguous, potentially misleading information but presented it in the second sentence of the story. These stories, then, required only a simpler bridging inference rather than the full revision of assumptions required when the misleading information came first (Clark, 1977). Consider the following example.

Johnny missed the wild pitch.
The windshield was shattered.

In this vignette, the second sentence in isolation suggests that there was a car accident that caused a broken windshield. This inference is not correct in light of the preceding sentence; in context, it is clear that the windshield was broken in a baseball game. This type of vignette, in which the potentially misleading information appeared later in the discourse, provided a baseline to assess subjects' ability to make simpler inferences and a control for unconstrained tangentiality apart from a specific deficit in revision.

The results of the study indicated that RHD patients again demonstrated a selective impairment in their ability to revise their assumptions. That is, on trials in which the misleading information occurred in the first sentence, they were significantly *more* likely than normal controls to affirm the incorrect inference and significantly *less* likely to affirm the correct inference. In contrast, they performed much better on fact statements and on the inference questions on the trials that only required the simpler bridging inferences (i.e., trials in which misleading information appeared in the second of the story sentences). As before, RHD patients demonstrated a significant impairment in their ability to revise their assumptions about even the briefest of narratives.

Discourse Deficits in the Context of Other Research

Together, these studies provide evidence for deficits in discourse comprehension that result from damage to the right hemisphere. They have shown that RHD patients are impaired in their ability to interpret new information in the light of what has come before and that they are also impaired in their ability to use new information to alter their initial assumptions.

These results are not surprising, given some of the clinical changes that have been shown to result from right-hemisphere disease—tangential conversation, for example. In themselves, however, they are not satisfying explanations for the clinical observations. For this one would need a better understanding of how linguistic information flows in the brain during the course of a conversation, and of how right-hemisphere damage can interrupt that flow. In trying to move toward such an understanding, we can examine to what extent the discourse impairments just described are specific to right-sided pathology, and whether they can be explained wholly or partially in terms of other, more basic processing disruptions.

Perhaps the most basic distinction to consider, then, is that between the effects of left- and right-hemisphere damage. Including LHD patients in studies of discourse is the most stringent way to control for whatever disabilities may affect brain-damaged patients as a class and not RHD patients only. However, in order to control for the perceptual problems that can result from right-hemisphere disease, the studies cited have relied heavily on verbal tasks. It has, for this reason, proven difficult to include aphasic patients as subjects; this has been done in two of the studies we have discussed.

The first of these was the study of indirect request comprehension (Weylman et al., 1989). As noted, Hirst et al. (1984) and Foldi (1987) demonstrated that LHD and RHD patients gave significantly different responses in a study of indirect requests that used videotaped or graphically depicted skits as stimuli. Weylman et al. failed to find marked differences between the patient groups in a purely verbal task. These authors found instead that both groups were similarly impaired in their ability to determine when an indirect request was appropriate. Given the task differences, the discrepancy in results across studies is perhaps not so great as it initially appears. Since stories in the Weylman et al. study were narrated, aphasics were unable to use visual cues that undoubtedly helped them in the Hirst et al. and Foldi studies.

The best evidence obtained for a discourse comprehension deficit specific to right-sided brain injury came from the nonverbal cartoon completion section of the Bihrle et al. joke study, the second study to include both major patient groups. Here, LHD and RHD patients did differ qualitatively in their responses.

Although the available results lend support to the idea that an intact right hemisphere is required for successful discourse comprehension, we have not to date found a way to distinguish reliably by lesion site within the right hemisphere. This is true in part because the majority of the patients tested have suffered strokes in the branches of the middle cerebral artery. The areas implicated are essentially portions of the frontal, parietal, and temporal lobes that are closest to the central sulcus and sylvian fissure. The resultant lesions often extend both anterior and posterior to the central sulcus; this makes even the most basic comparison between anterior and posterior patients difficult. One would expect, for example, that a patient with purely occipital lobe damage would have little difficulty on these tasks except perhaps the cartoon section of the joke study. In the absence of more precise information on the localization of these deficits, it seems best to consider right-hemisphere damage in terms of the kinds of information flow it may disrupt.

Broadly stated, the essential discourse impairment discussed here is an inability to combine old information and new. The findings presented are, in addition, remarkably similar to data from a different area of research on the role of right hemisphere in language comprehension. This set of results comes from research with unimpaired subjects on right- and left-hemisphere processing of single words. Chiarello (1988) reviews the processing differences that obtain when single words are projected to one hemisphere or the other through lateralized visual field presentation. She suggests that the right hemisphere maintains the ability to hold different meanings of a word available for use, whereas the left hemisphere is more inclined to select a single meaning quickly. The left hemisphere, then, directs the selection of a single meaning for further analysis and also inhibits other options. Chiarello hypothesizes that the function of the right hemisphere as a memory buffer for alternative meanings may provide an account for many of our own findings with units of language larger than a single word, including those presented here. We are inclined to agree. Inability to retain alternative interpretations—both literal and figurative—would crucially limit the capacity to evaluate ambiguous utterances or to revise assumptions (see also Brownell, Simpson, Bihrle, Potter, and Gardner, in press).

Consideration of both sets of research together raises two further questions: (1) how, exactly, does this maintenance, initial selection, and revision occur computationally; and (2) how do the left and right hemispheres coordinate their different treatment of available meaning? Although some progress has been made toward this goal in other areas of cognition (Kosslyn, 1988), a similar knowledge of discourse comprehension is a project for the future. However, some initial speculations can be offered here.

In a recent summary of research on the frontal lobes, neurobiologist Patricia Goldman-Rakic (1987, 1988) has noted that the tissue defining the principal sulcus in macaque monkeys—an area of prefrontal cortex homologous to Brodman's area 46 in human beings—is necessary for the successful maintenance of visuospatial information in the absence of external stimulation. The maintenance of information she describes, a goal-directed, short-term memory, is thought to be accomplished by way of connections between the principal sulcus and portions of the superior parietal lobule and also by way of connections between the principal sulcus and the hippocampus. Goldman-Rakic has suggested that other portions of the frontal lobes may play a similar role in the maintenance of different kinds of linguistic information. One possible explanation for the lack of localization we have found, then, may be that the component processes involved in maintaining semantic information involve both anterior and posterior regions and their interconnections.

One can also ask how these structures might figure in the coordination of the different meanings available to the left and right hemispheres. Interestingly, portions of the principal sulcus in monkeys that are connected to parietal structures are intercalated with fibers that cross the corpus callosum from the contralateral prefrontal cortex. An analogous pattern of contralateral connections in humans intercalated with parietal or temporal afferents would be well suited for this kind of interhemispheric communication and inhibition.

In order to determine whether these hypotheses about the discourse impairments we have described and their relationship to other findings are in any sense correct, we will need to do much work. We will need, in short, a more precise analysis of discourse comprehension and an understanding of how the functional components of that analysis can be neurally embodied. Such a project would indeed allow us to take the first steps toward a cognitive neuroscience of discourse.

Acknowledgments. The preparation of this chapter was supported by NIH grants NS11408 and 06209, by the Research Service of the Veterans Administration, and by Harvard Project Zero. We thank Nancy Lefkowitz, Director of Speech and Language Pathology, and other personnel of the Spaulding Rehabilitation Hospital for their support of the research described in this chapter. We also thank Alexandra Rehak for her comments on an earlier draft of this chapter.

References

Benson, D.F., & Geschwind, N. (1985). Aphasia and related disorders: A clinical approach. In M-Marsel Mesulam (Ed.), *Principles of behavioral neurology* (pp. 193–238). Philadelphia: F.A. Davis.

Bihrle, A.M. Brownell, H.H., Powelson, J.A., & Gardner, H. (1986). Comprehension of humorous and non-humorous materials by left and right brain-damaged patients. *Brain and Cognition, 5,* 399–411.

Brownell, H.H., & Gardner, H. (1988). Neuropsychological insights into humour. In J. Durant & J. Miller (Eds.), *Laughing matters* (pp. 17–34). Essex: Longman Scientific.

Brownell, H.H., Michel, D., Powelson, J.A., & Gardner, H. (1983). Surprise but not coherence: Sensitivity to verbal humor in right hemisphere patients. *Brain and Language, 18,* 20–27.

Brownell, H.H., Potter, H.H., Bihrle, A.M., & Gardner, H. (1986). Inference deficits in right brain-damaged patients. *Brain and Language, 27,* 310–321.

Brownell, H.H., Simpson, T.L., Bihrle, A.M., Potter, H.H., & Gardner, H. (in press). Appreciation of metaphoric alternative word meanings by left and right brain-damaged patients. *Neuropsychologia.*

Chiarello, C. (1988). Semantic priming in the intact brain: Separate roles for the right and left hemispheres? In C. Chiarello (Ed.), *Right hemisphere contributions to lexical semantics* (pp. 59–69). Heidelberg: Springer-Verlag.

Clark, H.H. (1977). Bridging. In P.N. Johnson-Laird & R.C. Wason (Eds.), *Thinking: Readings in cognitive science* (pp. 411–420). Cambridge: Cambridge University Press.

Clark, H.H. (1979). Responding to indirect speech acts. *Cognitive Psychology, 11,* 430–477.

Clark, H.H., & Gerrig., R.J. (1984). On the pretense theory of irony. *Journal of Experimental Psychology: General, 113,* 121–126.

Clark, H.H., & Lucy, P. (1975). Understanding what is meant from what is said: A study in conversationally conveyed requests. *Journal of Verbal Learning and Verbal Behavior, 14,* 56–72.

Clark, H.H., & Marshall, C.R. (1981). Definite reference and mutual knowledge. In A.K. Joshi, B.L. Webber, & I.A. Sag (Eds.), *Elements of discourse understanding* (pp. 10–63). Cambridge: Cambridge University Press.

Delis, D.C., Wapner, W., Gardner, H., & Moses, J.A. (1983). The contribution of the right hemisphere to the organization of paragraphs. *Cortex, 19,* 43–50.

Foldi, N.S. (1987). Appreciation of pragmatic interpretations of indirect commands: Comparison of right and left hemisphere brain-damaged patients. *Brain and Language, 31,* 88–108.

Gainotti, G. (1972). Emotional behavior and hemispheric side of the lesion. *Cortex, 8,* 41–55.

Gardner, H., Brownell, H.H., Wapner, W., & Michelow, D. (1983). Missing the point: The role of the right hemisphere in the processing of complex linguistic materials. In E. Perecman (Ed.), *Cognitive processing in the right hemisphere* (pp. 169–191). New York: Academic.

Gibbs, R.W. (1986). On the psycholinguistics of sarcasm. *Journal of Experimental Psychology: General, 115*, 3–15.

Goldman-Rakic, P.G. (1987). Circuitry of the prefrontal cortex and the regulation of behavior by representational memory. *Handbook of Physiology, 5*, (Part 1, Chapter 9), 373–417.

Goldman-Rakic, P.G. (1988). Topography of cognition: Parallel distributed networks in primate association cortex. *Annual Review of Neuroscience, 11*, 137–156.

Heilman, K.M., Bowers, D., Speedie, L., & Coslett, H.B. (1984). Comprehension of affective and nonaffective prosody. *Neurology, 34*, 917–921.

Heilman, K.M., Bowers, D., & Valenstein, E. (1985). Emotional disorders associated with neurological diseases. In K. Heilman & E. Valenstein (Eds.), *Clinical Neuropsychology*, second edition (pp. 377–402, esp. pp. 378–385). Oxford: Oxford University Press.

Heilman, K.M., Watson, R.T., & Valenstein, E. (1985). Neglect and related disorders. In K. Heilman & E. Valenstein (Eds.), *Clinical neuropsychology*, second edition (pp. 243–294). Oxford: Oxford University Press.

Hirst, W., LeDoux, J., & Stein, S. (1984). Constraints on the processing of indirect speech acts: Evidence from aphasiology. *Brain and Language, 23*, 26–33.

Huber, W., & Gleber, J. (1982). Linguistic and nonlinguistic processing of narratives in aphasia. *Brain and Language, 16*, 1–18.

Hughes, C.P., Chan, J.L., & Su, M.S. (1983). Aprosodia in chinese patients with right cerebral hemisphere lesions. *Archives of Neurology, 40*, 732–736.

Joanette, Y., Goulet, P., Ska, B., & Nespoulous, J.-L. (1986). Informative content of narrative discourse in right-brain-damaged right-handers. *Brain and Language, 29*, 81–105.

Jorgensen, J., Miller G.A., & Sperber, D. (1984). Test of the mention theory of irony. *Journal of Experimental Psychology: General, 113*, 112–120.

Kaplan, J.A., Brownell, H.H., Jacobs, J.R., & Gardner, H. (in press). The effects of right hemisphere damage on the pragmatic interpretation of conversational remarks. *Brain and Language.*

Kosslyn, S.M. (1988). Aspects of a cognitive neuroscience of mental imagery. *Science, 240*, 1621–1626.

Millikan, R.G. (1984). *Language, thought, and other biological categories.* Cambridge, Mass.: MIT Press.

Moya, K.L., Benowitz, L.I., Levine, D.N., & Finklestein, S. (1986). Covariant deficits in visuospatial abilities and recall of verbal narrative after right hemisphere stroke. *Cortex, 22*, 381–397.

Myers, P.S., & Linebaugh, C. (1981). Comprehension of idiomatic expressions by right hemisphere damaged adults. In R.H. Brookshire (Ed.), *Clinical aphasiology: Proceedings of the conference* (pp. 254–261). Minneapolis, Minn.: BRK.

Perrine, L. (1977). *Sound and sense: An introduction to poetry* (pp. 104–106). New York: Harcourt Brace Jovanavich.

Robinson, R.G., & Benson, D.F. (1981). Depression in aphasic patients: Frequency, severity and clinical-pathological correlations. *Brain and Language, 14*, 282–291.

Robinson, R.G., Kubos, K.L., Starr, L.B., Rao, K., & Price, T.R. (1984). Mood disorders in stroke patients: Importance of location of lesion. *Brain, 107*, 81–93.

Ross, E.D. (1981). The aprosodias: Functional-anatomic organization of the affective components of language in the right hemisphere. *Archives of Neurology, 38*, 561–569.

Stachowiak, F.-J., Huber, W., Poeck, K., & Kerschensteiner, M. (1977). Text comprehension in aphasia. *Brain and Language, 4*, 177–195.

Suls, J.M. (1983). Cognitive processes in humor comprehension. In P.E. McGhee & J.H. Goldstein (Eds.), *Handbook of humor research* (pp. 39–57). New York: Springer-Verlag.

Tompkins, C.A., & Mateer, C.A. (1985). Right hemispheric appreciation of prosodic and linguistic indications of implicit attitude. *Brain and Language, 24*, 185–203.

Tucker, D.M. (1981). Lateral brain function, emotion and conceptualization. *Psychological Bulletin, 89*, 19–46.

Tucker, D.M., & Frederick, S.L. (1988). Emotion and brain lateralization. In H. Wagner & T. Manstead (Eds.), *Social psychophysiology and emotion: Theory and clinical application*, Chapter 2. New York: Wiley.

Van Lancker, D.R. & Kempler, D. (1987). Comprehension of familiar phrases by left- but not by right-hemisphere damaged patients. *Brain and Language, 32*, 265–277.

Wecshler, A. (1973). The effect of organic brain disease on recall of emotionally charged versus neutral texts. *Neurology, 23*, 130–135.

Weinstein, E.A., & Kahn, R.C. (1955). *Denial of illness, symbolic and physiological aspects.* Springfield, Ill.: Charles C. Thomas.

Weylman, S.T., Brownell, H.H., Roman, M., & Gardner, H. (1989). Appreciation of indirect requests by left and right brain-damaged patients: The effects of verbal context and conventionality of wording. *Brain and Language, 36*, 580–591.

Winner, E., & Gardner, H. (1977). The comprehension of metaphor in brain-damaged patients. *Brain, 100*, 717–727.

6
Narrative Discourse in Right-Brain-Damaged Right-Handers

YVES JOANETTE and PIERRE GOULET

The interest in a possible contribution of the right "nondominant" hemisphere of right-handers to verbal communication has been popularized by the split-brain studies more than 20 years ago (Gazzaniga, 1971; Gazzaniga and Hillyard, 1971; Gazzaniga and Sperry, 1967; Sperry and Gazzaniga, 1967). This interest followed a long dark period for the right hemisphere, having begun with the contributions of Dax (1865) and Broca (1865) some 100 years before, and during which the verbal communication of right-handers was essentially attributed to the left-hemisphere functioning. The split-brain data came at the time when some clinicians were beginning to describe a certain number of "subtle" changes in the communicative behavior of right-handers having sustained an acquired lesion of the right hemisphere (RBD subjects) (Critchley, 1970; Eisenson, 1959, 1962; Weinstein, 1964). All these data pointed to either a certain potential of the right hemisphere of right-handers for verbal communication, or to a real and effective contribution of this hemisphere to verbal communication in right-handers, these two alternatives still being under discussion (Hannequin, Goulet, and Joanette, 1987; Joanette, Goulet, and Hannequin, 1989). Despite differences in results and some controversies, these studies as well as numerous other studies made since, both with these two experimental populations (split-brain and right-brain-damaged subjects) and normal subjects, using techniques such as divided field studies, seem to converge toward the following characteristic: if the right hemisphere does contribute to verbal communication, or if it does have a certain potential for it, this contribution, or this potential, pertains to aspects linked with the content of language rather than with its formal output or input. This widely accepted conclusion has been drawn essentially from a series of studies made at the word level and showing that the right hemisphere can process the semantic component of words, but not their phonological one (Levy and Trevarthen, 1977). In line with these results, other studies, such as those of Lesser (1974) as well as Gainotti, Caltagirone, Miceli, and Masullo (1981), have shown that the occurrence of a right-hemisphere lesion in a right-hander affects the properly *semantic* aspects of word processing more than syntactic, phonological, or phonetic aspects.

Given these indications at the word level, one can hypothesize that a similar tendency could be found at the discourse level. It has been shown that RBD subjects have difficulties in linguistic tasks requiring text-level processing. For instance, RBD subjects have difficulties interpreting metaphors (Winner and Gardner, 1977) and indirect speech acts (Heeschen and Reisches, 1979). However, most of these studies focused on *decoding* performances and only a few focused on sentence- or text-level processing in the context of a "production task."

Thus, it is legitimate to ask whether the occurrence of a right-hemisphere lesion may interfere with some of the cognitive processings necessary for discourse production. Expressed discourse allows a comparison between text-level processing necessary for the organization of the message "content," and those that are necessary for the "actualization" of the message. Among all types of discourse, "narrative discourse" on the basis of a visually presented set of pictures representing an original story has some advantages; among these are the fact that it is (more) comparable from one subject to another, that it can be accounted for by a text grammar in terms of narrative's macrostructure and, given that the story is not a previously known one, that it does not reflect an already internalized and routinized discourse. Such a task, of course, also has some disadvantages: for example, this task is not a purely "production" task since the subject has first to extract the content of the story from its iconographic representation. Despite these limitations — and no such tasks are without them — the purpose of this chapter is to report on a multiple-analyses study that has looked at different aspects of narratives produced by right-brain-damaged right-handers as compared to normal control subjects. More specifically, we were interested in comparing formal aspects of narrative discourse (properly lexical and syntactic aspects) with other aspects essentially representative of its content (story schema and informative content), considering at the same time aspects of discourse that proceed both from its form *and* its content (cohesion and coherence).

General Methodology

In order to do so, we analyzed the narrative production of fifty-six French-speaking literate adults whose native and daily language was French; some were bilinguals, and the second language in all cases was English. All subjects had score a higher than +80 at the Edinburgh Handedness Inventory (Oldfield, 1971), and all could therefore be considered strongly right-handed. Among the fifty-six experimental subjects, thirty-six of them (RBD subjects; RBD group) had suffered, without any previous history of neurological disease, a single stroke resulting in a unilateral focal lesion in the right hemisphere. None of the RBD subjects showed evidence either of a clinically labeled "crossed" aphasia (Joanette, Puel, Nespoulous, Rascol, and Lecours, 1982; Joanette, in press) or of a clinically detected dementia; moreover, none of these subjects had a clinically documented agnosia or amnesia. The other twenty subjects (C subjects; C group) were nonneurological patients who served as controls. Both C and RBD subjects

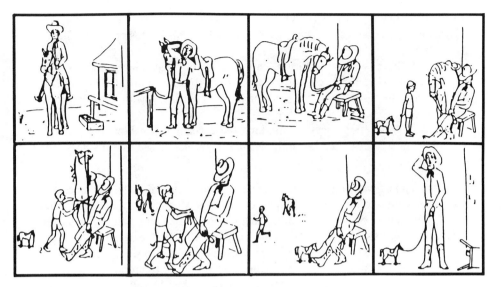

FIGURE 6.1. The "Cowboy Story": see text for further comments.

were ill and hospitalized, but their general condition was such that they could be submitted to testing without discomfort. Each subject received an explanation of the general purpose of our research and readily agreed to participate.

There were no statistically significant difference between C and RBD subjects with regard to age (mean = 57 years; n.s. using a Mann-Whitney test), sex (male/female ratio = 2; n.s. using a chi-square), family history of ambidextrality and/or left-handedness (presence/absence ratio = 1; n.s. using a chi-square), number of years of school attendance (mean = 8 years; n.s. using a Mann-Whitney test), and second language abilities (presence/absence ratio = 1; n.s. using a chi-square). RBD subjects were tested approximately 3 months after the onset of their right-hemisphere lesion (mean = 90.4 days; SD = 151.7 days).

In order to obtain narrative discourse production, each subject was submitted to a story narration task in the context of a protocol devised to document a large number of aspects of linguistic functioning in right-brain-damaged right-handers (Joanette, 1980; Joanette, Lecours, Lepage, and Lamoureux, 1983). Thus, subjects were shown an eight-frame drawing (Figure 6.1) presented on a single cardboard, and representing the illustrated version of a trivial story pertaining to a cowboy's misadventure, and referred to as the "Cowboy Story." This story is a modified version of one appearing in Ombredane's "The Miracle" (1951, pp. 25–26).

The "Cowboy Story" used here can be segmented into some of the basic components of a narrative structure (van Dijk, 1977); namely, a "setting," followed by a "complication" and a final "resolution." Thus, the "Cowboy Story" can be described as follows.

- First, there is a "setting," in which a tired cowboy comes into a small town, gets off his horse, and rests, sitting on a bench, holding his horse's bridle (frames 1, 2, and 3).
- Second, there is a "complication," in which a tricky young boy passes by with a small wooden horse, cuts off (with scissors) the horse's bridle and, having replaced the horse with his wooden horse, runs away with the real horse (frames 4, 5, 6, and 7).
- Third, a "resolution" occurs, in which the awakening cowboy finds himself holding a small wooden horse; he is quite surprised to see that his horse has changed (frame 8).

Each subject was presented with the cardboard in its midsaggital plane. The subjects were told that they would have to tell the story illustrated on the eight different frames of the cardboard. Each of the frames was pointed to by the experimenter to be sure that each of the subjects had indeed seen each of the eight frames. Subjects were then asked to look carefully at the eight-frame drawing and to tell the story. In order to minimize memory effects, the cardboard was left in front of them. Oral narratives were recorded on a Uher 4400 Report Stereo tape recorder and afterward were transcribed.

The following will report and discuss data pertaining to three different analyses. The first analysis (Analysis I) focuses on lexical and syntactic aspects of narratives and should thus give indications as to its formal aspects. The second analysis (Analysis II) bears on the cohesion and the coherence of the same narratives. This second analysis should give indications both on the form and the content of the narratives. The third analysis (Analysis III) pertains to story schema as well as informative content and thus is indicative of the content of these narratives. For each analysis, we will first give some indications as to the specific methodology; then, we will report results and discuss them specifically for each of them. Finally, a general discussion will address the meaning of all this information.

Analysis I: Formal Aspects

As stated earlier, the first analysis bears on some formal aspects of narratives produced by RBD subjects as compared to C-subjects' performance. In order to do so, transcripts of narratives were submitted to a series of descriptive measures frequently used in order to characterize the formal aspects of mild aphasics' narratives. For instance, Berko-Gleason, Goodlass, Obler, Green, Hyde, and Weintraub (1980) reported that Broca's aphasics show elevated noun/verb ratio whereas Wernicke's aphasics exhibit a lowered ratio. Similar features were reported in narratives of mild aphasics and even of elderly normals (Obler, 1980; Ulatowska, Freedman-Stern, Weiss-Doyel, Malacuso-Haynes, and North, 1983). As it is the case in the studies that have just been referred to, the measures retained here are focused on aspects of the lexical elements of the narratives, on the one hand, (e.g., verb/noun ratio) and, on the other hand, on some general descriptives of the sentential organization of these elements (e.g., percentages of subordinate clauses).

Methodology

Broad transcriptions of narratives produced by RBD and C subjects were first submitted to a series of lexical measures. *Total number of words* was counted on the basis of discrete units as they appeared on the transcripts, with the exception of reiterations. Then, transcriptions were analyzed in order to yield the following indexes.

- *Percentages of nouns*, calculated as the total number of substantives on the total number of words.
- *Percentages of verbs*, calculated as the total number of content verbs, excluding copulas, modal and auxiliary verbs, on the total number of words.
- *Percentages of adjectives*, calculated as the total number of "qualificative" adjectives on the total number of words.
- *Percentages of adverbs*, calculated as the total number of adverbs on the total number of words.
- *Verb/noun ratio*, corresponding to the number of content verbs divided by the number of substantives.
- *Adjective/noun ratio*, corresponding to the number of qualificative adjectives divided by the number of nouns.
- *Pronoun/concept ratio*, corresponding to the number of pronouns used by the subject in order to refer to a given concept. In the present study, only two concepts were examined in this manner, namely the concept "Cowboy" and the concept "Boy." Thus, two pronoun/concept ratios were obtained, one for each of these two concepts.

Apart from these basic indexes, lexicalization measures were also taken in order to compare the number of different lexical items used by each group for expressing a given set of concepts. Five semantic units to be found in the narratives were retained for this analysis: cowboy, horse, boy, wooden horse, and bridle. For each of these concepts, the following measures were taken.

- Percentages of subjects who verbalize the expected lexical item for each of the previously mentioned concepts.
- Number of different lexical items used by each "group" in order to express each of these concepts in their narratives.

Finally, an inventory of the lexical items used by each group of subjects in order to express each of the concepts was made.

In the second part of the so-called "formal" analysis, narratives were looked at in order to document a limited number of gross syntactic indexes. Given the relative simplicity of syntactical organization used by our subjects in their narratives, the only indexes that could be looked at was the percentage of subordinate

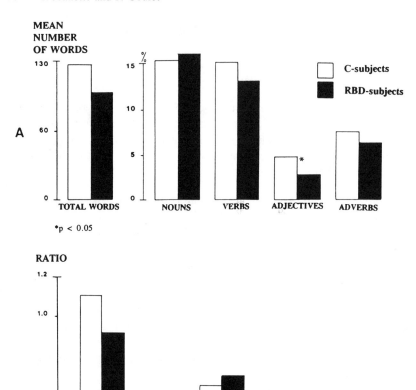

FIGURE 6.2. Total number of words, percentages of nouns, verbs, or adverbs.

clauses, calculated as the absolute number of subordinate clauses divided by the total number of clauses in the narratives.

Results

As it appears on Figure 6.2, there were no differences between RBD- and C-subjects' narratives with regard to total number of words, nor to percentages of nouns, verbs, or adverbs. Only percentages of adjectives yielded a significant difference between groups, RBD-subjects' narratives containing a smaller per-

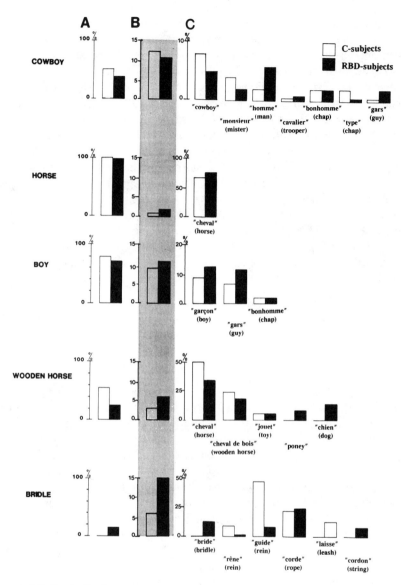

FIGURE 6.3. Lexicalization.

centage of qualificative adjectives. A similar tendency is to be found for the different ratios that were calculated (see Figure 6.2). Indeed, whereas there is no significant difference between RBD- and C-subjects' narratives for the verb/noun ratio and for the two pronoun/concept ratios ("cowboy" and "boy"), the adjective/noun ratio is significantly lower for RBD subjects.

As far as lexicalization is concerned, Figure 6.3 shows the following despite the absence of statistical support due to the nature of the data.

- The percentage of subjects who verbalized the expected lexical target depends on the concept; it is high for the concepts "horse" and "boy," very low for the concept "bridle," and somewhat in between for the concepts "cowboy" and "wooden horse." However, in general, percentages of RBD and C subjects are somewhat similar, except for the concept "wooden horse," which has been verbalized by fewer RBD than C subjects, and the concept "bridle," which has been lexicalized with this specific lexeme only by some RBD subjects.
- As for the number of different lexical items used by each group for each concept, there seems to be a certain tendency for RBD subjects to use, as a group, a greater number of different lexical forms for the same concept, with the exception of the concept "cowboy." This tendency is present despite the fact that there are more RBD than C subjects.
- When looking at the percentages of use of the most prevalent lexical items other than the expected one for each concept, one also has the feeling that RBD subjects may tend to use, as a group, more frequently different lexical items in order to express a given concept. This is most exemplified for the concepts "wooden horse" and "bridle" and, to a minor degree, for the concept "cowboy."

As for the only syntactical index that was calculated, no difference was found between RBD- and C-subjects' narratives in relation to the percentage of relative clauses.

Summary and Discussion

In summary, narratives produced by RBD subjects are not very different from narratives produced by C subjects with regard to lexical and syntactic aspects that were analyzed here. The most important difference is the slightly lower amount of qualification in RBD-subjects' narratives as expressed through lowered percentages of adjectives as well as through the smaller adjective/noun ratio. This result is relatively meaningless here, but it will reach its full significance when it will be put in relation with the results of the informative content analysis (see the section discussing Analysis III). Apart from that, there seems to be a tendency for RBD subjects to use, as a group, a greater number of different lexical items in order to express their underlying conceptual elements. If such a tendency is to be confirmed by other studies, then it could be interpreted as the manifestation of a certain impairment at the lexicosemantic level; indeed, the identification and/or the retrieval of specific lexical items being difficult or impossible, subjects would identify and retrieve a related but still acceptable item. Thus, the number of different items used by the RBD group, as a whole, could be larger. Such a tendency would be compatible with the now widely acknowledged effects of a right-brain damage onto the semantic aspect of lexicosemantic functioning in right-handers (Hannequin et al., 1987). However, the limits of the present results do not allow to conclude in such a way. The only thing that is to be retained is the fact that, on the whole, formal aspects do not seem to distinguish between narratives produced by RBD subjects and controls. This result is in contrast with those of similar analyses in left-brain-damaged mild aphasics, for instance, as reported by Berko-Gleason et al. (1980). It certainly supports the clinical impression that, with the exception of those rare cases of crossed aphasia (Joanette, 1989; Joanette et al., 1982), formal aspects of verbal communication are relatively well preserved in RBD patients, despite the fact that a very systematic and precise comparison with control subjects' performance can yield some small differences (Joanette et al., 1983).

Analysis II: Cohesion and Coherence

As mentioned earlier, another kind of analysis that seemed at first glance promising with regard to right-brain-damaged right-handers' narratives pertains to cohesion and coherence. Both these aspects refer to the relations of meaning between different segments of a connected discourse. However, whereas "cohesion" specifically corresponds to the semantic relations that are expressed through specific content or function words such as the use of pronouns (Halliday and Hasan, 1976), "coherence" corresponds to the semantic relations that are not expressed through the specific use of elements of the discourse, such as the non-contradiction rule (van Dijk, 1977; Charolles, 1983). Cohesion has been studied in a number of brain-damaged populations including aphasics (e.g., Ulatowska and Bond, 1983; Ulatowska et al., 1983; see also Chapter 8), patients with Alzheimer's disease (e.g., Ripich, Terrell, and Spinelli, 1983) as well as Sturge-Weber syndromes in children (Lovett, Dennis, and Newman, 1986). Coherence has been less extensively studied than cohesion in brain-damaged populations, probably because of the methodological difficulties associated with such studies. Lesser (1986) did look at aspects of both cohesion and coherence in a group of nine right-brain-damaged subjects, by reference to a group of paired controls submitted to a reading task. This study indicates that RBD subjects are impaired on the assignment of pronouns in coordinated sentences as well as on the proper-selection of cohesive markers, when cohesion is dependent on verbs or content words.

In order to see if RBD subjects do evidence cohesive and/or coherent impairments in the production of narratives, the four rules of Charolles (1978) were retained. Charolles suggests what he calls "meta-rules" that have to be respected in connected discourse in order that it is cohesive and coherent. The first meta-rule is that of "repetition" and corresponds, in fact, to an index of cohesion since it refers to the proper repetition of substantives and the use of pronouns. The three other rules relate to coherence as defined before. The second meta-rule is that of "progression," asking for a constant progression of the meaning with the advance of discourse (e.g., a new segment must bring some new information). The third one is the meta-rule of "noncontradiction," stating that a new information cannot contradict a previously given one. And the fourth meta-rule is that of "relation," asking for a new information to be related in one way or another to previously given implicit or explicit information. The way RBD subjects respect these four meta-rules in the production of narratives was here sought for.

Methodology

Transcriptions of narratives produced by RBD and C subjects were analyzed by reference to the following four cohesion-coherence errors derived from the model of Charolles (1978).

1. *Repetition Errors*. Errors in semantic relations between different segments of narratives that are expressed through specific content or function words (e.g., undetermined pronouns, inadequate lexical reiterations). This first class of error corresponds to "cohesive" errors.
2. *Nonprogression Errors*. Transgression of the progression meta-rule like the irrelevant repetition of a given information without the addition of new information.
3. *Contradiction Errors*. As self-explicit, the fact that new information is in contradiction with some previously given one.
4. *Relation Errors*. Transgression of the relation meta-rule, an example of which is the fact that some new information is given without any relation to previously given one, either explicitly or implicitly.

Results

Results are not very exciting since, when taken separately, there is no difference in the number of errors between groups for each of the four error types just described. However, considering the four types of errors together, the following emerges. Whereas both RBD and C subjects tend to make one of the four cohesion-coherence errors in their narratives, only RBD subjects show a significant tendency to make more often *two or more than two* cohesion-coherence errors of either type. More specifically, this significant tendency is to be attributed to approximately half of the RBD subjects, the other half being comparable to C subjects.

Discussion

Results reported in this analysis are not very striking. Indeed, only the summation of the four types of cohesion-coherence errors allowed a distinction between RBD and C subjects. This may mean, among other things, that the conceptual frame that was used here might not be sensitive enough. Indeed, only patent transgression of a certain number of so-called meta-rules of cohesion and coherence was sought for. The present results seem to contrast with those of Lesser (1986), who showed RBD subjects to have specific cohesive problems manifested through pronoun assignment, for example. However, there are differences between Lesser's study (1986) and the present one; for example, the present study examined cohesion and coherence in production, whereas Lesser (1986) studied RBD subjects in a decoding task (reading texts). Either the kind of problems unveiled by Lesser (1986) in a reception task is not present in production, or it is much more difficult to unveil cohesive and/or coherence errors in a production task given that it is not possible to refer to the precise communicative target subjects have in mind.

It remains that, on the whole, RBD-subjects' narratives do seem to have some degree of cohesion and/or coherence impairment given that their narratives contain significantly more often two or more than two errors—as defined in the present study—as compared to C subjects. However, one of the most interesting findings might be that not all RBD subjects tend to show this tendency; as reported, only half of RBD subjects seem to be so characterized. This result could mean that if a right-hemisphere lesion does affect narrative abilities, it may not be the case for all RBD subjects. If such a tendency was confirmed by other levels of analysis, it could mean that the effects of a right-hemisphere lesion on language, or on communicative skills in general, should not be looked for in each and every RBD subject but essentially in a subgroup of them, here corresponding approximately to half of them. As it will appear later, these results are converging toward those of the next level of analysis.

Analysis III: Story Schema and Informative Content

Narratives can be described as a series of pieces of information, captured through its microstructure and organized according to a general schema that determines the gross architecture of the macrostructure (van Dijk, 1977; Kintsch and van Dijk, 1978). Thus, the story schema as well as the amount of information conveyed by a narrative represent an opened window on how a given group of subjects organizes the content of his narratives.

For instance, studies have shown that narratives produced by left-brain-damaged aphasic patients conveyed less informative content (e.g., Berko-Gleason et al., 1980; Ulatowska et al. 1983; Yorkston and Beukelman, 1980). According to Berko-Gleason et al. (1980), this tendency is even present in Wernicke's aphasics, despite the fact that narratives are made of a number of words comparable to those of normal controls. However, in these studies, informative content is only approximated grossly. For example, in Berko-Gleason et al.'s study (1980), informative content is evaluated through counting of target lexemes and "meaningful" themes.

Narrative abilities of RBD subjects have also been studied by some authors. For example, Huber and Gleber (1982) required RBD subjects to rearrange a set of pictures and a set of sentences into a narrative. Left-brain-damaged (LBD) subjects were also submitted to the same task. It was found, not unexpectedly, that RBD subjects had more problems rearranging pictures, whereas LBD subjects had more problems rearranging sentences. However, it is interesting to note that both RBD and LBD subjects had more problems executing both tasks when compared to normals. Similar results were obtained by Delis, Wapner, Gardner, and Moses (1983), who showed RBD subjects to have difficulties rearranging written sentences into a story. Other studies have looked at the ability of RBD subjects to extract the informative content at the supraword level (Brownell, Michel, Powelson, and Gardner, 1983; Wapner, Hamby, and Gardner, 1981). These studies claim that RBD subjects have difficulty "in integrating specific information, in drawing proper inferences and morals, and in assessing the appropriateness of various facts, situations, and characterizations" (Wapner et al., 1981, p. 29).

Taken together, these studies indicated that RBD subjects may have problems with the extraction of informative content from connected speech, including narratives. However, it remains to know if RBD subjects do have problems when asked to *produce* narratives. Thus, this third analysis will look at the story schema as well as the specific (microstructure) informative content of narratives produced by RBD subjects. A detailed description of this study is to be found in Joanette, Goulet, Ska, and Nespoulous (1986).

Methodology

The transcript of each subject's narratives was submitted to a "propositional analysis." Before submitting the narratives to this analysis, two essential components of discourse were identified and separated: the *referential* and the *modalizing* components of discourse (Nespoulous, 1979).[1] Since only the former and not the latter corresponds to that part of discourse that is specifically related to the story, the modalizing component of narrative discourse was identified in the transcripts and discarded. Thus, the "propositional analysis" performed here bears only on the explicit referential narrative discourse.

Before undertaking the propositional analysis per se, the story schema of each narrative was evaluated. In order to achieve that, the presence of complete or partial information representative of each of the main components of a narrative story schema—the setting, the complication, and the resolution—was looked for. Given that the sequence was adequate, any narrative containing at least partial informative content related to these three parts was considered as respecting the general story schema.

The propositional analysis used in this study is adapted from those of Kintsch (Kintsch, 1974; Kintsch and van Dijk, 1978) and of Le Ny (1979). However, only the microstructural aspect of the propositional analysis has been retained, as it permits the extraction of the informative content from the surface text. According to this type of analysis, the information contained in a given segment of discourse is extracted piece by piece, or more precisely, "proposition" by "proposition," independently of the surface form of the discourse. Each proposition (P) consists of one "predicate" and usually one or more "arguments" (Kintsch and van Dijk, 1978; see Chapter 3 for more details). When none of the arguments corresponds to another P, the proposition is said to be "simple" (simple P). However, when one of the arguments corresponds to another P, then the proposition is said to be "complex" (complex P).

---

[1]Nespoulous (1979), in accordance with Halliday (1975) defines the referential component of discourse as the one containing specific reference to persons, objects, and ideas (in this context, the components of the "Cowboy Story"). The modalizing component of discourse is defined as the part of discourse that corresponds to the locutor's personal attitude toward what he is saying.

Results

Results will be presented as follows. First, a comparison will be made between narratives produced by RBD and C subjects. This comparison will focus on (1) story schema, (2) amount of information, and (3) nature of information. However, given that there can be many different narrative styles among normal subjects (Obler, 1980), on the one hand and, on the other hand, given that not all RBD subjects may show "deviant" narratives, a grouping of all RBD and C subjects has been made on the sole basis of the informative content of their narratives. Thus, all subjects were redistributed into two groups, groups I and II. These two groups were then compared as to (1) amount and (2) nature of informative content of their narratives.

Comparison Between RBD and C Subjects

Story Schema. Each narrative was analyzed grossly in order to see if the macrostructure of the story contained the minimal schema of a story, namely, its three parts: an introduction, a complication, and a resolution. The analysis was made by two independent judges. It seems that nearly all narratives produced by RBD and C subjects did contain an introduction, a complication, and a resolution. In other words, the presence of a story schema does not seem to distinguish RBD and C subjects' narratives.

Amount of Information. Total number of Ps contained in each subject's narratives (referential component only) was compiled. RBD-subjects' discourse contains a mean of 33.8 Ps, ranging from 14 to 96, whereas C-subjects' discourse is made up of a mean of 46.4 Ps, ranging from 24 to 106. The results of a Mann-Whitney test (Siegel, 1956) show that RBD-subjects' narratives contain a significantly smaller number of Ps ($p < 0.01$), i.e., less overall information. Complex Ps were extracted from total Ps and compiled separately; RBD-subjects' narratives contain a statistically significant smaller number of complex Ps ($p < 0.002$ using a Mann-Whitney test). RBD-subjects' narratives had a mean number of 11.3 complex Ps, ranging from 2 to 44, whereas C-subjects' narratives contained a mean number of 17.6 complex Ps, ranging from 7 to 39. Thus, narrative discourse of RBD subjects not only contains overall less verbalized information than that of C subjects but, moreover, this information may be described as being less complexly organized overall.

In order to allow a comparison of the informative content of RBD-subjects' narratives *by reference to the one of C-subjects'* narratives, a certain number of relatively invariant pieces of information (simple or complex Ps) had to be identified. These pieces of either simple or complex information are referred to as "core Ps"; they incorporate the expected informative content according to a canonical and expected version of the "Cowboy Story" on the basis of the authors' narratives. However, any piece of information that was not emitted by at least 20 percent of either group subjects was eliminated; on the other hand, unexpected pieces of information emitted by at least 20 percent of either group subjects were also incorporated. The final checklist thus comprises a set of 32 core Ps (see Appendix I for the list).

Number of core Ps was significantly different in both groups' narratives ($p <$ 0.05 using a Mann-Whitney test): C-subjects' narratives contained a mean number of 16.4 core Ps, ranging from 9 to 24, whereas RBD-subjects' narratives contained a mean number of only 12.0 core Ps, ranging from 0^2 to 20. This smaller number of core Ps in RBD-subjects' narratives has been shown not to be the mere reflection of some problems in visual signal processing, such as a left visual neglect. Indeed, a comparison between the number of Ps specifically related to visual information contained in the left or right half of the iconographic representation of the narrative showed that lowered informative content is equally distributed on both sides.

Nature of Information. The main goal of this section is to look for possible differences between pieces of information that characterize each group's narratives. Two complementary analyses were made: one focused on the frequency of occurrence of each core P, the second looking at the co-occurrence and/or co-nonoccurrence of subsets of core Ps.

In accordance with the first goal, the frequency of occurrence of each core P was individually compared among C and RBD subjects. It seems that a significant difference is obtained for only 3 out of the 32 core Ps. Core Ps numbers 7, 15, and 29 (see Appendix I) were significantly less frequent ($p < 0.01$ using a Fisher Exact test) in RBD-subjects' narratives. It is interesting to note that two of these core Ps, core Ps number 7 and 29, correspond to pieces of information that have to be *inferred* from the eight-frame drawing by reference to the story structure: namely, that the cowboy is tired (core P 7) and that he wakes up (core P 29). This result is to be interpreted with caution, since other core Ps also corresponding to inferred pieces of information were emitted as frequently by both groups of subjects.

Emitted core Ps of C- and RBD-subjects' narratives were then separately submitted to a set of cluster analyses. The procedure used was derived from CLUSTAN (Wishart, 1978). First, we computed similarities between propositions using a simple matching coefficient (i.e., the proportion of matches for the emitted/nonemitted pattern over the subjects). Then, we applied the Ward's method (Wishart, 1978) on the resulting similarity matrices. Figure 6.4 shows the resulting clusters for C and RBD subjects.

Two different clusters can be identified for each of the C and RBD groups. In both cases, the cluster on the left consists of the most frequently emitted set of core Ps as opposed to the cluster on the right, which consists of the less frequently emitted set of core Ps. In other words, core Ps appearing on the left side are characteristic of the part of the narrative that is verbalized, as a whole, by the greatest number of subjects. Core Ps appearing on the right side of the cluster

---

^{2}Only one RBD subject emitted 0 core Ps; this surprising result indicates that he did tell a story but without any element of information specifically linked with one or the other core Ps.

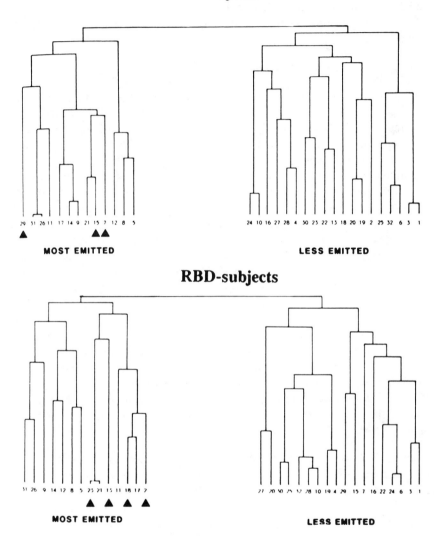

FIGURE 6.4. Core Ps clustering according to their co-occurring absence or presence in C- and RBD-subjects' narratives; arrows indicate core Ps, which are exclusive to either C- or RBD-subjects' most emitted cluster; see text for comments.

characterize the part of the narrative that was produced, as a whole, less frequently.

As a general comment, the same core Ps are to be found in the most frequently emitted cluster of C- as well as RBD-subjects' narratives. However, a certain number of core Ps are exclusive to C or RBD subjects' most frequently emitted cluster, respectively. In the case of C subjects, these core Ps correspond to those that were found to be less frequently emitted in the previous analysis (7, 15, and 29). For RBD subjects, these exclusive core Ps (2, 13, 18, and 23) pertain to some pieces of information that do not need to be inferred from the eight-frame drawing.

Homogeneity of C and RBD Groups

The second part of this analysis aimed at a description of the homogeneity of the two groups. In order to determine whether the amount, as well as the nature of information described previously, was representative of all RBD subjects, and in order to reassure ourselves that the right-hemisphere lesion was, in fact, a relevant and distinguishing factor between C and RBD subjects, the whole subject population was submitted to a hierarchical cluster analysis based on the proportion of matches in the presence/absence pattern across the 32 core Ps. Results show C and RBD subjects to redistribute themselves into two groups: groups I (31 subjects) and II (25 subjects). Of the 20 C subjects, 15 (75 percent) are to be found in group I, whereas only 5 (25 percent) fall into group II. As far as the 36 RBD subjects are concerned, they are relatively equally distributed between groups I and II, although slightly favoring group II ($n = 20$; 56 percent) over group I ($n = 16$; 44 percent). As a consequence, group II contains significantly more RBD subjects than C subjects as compared to group I, despite the fact that both groups contain both RBD and C subjects. Given that groups I and II are not different with regard to age, sex, schooling, stock handedness, or knowledge of a second language, this result probably reflects the existence of at least *two* different core versions of the "Cowboy Story." The version characteristic of group II subjects may correspond to a particular narrative strategy in C subjects. However, the fact that there are significantly more RBD subjects in group II may indicate that this type of narrative strategy may be more characteristic of right-brain-damaged subjects.

Amount of Information. Group I subjects' discourse comprises a mean of 46.4 Ps, ranging from 19 to 106, whereas group II subjects' discourse was made up of a mean of 28.3 Ps, ranging from 14 to 58. A Mann-Whitney test showed that group II narratives were made up of a significantly smaller number of Ps than group I narratives ($p < 0.001$), i.e., it contains less verbalized information. Group II narratives also contain a smaller mean number of complex Ps (17.2 for group I versus 9.0 for group II; $p < 0.001$ using a Mann-Whitney test). Contrary to the comparison between C and RBD subjects (see section entitled "Results"), however, group II narratives were made up of a significantly smaller mean number of words (126.5 for group I versus 90.4 for group II; $p < 0.01$ using a Mann-Whitney test). These differences between groups I and II are not to be attributed to the existence of a gross visuoperceptive impairment. Indeed, none of the RBD subjects had evidence of a visual agnosia as tested in a routine neuroclinical neuropsychological examination.

Nature of Information. A clustering procedure similar to the one used previously for C and RBD subjects was applied to groups I and II. Figure 6.5 presents the

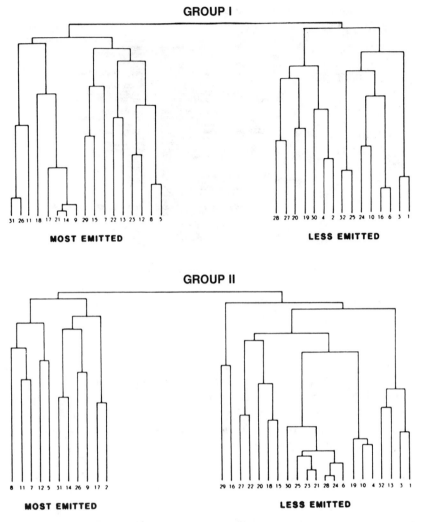

FIGURE 6.5. Core Ps clustering according to their co-occurring absence or presence in groups I and II subjects' narratives; see text for comments.

results of this clustering procedure for groups I and II. Two clusters of core Ps can be identified; the first one contains the most emitted core Ps and the second one, the less emitted ones. One of the most interesting points here is that the group II most emitted cluster of core Ps represents a *subset* of group I most emitted ones. Moreover, this subset pertains largely to the first and the last parts of the story, i.e., the setting and the resolution. In other words, the missing core Ps in group II most emitted cluster is to be found much more in the "complication" part of the story than in either of the two other parts.

A representation of the frequency of occurrence of each of the individual core Ps (Figure 6.6) — analyzed with respect to chronological occurrence within the

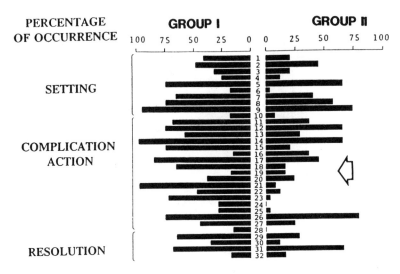

FIGURE 6.6. Frequency of occurrence of each one of the thirty-two core Ps in groups I and II chronologically presented, from top to bottom, according to the "Cowboy Story" three parts; see text for further comments.

"Cowboy Story"'s macrostructure – shows that, within group II narratives, there is a lower incidence of core Ps related to the "complication" than to other parts of the story. At the same time, one core P of the "complication" is *more* frequent in group II than in group I subjects' narratives; this core P (16) corresponds to the piece of information "The boy plays a trick." This piece of information can be considered as the gist, or the *substance*, of the "complication" part of the story and, in fact, of the story as a whole.

Summary and Discussion

In summary, results showed that the referential component (Nespoulous, 1979) of RBD-subjects narratives contained on the whole less information, either simple or complex. Moreover, the nature of the information contained in RBD-subjects' narratives was shown to be different from that of C subjects. Each group of subjects was then shown not to be homogeneous and was redistributed into two groups (groups I and II), on the sole basis of the informative content of their narratives. Even though both C and RBD subjects are to be found in both groups I and II, the nonrandom redistribution of subjects is the only statistically significant result. Group II is made up of a majority of RBD subjects. Again, a comparison between those two groups revealed different amounts and nature of information conveyed: group II subjects' narratives were characterized by a lack of information mostly pertaining to the "complication" part of the story.

   These results show that the integrity of the right hemisphere is needed for "normal" discourse abilities. If these results are taken along with those having shown left-brain-damaged aphasics, demented, or even normal aging subjects to show such a lowering in informative content, then it can be said that the integrity of the encephalon is needed for the full use of human communicative abilities, such as assessed through narrative discourse. However, these results also show that not every right-brain-damaged patient does show such a deficit. Even though it was not possible to identify either anatomic, genetic, or environmental factors that could have accounted for this, the lowering in informative content as well as its particular organization was only characteristic of a subgroup of RBD subjects (group II). Moreover, the same characteristics also apply to a subgroup of normal controls, even though in a smaller proportion. This might indicate that a particular narrative style that can be used by normal subjects is, for unknown reasons, used more frequently by RBD subjects. If this is so, then the lack of informative content per se could only represent a surface-level manifestation of a more basic effect of a right-hemisphere lesion on cognitive functioning and/or strategies.

The next step, in this respect, would be to characterize further the specificity of narrative strategies used by RBD subjects versus other populations, left-brain-damaged nonaphasics being among the first of them. In doing so, it might be important not only to focus on the core of the narrative, but also on the information provided by subjects that are not relevant to the story. Indeed, RBD subjects are known to have a tendency toward tangential speech. Such manifestations were not evaluated in the present study, since we focused on core Ps, that is, this information directly related to the story. We did note, however, a certain number of RBD subjects with such tangential speech. Another interesting aspect would be to analyze the *modalizing* aspect of discourse, which was discarded here in favor of the *referential* aspects of discourse. Modalizing components of discourse—that part of discourse that is the discourse on the discourse, that is, subjects' comments on their own discourse or on the task itself—might be a revelator of the particular strategies some RBD subjects use when confronted with narratives. However, these aspects of discourse seem to be more difficult to circumscribe, since interindividual differences may play an important role here. It is probable that only systematic case reports focused on those RBD subjects that do exhibit "impaired" discourse will allow such an understanding.

As far as the story schema is concerned, it is interesting to note that it seemed to be present in nearly all RBD and C subjects. This could either mean that the story schema is more robust and less affected by a brain lesion, or that it remains a very gross level of analysis and is not sensitive enough. However, the fact that story schema can be affected in dementia, for instance, might favor the first of these alternative explanations.

General Discussion

This series of analyses of narratives produced by right-brain-damaged patients shows that the occurrence of a right-hemisphere lesion affects more the content than the form of narrative discourse. Indeed, whereas only minimal differences were noted in the lexical and syntactic analyses, analysis of informative content showed relatively important differences between narratives produced by RBD subjects and those produced by normal controls. In fact, the only formal measure that yielded significant differences pertains to the amount of qualification as measured through the proportion of adjectives and the adjective/noun ratio. This formal measure may only reflect the lowering of informative content, since qualification is one vector of information.

The second important result is the fact that the characterization of RBD-subjects' discourse may not be specific to that population, nor did all RBD patients show these characteristics. The first of these points suggests that descriptions such as that of informative content are still very gross and general and should not be considered as the specific expression of one particular under-lying impairment process or set of processes. Moreover, lack of informative content may not be the expression of a cognitive impairment per se, but in-stead the expression of a particular communicative strategy. We know, for instance, that RBD patients tend to have difficulties in taking into account all aspects of their spatial context. It may be that, for some unknown reasons, they also have problems with their communicative context. Given such a difficulty, they may choose a certain narrative strategy that can sometimes be found among normal controls, but in this case now much more frequently. The second point alluded to earlier—the fact that not all RBD patients did show "impaired" narratives—may hint to us to focus our efforts toward those patients who show a communicative deficit after the occurrence of a right-hemisphere lesion, just like aphasiology focuses on those patients presenting communicative impairment after a—usually—left-hemisphere lesion. Only further descriptions, namely at the discourse level, will allow to identify those patients. At that point, it might be easier to characterize in more detail their communicative impairment.

Another challenging aspect of the problem will be to understand the exact reasons for this possible change in communicative attitude in RBD patients. Again, it might be, at one point, that there will be some correlations between the occur-rence of such a change in communicative attitude and changes in other attitudes toward the external world, such as anosognosia. In both cases, the change can be described as one toward a less "pragmatic" attitude, not to say a more "aprag-matic" one. It will remain to see if one is the cause of the other, or vice versa, or if both are the expression of a more basic problem toward the relation with the exterior world.

Finally, it will be important to compare the kind of discourse changes to occur in RBD patients with those occurring in left-brain-damaged nonaphasics, or even mild aphasics. Results such as those obtained by Ulatowska and her collaborators (see Chapter 8) seem to point to changes in discourse that are somewhat similar to the ones we have been reporting. If this is the case, it could mean that the integrity of both left and right hemispheres is necessary for full discourse abili-ties. However, it is also possible that the measures used up to this point are not specific enough to allow a distinction between the effects of a right- versus left-hemisphere lesion.

However, one thing remains, and this is the importance of the description of discourse abilities for the better understanding of the effect of a right-hemisphere lesion on verbal communication. In doing so, it opens a window on the "real" – versus the "potential" – contribution of the right hemisphere to verbal communication. The kind of analyses outlined in some of the chapters in the first section of this book may provide examples of the kind of approach and analyses that should now be used in order to tackle this problem further.

Acknowledgments. Yves Joanette is Scientist of the *Conseil de recherches médicales du Canada*. We thank Francois Dehaut for the data analyses and Louise Bourret for the illustrations. This research was supported by Program Grant PG-28 of the *Conseil de recherches médicales du Canada*. It was also supported by a grant from the *Fonds de la recherche en santé du Québec*. Requests for reprint should be sent to Yves Joanette, Ph.D., Laboratoire Théophile-Alajouanine, CHCN, 4565 chemin de la Reine-Marie, Montréal, Québec, Canada H3W 1W5.

Appendix I
List of the 32 Core Ps[3] of the "Cowboy Story"

1. (ARRIVE, COWBOY)
2. (ON, COWBOY, HORSE)
3. (IN, P1, VILLAGE)
4. (GET OFF, COWBOY, HORSE 1)
5. (OF, HORSE 1, COWBOY)
6. (TIE, COWBOY, HORSE 1)
7. (TIRED, COWBOY)
8. (SIT, COWBOY, BENCH)
9. (SLEEP, COWBOY)
10. (HOLD, COWBOY, HORSE 1)
11. (ARRIVE, BOY)
12. (SMALL, BOY)
13. (HOLD, BOY, HORSE 2)
14. (SMALL, HORSE 2)
15. (OF, HORSE 2, WOOD)
16. (PLAY TRICK, BOY)
17. (CUT, BOY, BRIDLE)
18. (OF, BRIDLE, HORSE 1)
19. (WITH, P17, SCISSORS)
20. (SLEEP, COWBOY)
21. (TIE, BOY, HORSE 2)
22. (OF, HORSE 2, BOY)
23. (TO, P21, HAND)
24. (OF, HAND, COWBOY)
25. (INSTEAD OF, P21, HORSE 1)
26. (RUN AWAY, HORSE 1)
27. (RUN AWAY, BOY)
28. (AND, P27, P26)
29. (WAKE UP, COWBOY)
30. (NOTICE, COWBOY, P31)
31. (HAVE, COWBOY, HORSE 2)
32. (OVERTURN, COWBOY, BENCH)

References

Berko-Gleason, J., Goodglass, H., Obler, L., Green, E., Hyde, M.R., & Weintraub, S. (1980). Narrative strategies of aphasic and normal-speaking subjects. *Journal of Speech and Hearing Research, 23,* 370–382.

[3]Free and literal translation of core Ps originally defined in French.

Broca, P. (1865). Sur la faculté du langage articulé. *Bulletin de la Société d'Anthropologie*, *6*, 337–393.

Brownell, H.H., Michel, D., Powelson, J., & Gardner, H. (1983). Surprise but not coherence: Sensitivity to verbal humor in right-hemisphere patients. *Brain and Language*, *18*, 20–27.

Charolles, M. (1978). Introduction aux problèmes de la cohérence des textes. *Langue française*, *38*, 7–41.

Charolles, M. (1983). Coherence as a principle in the interpretation of discourse. *Text*, *3*, 71–97.

Critchley, M. (1970). *Aphasiology and other aspects of language*. London: Arnold.

Dax, M. (1865). Lésions de la moitié gauche de l'encéphale coïncidant avec l'oubli de signes de la pensée. Lu au Congrès méridional de Montpellier en 1836, par le Docteur Marc Dax. *Gazette hebdomadaire de médecine et de chirurgie*, *23*, 259–262.

Delis, D.C., Wapner, W., Gardner, H., & Moses, J.A. (1983). The contribution of the right hemisphere to the organization of paragraphs. *Cortex*, *19*, 43–50.

Eisenson, J. (1959). Language dysfunctions associated with right brain damage. *American Speech and Hearing Association*, *1*, 107.

Eisenson, J. (1962). Language and intellectual modifications associated with right cerebral damage. *Language and Speech*, *5*, 49.

Gainotti, G., Caltagirone, C., Miceli, G., & Masullo, C. (1981). Selective semantic-lexical impairment of language comprehension in right-brain-damaged patients. *Brain and Language*, *13*, 201.

Gazzaniga, M.S. (1971). Right hemisphere language. *Neuropsychologia*, *9*, 479–482.

Gazzaniga, M.S., & Hillyard, S.A. (1971). Language and speech capacity of the right hemisphere. *Neuropsychologia*, *9*, 273–280.

Gazzaniga, M.S., & Sperry, R.W. (1967). Language after section of the cerebral commissures. *Brain*, *90*, 131–148.

Halliday, M.A.K. (1975). *Learning how to mean: Explorations in the development of language*. London: Arnold.

Halliday, M.A.K., & Hasan, R. (1976). *Cohesion in English*. London: Longman.

Hannequin, D., Goulet, P., & Joanette, Y. (1987). *Hémisphère droit et langage*. Paris: Masson.

Heeschen, C., & Reisches, F. (1979). Cited by Foldi, Cicone, & Gardner (1983) as an unpublished manuscript.

Huber, W., & Gleber, J. (1982). Linguistic and nonlinguistic processing of narratives in aphasia. *Brain and Language*, *16*, 1–18.

Joanette, Y. (1989). Aphasia in left-handers and crossed aphasia. In F. Boller & J. Grafman (Eds.), *Handbook of neuropsychology* (pp. 173–183). Amsterdam: Elsevier.

Joanette, Y. (1980). Contribution à l'étude anatomo-clinique des troubles du langage dans les lésions cérébrales droites du droitier. Ph.D. dissertation, Montréal, Université de Montréal.

Joanette, Y., Goulet, P., & Hannequin, D. (1990). *Right hemisphere and verbal communication*. New York: Springer-Verlag.

Joanette, Y., Goulet, P., Ska, B., & Nespoulous, J.-L. (1986). Informative content of narrative discourse in right-brain-damaged right-handers. *Brain and Language*, *29*, 81–105.

Joanette, Y., Lecours, A.R., Lepage, Y., & Lamoureux, M. (1983). Language in right-handers with right-hemisphere lesions: A preliminary study including anatomical, genetic, and social factors. *Brain and Language*, *20*, 217–248.

Joanette, Y., Puel, M., Nespoulous, J.-L., Rascol, A., & Lecours, A.R. (1982). Aphasie croisée chez les droitiers. I. Revue de la litterature. *Revue neurologique, 138*, 575–586.

Kintsch, W. (1974). *The representation of meaning in memory.* Hillsdale, N.J.: Erlbaum.

Kintsch, W., & van Dijk, T.A. (1978). Toward a model of text comprehension and production. *Psychological Review, 85*, 363–394.

Le Ny, J.-F. (1979). *La sémantique psychologique.* Paris: Presses Universitaires de France.

Lesser, R. (1974). Verbal comprehension in aphasia: An English version of three Italian tests. *Cortex, 10*, 247–263.

Lesser, R. (1986). Comprehension of linguistic cohesion after right brain-damage. Paper presented at the 9th European Conference of the International Neuropsychological Society, Veldhoven.

Levy, J., & Trevarthen, C. (1977). Perceptual, semantic and phonetic aspects of elementary language processes in split-brain patients. *Brain, 100*, 105–118.

Lovett, M.W., Dennis, M., & Newman, J.E. (1986). Making reference: The cohesive use of pronouns in the narrative discourse of hemidecorticate adolescents. *Brain and Language, 29*, 224–251.

Nespoulous, J.-L. (1979). De deux comportements verbaux de base: Référentiel et modalisateur. Paper presented at the Société de Neuropsychologie de Langue française, Paris.

Obler, L. (1980). Narrative discourse style in the elderly. In L.K. Obler & M.L. Albert (Eds.), *Language and communication in the elderly* (pp. 75–90). Lexington, Mass.: Lexington Books.

Oldfield, O.D. (1971). The assessment and analysis of handedness: The Edinburgh Inventory. *Neuropsychologia, 9*, 97–113.

Ombredane, A. (1951). *L'aphasie et l'élaboration de la pensée explicite.* Paris: Presses Universitaires de France.

Ripich, D.N., Terrell, B.Y., & Spinelli, F. (1983). Discourse cohesion in senile dementia of the Alzheimer type. In R.H. Brookshire (Ed.), *Clinical aphasiology: Conference proceedings* (pp. 316–321). Minneapolis, Minn.: BRK Publishers.

Siegel, S. (1956). *Nonparametric statistics for the behavioral sciences.* New York: McGraw-Hill.

Sperry, R.W., & Gazzaniga, M.S. (1967). Language following surgical disconnection of the hemispheres. In C.H. Milikan & F.L. Darley (Eds.), *Brain mechanisms underlying speech and language* (pp. 108–121). New York: Grune & Stratton.

Ulatowska, H.K., & Bond, S.A. (1983). Aphasia: Discourse considerations. *Topics in Language Disorders, 3*, 21–34.

Ulatowska, H.K., Freedman-Stern, R., Weiss-Doyel, A., Macaluso-Haynes, S., & North, A.J. (1983). Production of narrative discourse in aphasia. *Brain and Language, 19*, 317–334.

van Dijk, T.A. (1977). *Text and context. Explorations in the semantics and pragmatics of discourse.* London: Longman.

Wapner, W., Hamby, S., & Gardner, H. (1981). The role of the right hemisphere in the apprehension of complex linguistic material. *Brain and Language, 14*, 15–33.

Weinstein, E.A. (1964). Affections of speech with lesions of the non-dominant hemisphere. *Research in Nervous and Mental Disease, 42*, 220.

Winner, E., & Gardner, H. (1977). Comprehension of metaphor in brain-damaged patients. *Brain, 100*, 719–727.

Wishart, D. (1978). *Clustan.* Inter-University/Research Council Series, Report number 47, Edinburgh University.

Yorkston, K.M., & Beukelman, D.R. (1980). An analysis of connected speech samples of aphasic and normal speakers. *Journal of Speech and Hearing Disorders, 45*, 27–36.

7
Text Comprehension and Production in Aphasia: Analysis in Terms of Micro- and Macroprocessing

WALTER HUBER

Introduction

During the last two decades, most psycholinguistic research on aphasia started from the assumption that only elementary linguistic units and regularities are worth studying. According to this view, only these units and regularities are expected to have a specific impact on language production and comprehension of aphasic patients. Furthermore, the study of text and discourse processing can be disregarded for both methodological and theoretical reasons. On one hand, in text there is always complex interaction between numerous elementary linguistic parameters, which prevents a precise specification of the underlying linguistic deficit. On the other hand, those parameters that are unique to text, such as stylistic cohesion, semantic coherence, and narrative form as represented in a story grammar, appear to be irrelevant for understanding aphasia.

For example, the stylistic cohesion device of coreference crucially depends on the knowledge of pronominal forms and of grammatical regularities that govern their occurrence. If this knowledge is affected in aphasia, it follows automatically that stylistic cohesion by means of coreference cannot be attended to either in comprehension or in production of texts. Conversely, semantic and pragmatic coherence of a text, when defined in terms of real-world context, should be unaffected as long as aphasia is viewed as an impairment of language and not of thinking. Likewise, knowing how to compose a good story should be preserved in aphasia as this is hardly tied to knowing the phonological, lexical, or syntactic units/regularities of one's native language.

However, despite undisputable elementary linguistic deficits, aphasic patients often do surprisingly well in everyday conversation. Their situational comprehension appears quite unimpaired, and they are able to convey their main ideas rather coherently using additional para- and extralinguistic means such as facial

I thank Klaus Willmes and Ralf Glindemann for many helpful suggestions on an earlier version of this chapter. The work reported was, in part, supported by the Deutsche Forschungsgemeinschaft.

expression, gesture, pantomime or drawing (cf. e.g., Wilcox, Davis, and Leonard, 1978; De Bleser and Weismann, 1987).

Focussing on sentence comprehension, several recent studies have demonstrated that asphasic patients rely on perceptual strategies rather than on complete linguistic analysis (e.g., Blumstein, Goodglass, Statlender, and Biber, 1983; Caramazza and Zurif, 1976; Heeschen, 1980; Huber, Lüer, and Lass, 1988; Lonzi and Zanobio, 1983; Saffran, Schwartz, and Marin, 1980; Scholes, 1978; Schwartz, Saffran, and Marin, 1980). Aphasic patients rely on semantic information derived from individual lexical items or on simple string information (such as the first noun phrase followed by a verb) and match this kind of information to situational expectations and general world knowledge. In this way, they arrive at plausible, but not necessarily correct interpretations. Therefore, a full understanding of aphasic performance forces one to consider not only what aphasic patients cannot do but also what they still can do when they are confronted with a language task. Text processing seems to be particularly suited as it requires the processing of both linguistic and situational information even by normal subjects.

In Figure 7.1, two modes of normal text processing are contrasted schematically. Macroprocessing enables the speaker/hearer to deal primarily with the most important ideas in a text. Microprocessing, on the other hand, deals with individual propositions and their relationships as conveyed by various syntactic and stylistic cohesion devices such as coreference relations, attributive and

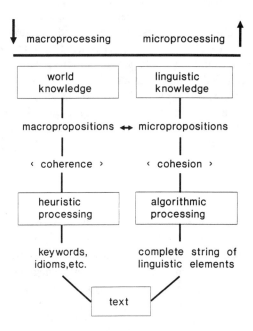

FIGURE 7.1. Two modes of text comprehension.

adverbal specifications, changes in word order, paraphrases, repetitions, and so on. Obviously, microprocessing of texts requires extensive linguistic knowledge and presumably an algorithmic processing mode which is fully rule governed and entails a complete analysis of all linguistic elements.

There are two competing theories on how macroprocessing takes place. (See also (this volume) the chapters by Frederiksen, Bracewell, Breleux, and Renaud and that by Mross.) Kintsch and van Dijk in their early work (e.g., 1978) proposed that macroprocesses generalize and summarize the contents of the micropropositions. But other authors (e.g., Johnson-Laird, 83) have suggested – and van Dijk and Kintsch in their more recent work (1983) seem to agree – that general world knowledge and pragmatic reasoning play a crucial role for macroprocessing. Macropropositions are considered as "fact units" constrained by referential continuity and general plausibility rather than as members of linguistically defined classes. The mode of processing is heuristic. Lexical information, such as key words and idioms, is picked up from the text and matched to experiential knowledge and expectations about persons, events, and situations. As soon as a plausible match is obtained, the interpretation process comes to an end.

What would be the consequences for text processing in conditions of aphasia? If the preferred mode is knowledge-based macroprocessing of key-word information, then even severely impaired aphasic patients can be expected to grasp the main ideas of texts, given that they still have some residual lexical knowledge and that their aphasia does not necessarily coincide with an impairment of nonlinguistic cognitive abilities. Microprocessing would, of course, be impaired – it may even be avoided. The aphasic's reliance on macrostructure information alone may lead to confusions of persons, events, and situations as long as these confusions do not contradict the main ideas gleaned from the text.

In contrast, normal subjects should achieve a more accurate understanding of texts as they are engaged in simultaneous macro- and microprocessing until an optimal match is obtained. However, even for normal subjects, due to limitations of working memory, a perfect understanding of all propositional elements cannot be expected in all circumstances. Nevertheless, normal text comprehension should clearly surpass that of aphasic patients.

Text–Picture Matching

In our first study on text comprehension (Stachowiak, Huber, Poeck, and Kerschensteiner, 1977), we obtained quite unexpected negative findings. Normal subjects' text comprehension did not significantly surpass that of aphasic subjects, not even of those patients who exhibited severe degrees of expressive and receptive language impairment as assessed by clinical examination.

The narrative structure of the text stimuli we used is exemplified in Table 7.1. We kept the narrative structure and the amount of stylistic cohesion parallel across all 26 text stimuli.

TABLE 7.1. Examples of text stimuli

Redundant text-5 picture matching (Stachowiak et al., 1977)	
Setting	Mr. Bauer works in an office.
Complication 1	He has volunteered to replace his colleagues during their holidays.
Complication 2	But, after having been ill himself for a week,
Resolution	Mr. Bauer is unable to cope with the piles of files on his desk.
Comment (idiom)	Germ.: Da hat er sich eine schöne Suppe eingebrockt.
	Fig. He got himself into a nice mess.
	Lit. He has filled his soup with pieces of bread.
Moral	That's what comes of his ambition.
Question	Which picture shows what situation he is in?
Nonredundant text-4 picture matching (Kohlert, 1979)	
Resolution	Mr. Drucks works on a big pile of files.
Complication	because he voluntarily took over too much paper work
Comment (idiom)	Germ.: Da hat er sich eine schöne Suppe eingebrockt.
	Fig. He got himself into a nice mess.
	Lit. He has filled his soup with pieces of bread.
Question	What is Mr. Drucks doing?

Each story was read aloud to the subject who was asked to choose one out of five multiple choice pictures. Figure 7.2 illustrates the kinds of pictures we used. The target picture (a) always represented the core event of the story. Three semantic distractor pictures misrepresented either the agent (b), the action (c), or the situation (d) expressed in each story. There was always a fourth distractor (e) that depicted the literal meaning of the metaphorical idioms which were used as a comment on the main event of each story. In the example given in Table 7.1 and Figure 7.2, the German idiom "Da hat er sich eine schöne Suppe ein-gebrockt" literally means "He filled his soup with pieces of bread." This literal meaning was depicted as a distractor; the figurative meaning "he got himself into a nice mess," of course, corresponded to the target picture.

The five pictures of each item were shown in a circular array while the text was read aloud. The order of the multiple choice pictures was randomized across items.

Neither aphasic patients of the standard syndromes, right hemisphere patients, nor normal controls ($n = 19$ in each group) consistently applied a precise linguistic analysis of the spoken text. On the average, in 25 percent of the items subjects pointed to the semantic distractor pictures and showed no differential attraction to misrepresentations of agent, action, or situation. Statistically, the groups were indistinguishable. We assumed that this similarity across groups was due to the redundancy of both the text and the picture stimuli used. Note that the agent of each story was referred to in each of the six sentences of each text. Furthermore, the core event was not only stated literally but also commented on by the figurative meaning of the idiom.

Since 1977, several other studies reported beneficial effects of linguistic context on comprehension in aphasia. This is so, most likely, because any themati-

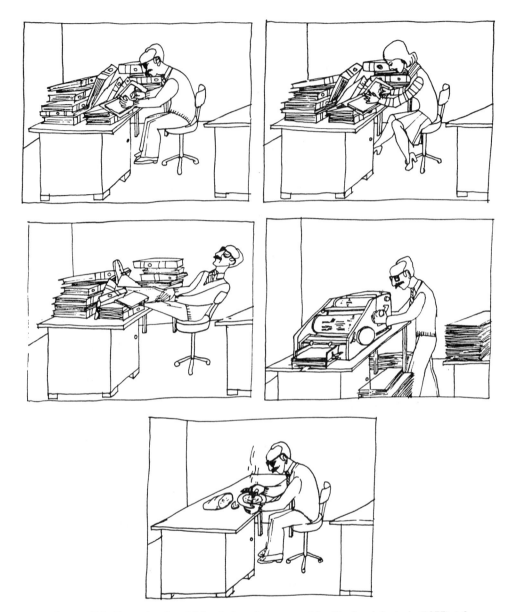

FIGURE 7.2. Example of multiple choice pictures used by Stachowiak et al. (1977) (cf. text).

cally coherent context creates redundancy of information (Cannito, Jarecki, and Pierce, 1986; Hough, Pierce, and Cannito, 1989; Waller and Darley, 1978). In contrast, some other studies support the more specific view that context is only favorable when it pragmatically predicts the forthcoming event (Nicholas and Brookshire, 1983; Pierce and Wagner, 1985; Pierce, 1989). It remains an unresolved question (cf. Boyle and Canter, 1986) whether predictive context helps aphasic listeners to understand difficult sentences (i.e., to enhance microprocessing) or if it merely provides enough information to make those sentences superfluous (i.e., to support macroprocessing).

In our own study (1977), predictability of the core event was not specifically controlled for. However, in order to examine the redundancy assumption, we carried through a second study (Kohlert, 1979). We reduced the contents of the original stories to only one complication and its resolution, leaving out the setting and the moral of each narrative (cf. Table 7.1). The multiple choice set of pictures was also reduced. Besides the target picture, only the action and idiom distractors (cf. Figure 2) were given together with a new, totally unrelated distractor picture.

This time, the expected group differences were found as shown in Table 7.2. Right-hemisphere, brain-damaged patients and normal controls exhibited only a few semantic errors as opposed to 17% to 30% in the aphasic groups. The other errors were metaphor errors which will be discussed in the next section. The reduced task demands obviously enabled only the nonaphasic subjects to apply more precise linguistic microprocessing.

Thus, the originally observed beneficial effect of redundant context on text comprehension of aphasic patients turns out to be a rather indirect one. With greater redundancy, aphasic patients do not necessarily show better comprehension, rather the non-aphasic control subjects obtain a lower accuracy of comprehension. When texts are more redundant, but also longer and more complex, normal listeners just like aphasics rely to a larger extent on macro- than on microprocessing.

The question arose whether the more severely impaired global and Wernicke's aphasics were engaged in linguistic processing at all. Maybe, these patients made their choice simply by comparing the contents of the pictures. However, in a third study, we were able to show that at least with respect to idioms some linguistic processing was going on.

Comprehension of Metaphorical Idioms

As already mentioned, the stories in the original and in the reduced version contained metaphorical idioms that commented on the core event. In half of the items, there was a remote relationship between the literal meaning of the idiom and the reference situation (cf. Figure 7.3). With the idiom "Da hat er sich eine schöne Suppe eingebrockt" ("He has filled his soup with pieces of bread"), the two actions—working on piles of files and eating a soup—have no features in common.

However, in the other half of the items, the idioms exhibited a close relationship between the literal meaning and the reference situation (cf. Figure 7.3). An example is the idiom "Die andern nehmen ihn bis aufs Hemd aus/The others strip him right down to his shirt," which has the figurative meaning "The others take all his money." This idiom is commonly used as in one of our stories in the context of gambling. Obviously, the figurative and the literal meaning have something in common: Things are taken away from somebody.

TABLE 7.2. Overall accuracy of performance in text-picture-matching (means of correct responses in percent)

Group size n = 19/17 each	Global	Wernicke	Broca	RH-Controls	Normals
Redundant text (26 items, 5-choice)	47.3	50.8	63.5	60.0	68.8
(Stachowiak et al., 1977)					
Nonredundant text (20 items, 4-choice)	42.0	45.5	67.5	80.5	95.5
(Kohlert, 1979)					

MANOVA multivariate analysis of variance (alpha = 5%) and post hoc pairwise comparisons (alpha-level adjusted).
_____ = nonsignificant group difference.

In both the Stachowiak et al. and Kohlert studies, all groups chose the depiction of the literal meaning significantly more often when there was a close than a remote relationship between the two pictures. The differences in frequencies of such literal responses are reported in Table 7.3. It was not clear whether these differences were the result of processing the idioms themselves or whether they were due to pictorial comparisons and reasoning on the basis of factual similarity among the multiple choice pictures.

We therefore conducted a further experiment (Freund, 1980), using an idiom-3 picture matching task in which each meaning of the idiom had to be understood separately. There was a total of 52 items with each idiom being presented twice. The multiple choice set contained a depiction of the literal meaning in one condition, and a depiction of the figurative meaning in the other condition. In both conditions, in addition to the target picture, there were the same two unrelated distractor pictures, which precluded any plausible inference with respect to either the literal or the figurative meaning of the idiom. Normal controls made practically no errors in this task. What did we expect for the aphasic subjects? If in this task the same close-remote relationship effect would show up as in the previous text–picture matching tasks, then this would have to be due to processing the idiom itself and not the multiple choice pictures presented.

The results are given in Table 7.4. They were remarkable in two respects: First, the relationship effect showed up only in global and Wernicke's aphasics and only when they had to understand the literal meaning. Second, choosing the depiction of the figurative meaning was more demanding than choosing the literal meaning in all groups.

How can these findings be reconciled with the previous ones obtained in the text picture matching experiments? In Figure 4, the possible steps of idiom comprehension are illustrated separately for idioms with a close and with a remote relationship between the two meanings. For both types of idioms, it is assumed

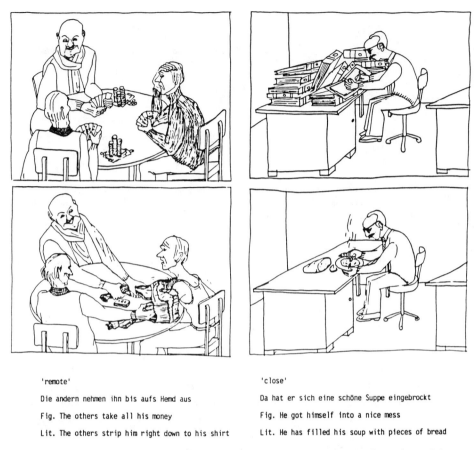

'remote'   'close'

Die andern nehmen ihn bis aufs Hemd aus   Da hat er sich eine schöne Suppe eingebrockt

Fig. The others take all his money   Fig. He got himself into a nice mess

Lit. The others strip him right down to his shirt Lit. He has filled his soup with pieces of bread

FIGURE 7.3. Examples of target and metaphor pictures representing the figurative and the literal meaning of idioms with a close and remote relationship between the two meanings.

that the figurative meaning is represented holistically in the lexicon and that this meaning is dominant over the literal meaning, which has to be derived via regular sentence comprehension (cf. Marschark and Hunt, 1985; Swinney and Cutler, 1979; Tourangeau and Sternberg, 1982). However, with the idioms we used (cf. Figure 3), the figurative meanings were always broader and less specific than the literal ones. Therefore in Figure 7.4, large "mental clouds" of possible reference situations are attached to the figurative meanings whereas a small "mental cloud" emerges from the literal meaning (i.e., the set of possible reference situations is more restricted). Within this model, closeness between figurative and literal meaning can be easily specified as degree of overlap between the two sets of possible reference situations. In Figure 7.4, only close idioms are characterized by an overlap between the large and the small "mental cloud," but no such overlap is assumed for remote idioms. Therefore, in terms of possible reference situa-

TABLE 7.3. Frequency of literal responses in text–picture matching (mean percentages)

Group size n = 19/17 each		Global	Wernicke	Broca	RH-Controls	Normals
Redundant text	Close	24.7⌐	27.6⌐	16.9⌐	26.2⌐	25.3⌐
(2 × 13 items, 5-choice)		s	s	s	s	s
(Stachowiak et al.,	Remote	4.6⌐	7.7⌐	3.8⌐	6.9⌐	4.6⌐
1977)						
Nonredundant text	Close	34.1⌐	51.8⌐	26.4⌐	21.2⌐	5.3⌐
(2 × 10 items, 4-choice)		s	s	s	s	s
(Kohlert, 1979)	Remote	17.6⌐	20.5⌐	5.3⌐	3.5⌐	1.2⌐

Split-plot MANOVA (alpha = 5%) and post hoc pairwise comparisons (alpha-level adjusted).
_____ = nonsignificant group difference.
s = significant difference between close/remote, Wilcoxon–sign test.

tions, figurative and literal interpretations of idioms may either facilitate or inhibit each other, depending on the degree of relatedness between the two meanings of the idiom given.

Our findings on comprehension of metaphorical idioms can now be interpreted in the following way (for quite different interpretations cf. Stachowiak, 1986):

1. All subjects, whether they are aphasic, right-hermisphere-brain-damaged patients, or whether they belong to the normal control group, are sensitive to overlap of possible reference situations. Therefore, in the text–picture matching tasks idioms with close relationships led to a higher frequency of pointing to a depiction of the literal meaning of the idiom (cf. Table 7.3). In fact, this happened at the cost of pointing to the target picture. The number of correct responses was lower to approximately the same degree as the number of literal responses was higher (cf. Kohlert, 1979; Stachowiak et al., 1977).

TABLE 7.4. Accuracy of response in idiom-picture matching (means of correct responses in percent)

Group size n = 15 each		Global	Wernicke	Broca	RH-Controls
Literal meaning	Close	82.3⌐	93.1⌐	96.2	96.2
(2 × 13 items, 3-choice)		s	s		
	Remote	71.5⌐	83.8⌐	93.1	95.4
Figurative meaning	Close	73.1	76.2	84.6	87.7
(2 × 13 items, 3-choice)					
	Remote	73.1	76.9	87.7	86.2

Split-split-plot-ANOVA (analysis of variance) (alpha = 5%) and post hoc pairwise comparisons (alpha-level adjusted).
s = significant simple simple main effect, _____ = nonsignificant group difference.

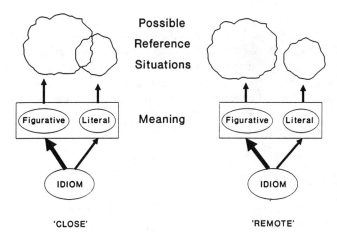

FIGURE 7.4. Modes of idiom comprehension.

2. When the two meanings are tested in isolation, nonaphasic, right-hemisphere patients as well as aphasic, left-hemisphere patients seem to have both alternatives available. But the literal meaning is easier to match to the appropriate picture (cf. Table 7.4) because the range of possible reference situations is more restricted than with the figurative meaning (cf. also Winner and Gardner (1977), who reported a tendency for right-hemisphere patients to select literal depictions of metaphorical noun phases such as "heavy heart," "colorful music").

3. Patients with global and Wernicke's aphasia have, as must be expected, more difficulties with both the figurative and the literal meaning. With respect to the figurative meaning, this indicates difficulties of lexical access and/or knowledge, assuming that idioms are holistically available like lexical units. Furthermore, in contrast to right-hemisphere controls and patients with Broca's aphasia, finding the literal meaning is not generally easier for global and Wernicke's aphasics. It requires the more demanding analytical processing of a sentence, which is particularly disturbed in patients with Wernicke's and global aphasia. This disturbance overrides the less demanding effort for referential reasoning, which can be only applied after the literal meaning is detected.

But why is it that these patients are significantly better when they have to find the literal meaning of idioms with a close relationship? Only in the case of a close relationship is the literal meaning partially activated by both top-down and bottom-up processing: The patients get some help from the possible reference situation due to their less impaired lexical understanding of the figurative meaning along with some help from the literal content as well. In the case of a remote relationship, there is no possibility for the literal meaning to be activated via the figurative meaning. Therefore, in these patients, the literal meaning is more difficult to understand when there is a remote as opposed to a close relationship between the two meanings of the idiom.

The results so far have shown that understanding of a text is clearly guided by nonlinguistic knowledge. If text comprehension is demanding, even normal subjects prefer macroprocessing over microprocessing (cf. Figure 7.1). This leads to an apparent advantage for aphasic patients. As the example of idiom comprehension showed, even severely impaired aphasic patients achieve surprisingly good comprehension when they can successfully rely on partial sentence information in combination with expectations derived from their general world knowledge (i.e., when they rely on macroprocessing).

Arrangement of Stories

A weak point of my argument so far is that I have not really shown whether or not aphasics attempt microprocessing as well as macroprocessing. Some evidence comes from another study (Huber and Gleber, 1982) in which we tried to find out whether high versus low linguistic cohesion among the sentences of a text would have a differential impact. If subjects predominantly rely on key-word information and pragmatic reasoning in order to grasp the main ideas of a text (i.e., on macroprocessing), then their level of performance should not be substantially changed when they are provided with texts of varying degrees of cohesion. If, on the other hand, subjects are also engaged in microprocessing, then they should gain a better understanding with texts of high cohesion. The more elaborate linguistic linkage between sentences should make it easier to gain a precise understanding of the temporal and causal sequences expressed in the texts. Aphasic subjects clearly should have more comprehension difficulties with high

TABLE 7.5. Examples of the two verbal versions of the story arrangement task (translated from the original German)

High Linguistic Cohesion
1. While walking down the street with his dog, an elderly gentleman was suddenly hit on the head by a flower pot falling from a balcony.
2. Both master and dog scolded the culprit on the balcony angrily at the top of their voices.
3. In order to teach the culprit a lesson, they entered the house purposefully.
4. They stopped on the second floor and the gentleman knocked on the apartment door with his cane.
5. An elderly lady opened the door and, full of sympathy, comforted the dog with a bone.
6. This made the elderly gentleman feel good and he gallantly kissed the ladies hand.

Low Linguistic Cohesion
1. A man is hit on the head by a flower pot.
2. The man scolds the woman on the balcony.
3. The man and his dog enter the house.
4 The man knocks on the apartment door.
5. The woman gives the dog a bone.
6. The man kisses the woman's hand.

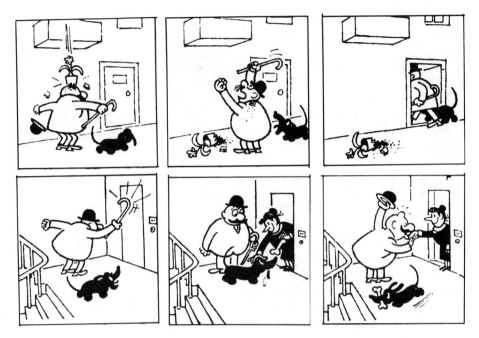

FIGURE 7.5. Example for the pictorial version of the story arrangement task (adapted from Kossatz (1972)).

cohesion texts because of the greater linguistic complexity involved in these texts. This, however, would be only the case if aphasic subjects indeed tried microprocessing at all.

We used an arrangement task (i.e., we asked subjects to arrange an unordered set of either sentences or pictures into a narrative). Two verbal versions of the target stories were constructed (cf. Table 7.5).

In the high-cohesion version, sentences were long and redundant because (1) they contained many attributive and adverbial specifications and (2) because the sentences were interconnected by many stylistic and semantic devices, such as topicalization of constituents and embedding temporal or causal clauses. On the basis of intact microprocessing, the correct order of sentences should be determined easily and unambiguously.

In the low-cohesion version, the sentences were rather nonredundant, expressing only the core events. The only cohesion devices used were repetition of content words and variation of the indefinite and definite articles marking new versus old information. In this version, determining the correct sequence should depend much more on general reasoning and would be less guided by linguistic cues.

There was a third version using the pictures of the original cartoon story (cf. Figure 7.5). As the individual sentences corresponded to the core events of each

TABLE 7.6. Mean error scores in the story arrangement tasks (max. score = 31, 9 items each)

Group size n = 18	Global	Wernicke	Broca	Amnesic	RH-Controls	Normals
Sentences						
High cohesion	20.3^a	19.6^a	11.0	6.0	7.0	1.6
Low cohesion	20.7^a	19.6^a	11.9	7.7	7.2	3.3
Pictures	13.1	15.6	8.6	7.6	11.8	5.1

ANOVA (alpha = 5%) and post-hoc-pairwise comparison (alpha-level adjusted).
⌋ = nonsignificant difference.
[a] No substantial reduction when compared to the maximum number of 31 (i.e., the total number of permutations given in all nine stimulus sequences) (binomial tables, alpha = 1%).

picture, logical and pragmatic coherence was kept as constant as possible across the three versions of the task. There were 9 items in each version. The order of presentation was, of course, systematically varied. For each item, we obtained an error score by counting the number of elements that were placed into a wrong position in the final solution given by the subject. The number of elements that had to be reordered for a correct solution was 3 or 4 per item and 31 total for all 9 items of one version. The mean error scores are presented in Table 7.6.

Contrary to expectation, the degree of linguistic cohesion had no significant influence on the performance of any of the groups. The largest numerical difference between scores of low- and high-cohesion texts was found in the group of normal subjects, which, however, did not reach the statistical significance. The smaller number of errors occurred in the high-cohesion version. This can be attributed to the additional microstructure information provided in this version. The brain-damaged groups, however, seem to have relied only on macrostructure information, which was essentially the same in the two verbal versions of the task.

There is the possibility that underlying differences in the processing of the two texts were obscured by the additional redundancy that compensated for the greater lexical and syntactic complexity of the high-cohesion texts. In a recent study, Caplan and Evans (in press) developed text stimuli that differed only in syntactic complexity whereas length, cohesion, and coherence were kept as parallel as possible between the two types of texts. But again, contrary to expectation, neither aphasics nor nonaphasics experienced greater difficulty with the syntactically complex stories than with the simple ones. Thus, this study further substantiates the view that variation in purely linguistic processing demands (i.e., in microprocessing) does not have a decisive influence on the outcome of text comprehension of aphasic patients.

Further evidence comes from correlational studies. In our two studies on text–picture matching as well as in the story arrangement experiment, we used the German version of the Token Test (Orgass, 1976) as a control task. The subject is required to point—on oral command—to a multiple choice set of geometric forms of varying size, shape, and color. The stimulus sentences are strictly nonredundant and abstract in the sense that situational and experiential reasoning is clearly irrelevant for a correct understanding. Since DeRenzi and Vignolo's pioneering study in 1962, it has been repeatedly demonstrated that aphasics are outstandingly impaired in this task (cf. Boller and Dennis, 1979). Therefore, the Token Test is generally considered to detect the severity of "aphasia proper." As its processing demands are very different from macroprocessing of texts, we expected no substantial correlation between the performance on texts and on the Token Test. This is exactly what we found. The majority of correlation coefficients was far below .40; none of them was significantly larger than zero (Huber and Gleber, 1982; Kohlert, 1979; Stachowiak et al., 1977). This was true for each aphasic subgroup without exception.

Two other studies (Brookshire and Nicolas, 1984; Wegner, Brookshire, and Nicholas, 1984) also found no relationship between text comprehension scores and the ability of aphasic patients to comprehend sentences as assessed by the Token Test. Even when sentences and texts contained precisely the same syntactic complexity, as in the study by Caplan and Evans (in press), the degree of correlation in the comprehension performances of aphasic patients was surprisingly low. It is safe to conclude that text comprehension in aphasia is determined by other factors than sentence comprehension and, furthermore, that performance on text comprehension does not directly reflect the kind and amount of underlying linguistic deficits in aphasia.

So far, the results obtained from the pictorial version of the story arrangement task (cf. Table 6) have not been mentioned. As one would expect, the right-hemisphere patient group performed better on both linguistic versions relative to their significantly greater difficulties with the pictorial version. This was predominantly due to right-hemisphere patients who had retrorolandic (posterior to Rolandic fissure) brain damage as assessed by computerized tomography (CT) (Huber and Gleber, 1982). Visual-spatial deficits caused by lesions in this area are well documented in the literature (Milner, 1974; Sperry, 1974). Quite surprisingly, patients with global and Wernicke's aphasia had the same amount of difficulty with the pictorial version (besides being unable to work purposefully on either linguistic version). How can this be explained? Processing of complex visual information seems to be affected by lesions in both hemispheres, especially in the retrorolandic areas (Basso, DeRenzi, Faglioni, Scotti, and Spinnler, 1973; Orgass, Hartje, Kerschensteiner, and Poeck, 1972). The CT lesions in most of the patients with global and Wernicke's aphasia also showed retrorolandic involvement.

Rather than difficulties specific to pictures, more general impairment of reasoning and/or sequencing may be responsible. This should influence the performance in the linguistic versions of the task in a similar way despite differences in level of performance. Therefore, my colleagues and I conducted correlational studies comparing all three versions of the story arrangement task. The results are shown in Table 7.7 (taken from Gleber, 1980).

The relationship between performance in the two linguistic versions was always strongest and its strength did not decrease when partial correlational coefficients were calculated (cf. first and last line in Table 7.7) (i.e., when any

TABLE 7.7. Intercorrelations between the three versions of the story arrangement task: (1) simple and (2) partial rank correlation coefficients (Kendall's tau)

Group size n = 18 each	Global	Wernicke	Broca	Amnesic	RH-Controls	Normals
Sentences (1)						
High × low cohesion	.47	.93[a]	.71[a]	.65[a]	.77[a]	.65[a]
Picture × sentences (1)						
High cohesion	.51[a]	.45	.58[a]	.43	.69[a]	.31
Low cohesion	.45	.57[a]	.58[a]	.28	.56[a]	.57[a]
Sentences (2)						
High × low cohesion	.31	.93[a]	.56[a]	.62[a]	.63[a]	.61[a]
Without picture						

[a] Significantly larger than zero (for partial correlation coefficients critical values taken from Maghsoodloo, 1975).

additional interrelations with the performances on the pictorial versions were eliminated statistically). Thus, constructing a coherent text from scrambled written sentences is clearly different from reordering the scrambled pictures of the corresponding cartoon story. However, many of the additional relationships between arranging pictures and sentences are also remarkably high (cf. the second and third lines in Table 7.7).

This pattern of correlations between the three versions of the arrangement task is quite compatible with the view that processing of texts in general — not only in aphasia — is determined by macroprocessing (cf. Figure 7.1). The strong relationship between the two linguistic versions appears to reflect the common effort in picking up lexical information such as carried by key words and idioms. This common effort of heuristic information processing is not much influenced by the degree of cohesion in a text. Low versus high cohesion is more likely to have an impact on the perceptual processes (e.g., visual scanning) until salient lexical elements are detected, but the succeeding mental decisions and plausibility judgments for constructing a coherent sequence of events are apparently based on information other than the linguistic cohesion cues of the text. Rather, it is the general and experiential knowledge of the listener that constrains macroprocessing. These nonlinguistic constraints are of course also effective when the subject tries to rearrange the pictures of cartoon stories.

Chapman and Ulatowska (1989) have recently argued that high versus low pragmatic plausibility determines text comprehension more than differences in linguistic cohesion. Patients with moderate aphasia had outstanding difficulties when the sentences were connected with pronominal coreference as opposed to recurrence of lexically fully specified nouns. The understanding of the pronoun versions of the texts were, however, significantly better when the reference could be inferred with high plausibility from the communicative situation expressed in the text. Unfortunately, the statistical analysis of the data was not completely reported. Therefore, it remains unclear whether aphasic subjects perform more poorly than nonaphasic controls even under the simplest conditions and whether pronominal coreference still causes significant residual difficulty even in the presence of high plausibility.

A return to the results from our story arrangement study suggests what appears to be an inevitable conclusion: The initial assumption that reasoning based on world knowledge is surprisingly intact in severe aphasia must be questioned. Apparently, macroprocessing is also impaired. As discussed above, patients with global and Wernicke's aphasia had considerable difficulties with the pictorial version of story arrangements. Also, their performances on the pictorial version were highly correlated—just as in all other groups—with their performances on the linguistic version of the same task. Difficulties in the cognitive planning of text were attributed by Luria and his school (cf. Luria, 1976) to "dynamic aphasia" caused by anterior cortical lesions. But in our study, patients with Wernicke's aphasia caused by posterior lesions performed equally poorly as patients with global aphasia with lesions extending over both anterior and posterior areas (Huber and Gleber, 1982).

Verbal Description of Cartoon Stories

An impairment in cognitive text planning should manifest itself in oral text production as well. Therefore, we asked the aphasic patients to verbally describe the correctly ordered cartoon stories after they had carried out the arrangement task (Hüttemann and Huber, 1986). Before this study is presented in detail, I would like to raise some critical issues for the evaluation of aphasic text production.

Normal text production also involves macro- and microprocesses (cf. van Dijk and Kintsch, 1983; Levelt, 1989), but these processes are not simply the reverse of those used in text comprehension. Instead, they are organized in a more hierarchical fashion. Message construction precedes linguistic formulation. During message construction, cognitive and emotional information as well as communicative intensions are coded into both macro- and micropropositions. For example, when subjects have to describe a cartoon story, they will first try to grasp the gist or the general theme of the cartoon before they plan and formulate one microproposition after another. This will most likely result in a pragmatically and semantically coherent text (i.e., the individual actions and events depicted in the stimulus pictures will be selected and ordered in a logical and plausible way with no intrusions of elaborations or comments on irrelevant details, task difficulties, etc.).

The propositional coherence of a text is not necessarily reflected in its stylistic "surface" organization. There are communicative situations where many colloquial speakers tell stories rather incoherently despite great stylistic and rhetorical skill. On the other hand, a telegraphic colloquial style can be very precise and coherent despite the lack of linguistic linkages. Cohesion refers to the syntactic, morphological and lexical means of connecting sentences within a text. Coherence refers to their semantic and pragmatic connectedness (cf. Beaugrande and Dressler, 1981).

Taking this distinction as a starting point, there are two crucial questions to be asked regarding aphasic text production:

1. Are there linguistic deviations that point to a specific impairment in applying text cohesion devices that do not necessarily follow from more elementary linguistic processing deficits on the word and sentence level?
2. What kind of linguistic data are available that allow unambiguous conclusions about whether the underlying propositional text base is affected or not?

One exploratory approach was undertaken by Berko-Gleason, Goodglass, Obler et al. (1980). They asked subjects to retell stories illustrated by series of cartoonlike pictures. Several distinguishing features were reported that can be divided into three sets depending on whether they reflect basic linguistic deficits, specific difficulties with cohesion, or coherence pattern of the texts. A more extensive collection of data with similar results for similar sets of features (except for the analysis of coherence) can be found in Dressler and Pléh (1988).

The first set of features following is related to the aphasic symptom-complex typically found either in Broca's or Wernicke's aphasia.

• Reduced speech output in Broca's aphasia
• High proportion of nouns in Broca's as opposed to verbs in Wernicke's aphasia
• Lack of complete syntactic constructions in Broca's aphasia and unexpected reduction of syntactic complexity in Wernicke's aphasia

These features clearly reflect lexical and syntactic impairment. They can be found independently of text production (e.g., in naming on confrontation, repetition, reading and writing of words and sentences, or in describing a picture with just one sentence).

Other features reported by Berko-Gleason et al. (1980) were more specific with respect to the cohesion demands of text production:

• High proportion of deictic pronouns ("this," "that," etc.) in Wernicke's aphasics.
• Normal proportion of pronouns in Wernicke's and reduced frequency in Broca's aphasia. However, in both groups, the majority of pronouns had no antecedent (so-called exophoric pronouns) in contrast to anaphoric pronouns (i.e., backward referring pronouns which were most frequently found in the narratives of normal controls).

Both features appear to violate a basic rule of discourse cohesion requiring the speaker to establish a chain of reference throughout the text. The most straightforward way to do this is labeling things by their name and then referring back to them by either a pronoun or by labeling them again.

These mechanisms for establishing reference and coreference do not function well in aphasia as shown by the lack of lexically specified noun phrases and anaphoric pronouns. However, when labeling is generally impaired—as can be seen from any naming to confrontation task—reference can only be established by compensatory devices such as use of deictic pronouns or by predication (i.e., by descriptions of function or property). Furthermore, establishing coreference by means of pronouns might not be impaired as such, but its failure may be the consequence of morphological deficits either at the lexical or syntactic level. It is definitional for both paragrammatism in Wernicke's aphasia and agrammatism in Broca's aphasia that "function words" including pronouns are affected, being either confused or omitted (cf. De Bleser, 1987). These symptoms occur not only in discourse but also in the production of isolated sentences. Therefore, they do not necessarily reflect a specific impairment in the knowledge and/or application of stylistic cohesion devices. (See Dressler and Pléh, 1988, for a somewhat different conclusion.) Recent work on text cohesion in aphasia (Armstrong, 1987; Mentis and Prutting, 1987) used the linguistic analysis procedures proposed in Halliday and Hasan (1976). From this work it is difficult to see at the moment whether cohesion patterns are specifically impaired in aphasia. Baseline data for a comparison with normal cohesion patterns are not yet available. It is not known to what extent variability in quantity and quality of cohesive ties must be expected among nonaphasic adults, within a single speaker, and across different discourse types and task demands.

Finally, two more features were reported by Berko-Gleason et al. (1980) that may indicate a disruption of the propositional planning of texts:

- Both Wernicke's and Broca's aphasics uttered only about 25 percent of the "target lexemes" as compared to normals. These target lexemes or key words were produced by nearly all control subjects for denoting the basic component of a series of stimulus pictures (e.g., "lunch," "drink," and "milk" in one of the stories).
- A similar reduction was found for "main themes" (between three and seven per story in normals). Patients of either group produced only one or two themes per story, and paraphrased the most salient one several times while neglecting less important parts of the story.

Unfortunately, no operational criteria were given for the distinction between "target lexemes" and "main themes." It also remained unclear how an aphasic utterance was mapped onto a "main theme." Nevertheless, these two features might reflect a reduction of the propositional text base underlying the text productions of the aphasic patients. If patients indeed adhere to the most salient theme only, then it is conceivable that they rely primarily on macroprocessing whereas generating a sequence of micropropositions is impaired.

The possibility that the cognitive planning of texts is affected in aphasia was most intensively studied by Ulatowska and her colleagues (Ulatowska, Freedman-Stern, Weiss-Doyal, Macaloso-Haynes, and North, 1983; Ulatowska, North, and Macaluso-Haynes, 1981; Ulatowska, Weiss-Doyel, Freedman-Stern, Macaluso-Haynes, and North, 1983). These researchers specifically investigated the availability of macro- or superstructures for the production of narrative and procedural discourse. Superstructures were defined either as categories of story grammar (setting, action, resolution, and evaluation) or as steps of instrumental scripts (e.g., steps required when changing a light bulb). Even in moderately impaired aphasics, the most essential elements of superstructure were well preserved and recognizable in spite of significant language reduction on the word and sentence level and in spite of low ratings (by normal listeners) for the content and clarity of the produced text.

Two other studies have recently demonstrated that knowledge of scripts for common situations (cf. Schank and Abelson, 1977) is not seriously compromised either by right hemisphere damage (Roman, Brownell, Potter, Seibold, and Gardner, 1987) or by left-hemisphere damage with aphasia, at least when the aphasia is only mild to moderate (Armus, Brookshire, and Nicolas, 1989).

Methodologically, the discovery of macropropositions is difficult to achieve. Script analysis in terms of general world knowledge is limited to those texts that describe a familiar, routinized activity. The categories of story grammar establish schemata of narration, but they do not specify the contents of macro- and micropropositions. A third possibility consists of segmenting given texts into propositions and establishing empirically which of them are essential and which are not. Ulatowska et al. (1983), in their study on narrative discourse in aphasia, took as essential those propositions that were present in "either explicit or implicit form" in the story productions of all normals ($n = 7$) and were mentioned most frequently in their summaries. None of the aphasics produced the complete set of essential propositions. However, nonessential propositions were left out even more often. This again seems to indicate that macroprocessing is the preferred mode of text planning in aphasia.

We now return to our study of verbal descriptions of cartoon stories by aphasic patients. For the evaluation of the propositional content of their descriptions, it was necessary to first establish a normal propositional text base. This procedure is illustrated with the story of the flower pot (cf. Figure 7.5).

As we were mainly interested in macroprocessing, we defined propositions as broadly as possible, referring only to basic facts as conveyed picture by picture. The format of propositions was specified as 1- to 3-place predicates, ignoring all lexical and syntactic variation as well as any semantic modification or quantification.

In Figure 7.6, the standardized propositional text base obtained from a group of 20 normal speakers is shown in forms of a matrix illustrating the sequence of pictures together with the "action space" of each of the three participants in the story. The solid circles identify essential propositions, and the dotted circles optional ones. The distinction was based on the frequency with which these propositions were produced by normal speakers. The cutoffs were set by means of the binomial model. Frequencies ($n \geq 15$) high enough to have a binomial 95 percent confidence interval falling completely above 0.50 were taken to indicate "essential" propositions; those frequencies ($n = 6$–14) with confidence intervals including 0.50 to indicate "optional" propositions; and frequencies ($n \leq 5$) with confidence intervals falling completely below 0.50 to indicate "idiosyncratic" propositions. The latter are not illustrated in Figure 7.6. They were either self-centered comments of the speaker or rhetorical and descriptive elaborations (e.g., "now it is happening," "the house apparently has got several balconies," etc.).

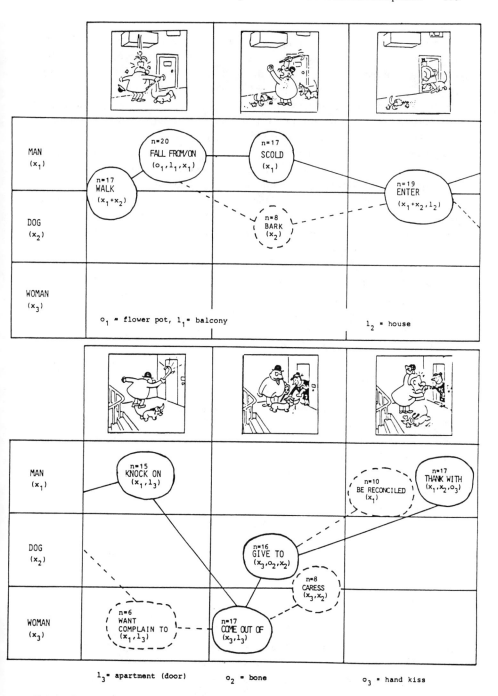

FIGURE 7.6. Standardized propositional textbase.

As a result of this procedure we had standards for the evaluation of the aphasic utterances. Even in severely paraphasic or agrammatic utterances, there may be single linguistic elements such as individual nouns or fragments of a verb phrase that express at least part of the standard propositions. In Table 7.8, the propositional text bases of six different aphasic speakers are presented in order to give an impression of the individual variation that has to be expected from aphasic text productions. In this table, all propositions derived from the aphasic utterances are coded as being either standard (O) or idiosyncratic (A). The arrows connecting the individual propositions illustrate how the patient proceeded from one picture to the other. Regressions are marked by backward arrows and elaborations (i.e., iterations of standard and/or idiosyncratic propositions with respect to the same event shown in the picture) by downward arrows. In the scoring, the number of different propositions as well as deviations from linear sequencing are counted. Gaps occurred when pictures were left out in the narrative or when they were described by idiosyncratic propositions only.

The first example in Table 7.8 is the text base of a patient with amnesic aphasia who tried to be extremely precise in his descriptions. The contents of the first two pictures were tied together by overextensive use of cohesion devices, such as formulating the same proposition in the main clause and in its embedded relative clause (i.e., thematic elaboration). Furthermore at the end of the description to picture 2, he referred back to this multiply expressed proposition again (i.e., regression). Besides his production of all essential and most optional propositions, this patient also introduced a few idiosyncratic propositions. Such occasional elaborations are also characteristic of normal descriptions, of course.

The second example is taken from a different patient with amnesic aphasia. This aphasic left out a few standard propositions. After description of the third picture, she made a regression back to pictures 2 and 1 and then immediately went on to the fifth picture and ended the story with the optional instead of the essential proposition. Again, the propositional organization of this patient's narrative is still within the normal range.

The next examples illustrate text production in Broca's aphasia. The patient of example 3 laboriously produced simple sentences that were morphologically complete. His propositional organization was, however, incomplete resulting in coherence gaps. Whether this reflects directly impaired propositional planning or whether it is brought about by a trade-off effect due to his great effort to produce complete syntactic structures cannot be answered at this level of analysis.

Example 4 presents data from a Broca's aphasic with classical agrammatism. His propositional organization was only slightly incomplete. However, several times he particularized standard propositions (i.e., he referred to details that are entailed by the standard proposition). An example is "Stock schmeiss/Walking stick throws" with reference to the scolding of the person on the balcony. The patient repeated this expression stereotypically in picture 4, which was, nevertheless, adequate as a description of the depicted situation.

TABLE 7.8. Variety of propositional text bases in patients with different aphasic syndromes

	PICT1 Walk Fall	PICT2 Scold (Bark)	PICT3 Enter	PICT4 Knock (Want to Complain)	PICT5 Come (Caress)	Give	(Reconciled) Thank	Proposition 0	0*	A	Sequence E	R	G
Amnesic M,65 yr CVA, 1 mo								10	1	2	3	1	0
Amnesic F,61 yr CVA,1 mo								5	1	0	0	2	1
Broca M,32 yr CVA,11 mo								4	0	0	0	0	2
Broca M,49 yr CVA,19 mo								2	6	0	1	0	0
Wernicke M,64 yr CVA,7 mo								7	3	4	2	0	1
Wernicke M,54 yr CVA (cerebral vascular accident), 18 mo duration								2	5	19	18	0	1

0 = essential/optional, 0* = particularized, A = additional idiosyncratic proposition, E = thematic elaboration/perseveration, R = regression, G = gap.

The last two examples illustrate text production by patients with Wernicke's aphasia. In the text base of example 5, there were many intrusions of idiosyncratic propositions in addition to particularizing of standard propositions. The final patient (example 6) produced predominantly semantic jargon. His propositional content was mainly idiosyncratic, and there were many interruptions of self-comments or comments on the events depicted. Most of the idiosyncratic propositions referred to the mental or psychological state of the main actor. Nevertheless, he was the only patient who missed the surprising resolution of the story in picture 5 – the comforting of the dog by the woman giving him (the dog) a bone. Obviously, the patient's semantic jargon corresponded to a dissolution of propositional planning.

Conclusions

The series of experiments reviewed in this chapter demonstrates that knowledge-based macroprocessing indeed seems to be the preferred mode of text processing in aphasia. Thus, in comprehension even severely impaired aphasic patients can successfully circumvent their elementary linguistic processing difficulties. This compensatory effect most clearly shows up under those task demands that require normal subjects to also rely more on macro- than microprocessing.

However, the knowledge-based macroprocessing of aphasic patients is far from being unimpaired both in comprehension and production tasks. We do not know very well what the underlying mechanisms of this disturbance are. Do aphasic patients have deficits in propositional thinking in general as one would claim in the tradition of Hughlings Jackson and Kurt Goldstein? Or are the propositional difficulties merely trade-off effects? Are aphasic patients so much involved in their linguistic difficulties that propositional reasoning and planning are impoverished as a result? In future research, it would be interesting to detect specific interactions between linguistic production errors and propositional errors such as coherence gaps or irrelevant elaborations.

References

Armstrong, E. (1987). Cohesive harmony in aphasic discourse and its significance to listener perception of coherence. In R.H. Brookshire (Ed.), *Clinical aphasiology*, Vol. 17. Minneapolis, MN: BRK Publishers.

Armus, S.R., Brookshire, R.H., & Nicolas, L.E. (1989). Aphasic and non-brain-damaged adults' knowledge of scripts for common situations. *Brain and Language*, 36: 518–528.

Basso, A., DeRenzi, E., Faglioni, P., Scotti, C., & Spinnler, H. (1973). Neuropsychological evidence for the existence of cerebral areas critical to the performance of intelligence tasks. *Brain*, 16: 715–728.

Beaugrande, R.-A. de, & Dressler, W.U. (1981). *Introduction to text linguistics*. London: Longman.

Berko-Gleason, J., Goodglass, H., Obler, L., Green, E., Hyde, M.R., & Weintraub, S. (1980). Narrative strategies of aphasic and normal speaking subjects. *Journal of Speech and Hearing Research, 23*: 370–382.

Blumstein, S.E., Goodglass, H., Statlender, S., & Biber, C. (1983). Comprehension strategies determining reference in aphasia: A study of reflexivization. *Brain and Language, 18*: 115–127.

Boller, F., Dennis, M. (Eds.) (1979). *Auditory comprehension. Clinical and experimental studies with the Token Test.* New York: Academic Press.

Boyle, M., & Canter, G.J. (1986). Verbal context and comprehension of difficult sentences by aphasic adults: A methodological problem. In R.H. Brookshire (Ed.), *Clinical aphasiology*, Vol. 16. Minneapolis, MN: BRK Publishers.

Brookshire, R.H., & Nicholas, L.E. (1984). Comprehension of directly and indirectly stated main ideas and details in discourse by brain-damaged and non-brain-damaged listeners. *Brain and Language, 21*: 21–36.

Cannito, M., Jarecki, J., & Pierce, R.S. (1986). Effects of thematic structure on syntactic comprehension in aphasia. *Brain and Language, 27*: 38–49.

Caplan, D.N., & Evans, K.L. (in press). The effect of syntactic complexity on discourse comprehension in aphasia. *Brain and Language.*

Caramazza, A., & Zurif, E. (1976). Dissociation of algorithmic and heuristic processes in comprehension: Evidence from aphasia. *Brain and Language, 3*: 572–582.

Chapman, S.B., & Ulatowska, H.K. (1989). Discourse in aphasia: Integration deficits in processing reference. *Brain and Language, 36*: 651–668.

De Bleser, R. (1987). From agrammatism to paragrammatism. German aphasiological traditions and grammatical disturbances. *Cognitive Neuropsychology, 4*: 187–256.

De Bleser, R., & Weismann, H. (1986). The communicative impact of non-fluent aphasia on the dialogue behavior of linguistically unimpaired partners. In F. Lowenthal, & F. Vandamme (Eds.), *Pragmatics and education.* New York: Plenum Press.

DeRenzi, E., & Vignolo, L.A. (1962). The Token Test: A sensitive test to detect receptive disturbances in aphasics. *Brain, 85*: 665–678.

Dijk, T.A. van, & Kintsch, W. (1983). *Strategies of discourse comprehension.* New York: Academic Press.

Dressler, W.U., & Pléh, C. (1988). On text disturbance in aphasia. In W.U. Dressler, & J.A. Stark (Eds.), *Linguistic analyses of aphasic language.* New York: Springer-Verlag.

Freund, G. (1980). Experimentelle Untersuchungen zum Sprachverständnis aphasischer Patienten. Med. Diss., RWTH Aachen.

Gleber, J. (1980). Sprachliches und nichtsprachliches Verarbeiten von Texten bei Aphasie. Med. Diss., RWTH Aachen.

Halliday, M.A.K., & Hasan, R. (1976). *Cohesion in English.* London: Longman.

Heeschen, C. (1980). Strategies of decoding actor–object relations by aphasic patients. *Cortex, 16*: 5–19.

Hough, M.S., Pierce, R.S., & Cannito, M.P. (1989). Contextual influences in aphasia: Effects of predictive versus nonpredictive narratives. *Brain and Language, 36*: 325–334.

Huber, W., & Gleber, J. (1982). Linguistic and nonlinguistic processing of narratives in aphasia. *Brain and Language, 16*: 1–18.

Huber, W., Lüer, G., & Lass, U. (1988). Eye movement behavior in aphasia. In C.W. Johnstone, & J.F. Pirozzolo (Eds.), *Neuropsychology of Eye Movements.* Hillsdale, NJ: Erlbaum.

Hüttemann, J., & Huber, W. (1986). Bildbeschreibungen aphasischer Patienten (unpublished manuscript), RWTH Aachen.

Johnson-Laird, P.N. (1983). *Mental models.* Cambridge, MA: Harvard University Press.

Kintsch, W., & van Dijk, T.A. (1978). Towards a model of text comprehension and production. *Psychological Review, 85:* 363–394.

Kohlert, P.O. (1979). Zur neurolinguistischen Diagnose von Sprachverständnisstörungen bei Aphasie. Med. Diss., RWTH Aachen.

Kossatz, H. (1972). *So ein Dackel! 22 Bildergeschichten für den Sprachunterricht.* Stuttgart: Klett.

Levelt, W.J.M. (1989). *Language production.* Cambridge, MA: MIT Press.

Lonzi, L., & Zanobio, E. (1983). Syntactic component in language responsible cognitive structure: Neurological evidence. *Brain and Language, 18:* 177–191.

Luria, A. (1976). *Basic problems of neurolinguistics.* The Hague: Mouton.

Maghsoodloo, S.M. (1975). Estimates of the quantiles of Kendall's partial rank correlation coefficient. *Journal of Statistical Computation and Simulation, 4:* 155–164.

Marschark, M., & Hunt, R.R. (1985). On memory for metaphor. *Memory and Cognition, 13:* 413–424.

Mentis, M., & Prutting, C.A. (1987). Cohesion in the discourse of normal- and head-injured adults. *Journal of Speech and Hearing Research, 30:* 88–98.

Milner, B. (1974). Hemispheric specialization: Scope and limits. In F.O. Schmitt, & F.G. Worden (Eds.), *The neurosciences. Third study program.* Cambridge, MA: MIT Press.

Nicholas, L., & Brookshire, R. (1983). Syntactic simplification and context. Effects on sentence comprehension by aphasic adults. In R. Brookshire (Ed.), *Clinical aphasiology conference proceedings.* Minneapolis, MN: BRK Publishers.

Orgass, B. (1976). Eine Revision des Token Tests. Part I & II. *Diagnostica, 22:* 70–87, 141–156.

Orgass, B., Hartje, W., Kerschensteiner, M., & Poeck, K. (1972). Aphasie und nicht-sprachliche Intelligenz. *Nervenarzt, 43:* 623–627.

Pierce, R. (in press). Influence of prior and subsequent context on comprehension in aphasia. *Aphasiology.*

Pierce, R.S., & Wagner, C. (1985). The role of context in facilitating syntactic decoding in aphasia. *Journal of Communication Disorders, 18:* 203–214.

Roman, M., Brownell, H.H., Potter, H.H., Seibold, M.S., & Gardner, H. (1987). Script knowledge in right hemisphere-damaged and in normal elderly adults. *Brain and Language, 31:* 151–170.

Saffran, E.M., Schwartz, M.F., & Marin, O.S.M. (1980). The word order problem in agrammatism, II. Production. *Brain and Language, 10:* 263–280.

Schank, R.C., & Abelson, R.P. (1977). *Scripts, plans, grals, and understanding.* Hillsdale, NJ: Erlbaum.

Scholes, R.J. (1978). Syntactic and lexical components of sentence comprehension. In A. Caramazza, & E.B. Zurif (Eds.), *Language acquisition and language breakdown.* Baltimore: The Johns Hopkins University Press.

Schwartz, M.F., Saffran, E.M., & Marin, O.S.M. (1980). The word order problem in agrammatism. I. Comprehension. *Brain and Language, 10:* 249–262.

Sperry, R.W. (1974). Lateral specialization in the surgically separated hemispheres. In F.O. Schmitt, & F.G. Worden (Eds.), *The neurosciences. Third study program.* Cambridge, MA: MIT Press.

Stachowiak, F.J. (1986). Metaphor comprehension and production. In W. Paprotte & R. Dirven (Eds.), *The ubiquity of metaphor: Metaphors in language and thought.* Philadelphia, PA: J. Benjamins North America.

Stachowiak, F.J., Huber, W., & Poeck, K., & Kerschensteiner, M. (1977). Text comprehension in aphasia. *Brain and Language*, *4*: 177–195.

Swinney, D.A., & Cutler, A. (1979). The access and processing of idiomatic expressions. *Journal of Verbal Learning and Verbal Behavior*, *18*: 523–534.

Tourangeau, R., & Sternberg, R.J. (1982). Understanding and appreciating metaphors. *Cognition*, *11*: 203–244.

Ulatowska, H.K., Doyel, A.W., Stern, R.F., Macaluso-Haynes, S.M., & North, A.J. (1983). Production of procedural discourse in aphasia. *Brain and Language*, *18*: 315–341.

Ulatowska, H.K., Freedman-Stern, R., Weiss-Doyel, A., Macaluso-Haynes, S., & North, A.J. (1983). Production of narrative discourse in aphasia. *Brain and Language*, *19*: 317–334.

Ulatowska, H.K., North, A.J., & Macaluso-Haynes, S. (1981). Production of narrative and procedural discourse in aphasia. *Brain and Language*, *13*: 345–371.

Waller, M.R., & Darley, F.L. (1978). The influence of context on the auditory comprehension of paragraphs by aphasic subjects. *Journal of Speech and Hearing Research*, *21*: 732–745.

Wegner, M.L., Brookshire, R.H., & Nicholas, L.E. (1984). Comprehension of main ideas and details in coherent and non-coherent discourse by aphasic and non-aphasic listeners. *Brain and Language*, *21*: 37–51.

Wilcox, M.J., Davis, G.A., & Leonard, L.B. (1978). Aphasics' comprehension of contextually conveyed meaning. *Brain and Language*, *6*: 362–377.

Winner, E., & Gardner, H. (1977). The comprehension of metaphor in brain-damaged patients. *Brain*, *100*: 717–729.

8
Narrative and Procedural Discourse in Aphasia

Hanna K. Ulatowska, Lee Allard, and Sandra Bond Chapman

Introduction

Current interest in discourse performance has been motivated by the explanatory power provided by recent developments in discourse grammar. Discourse, unlike sentences, does not have a strict set of rules that specify grammaticality. Nor does discourse have a specified length. Although discourse is often described as a series of connected sentences, it may be a single word, a phrase, a sentence, or an infinite combination of all these forms. The length is specified in terms of communicative function (i.e., discourse is a unit of language that conveys a message). Discourse grammar provides a linguistic description of the properties that contribute to acceptability or well-formedness of discourse. There are several discourse types (e.g., narrative, procedural, expository, and conversational) that differ in structure and information content.

Discourse performance entails a complex interaction between cognitive and linguistic factors, which may be differentially impaired in different neurological populations. Therefore, discourse studies can increase our knowledge regarding brain-behavior relationships. Specifically, discourse grammar provides a means for exploring patterns of behavioral disruption associated with particular focal or diffuse brain injuries. Discourse performance by aphasic patients is of particular interest, because this is the only population with a well-documented linguistic impairment in the presence of more intact cognitive functioning. It is of interest to investigate how aphasic patients with limited linguistic abilities can manipulate large chunks of information.

Currently, limited empirical data exist regarding effects of sentence-level language disruption on the ability to process discourse, although a dissociation between discourse- and sentence-level abilities can be observed in aphasia. Many aphasic patients can communicate effectively despite severe disruption in syntax and reduction in vocabulary. Perhaps the cognitive structures that underlie sentential processing are independent of, yet critical to, discourse processing. Discourse grammars provide a way of explaining communicative performance that is not tied to sentence-level performance.

Examining discourse performance in disordered populations can provide insights into normal discourse processing. In many disordered populations, certain mechanisms underlying discourse performance may be impaired, while other mechanisms may be intact. This dissociation can help reveal the contribution of particular processes to discourse performance.

In this chapter, we will summarize and interpret the most important findings from our studies of narrative and procedural discourse performance in aphasic patients at varying severity levels. We have been interested in what happens to discourse structure as linguistic resources become more impaired. We have also been concerned with the relationship and possible dissociation between sentence- and discourse-level performance, an issue that can be addressed using discourse grammar. While we have gained important information regarding aphasic patients' ability to organize linguistic information, we have also gained insight regarding methodological improvements for increased explanatory power. We will discuss these insights and suggest new directions for future research.

Perspectives on Discourse Genre

In our studies of discourse performance in disordered populations, we have examined both narrative and procedural genres. Use of both genres allows for a more precise characterization of discourse problems, since the cognitive and linguistic demands of these genres differ. From a neurolinguistic perspective, the different demands of narrative and procedural discourse may lead to different patterns of impairment in each genre. In our studies, narrative and procedural discourse were selected because both are important discourse types in normal communication and because they differ along a number of linguistic and cognitive parameters (Longacre, 1976a).

There are important differences between narrative and procedural discourse at a pragmatic level, insofar as the communicative functions of the two genres differ. A primary function of narrative is to entertain, whereas the primary function of procedural discourse is to inform or instruct. Consequently, there may be greater demands for explicitness and clarity in procedures.

There are also marked differences between narrative and procedural discourse in terms of information content. Narratives are typically oriented around characters and events, while procedures are action oriented. Although information content per se is not a linguistic parameter, these differences in information content across genres have linguistic implications, particularly in the areas of cohesion and superstructure, which are discussed next.

Cohesion involves relations between words, sentences, or larger units within a text. It binds together the parts of a text into a coherent whole. In a narrative, compared to a procedure, cohesion is likely to involve larger segments of text. For example, each episode of a narrative usually focuses on a particular character, so that a cohesive chain involving that character will extend across a relatively long stretch of discourse. In contrast, procedural discourse may involve primarily local cohesion (i.e., linkages between adjacent sentences but not across larger segments of text).

Narrative discourse conforms to a fairly conventional superstructure, consisting of elements such as a setting, complicating action, and resolution. More complex narratives will consist of multiple episodes, each containing some of these superstructure elements. Procedural discourse has a different type of superstructure, which is less well understood. A simple procedure may consist only of a series of steps culminating in a target step, which specifies the goal or end state of the procedure. More complex procedures may contain additional elements (e.g., a "setting" that specifies preconditions for performing the procedure, such as items needed or the location where the procedure is performed).

Some of the differences just described between narrative and procedural discourse may exert an influence at the level of syntax. Narrative discourse may be characterized by more complex syntax and by a wider range of syntactic structures, partly because of stylistic demands and partly because of the diversity of information types expressed. This increased complexity of syntax in narratives may result in a higher proportion of syntactic errors in narrative as opposed to procedural discourse.

Review of Research

Research conducted by us and our colleagues has focused on narrative and procedural discourse in aphasic patients, although some work has also been done with demented and normal elderly subjects. There were three general purposes for our studies. First, we wanted to describe the characteristics of discourse produced by disordered subjects at multiple linguistic levels, including the lexical-semantic, syntactic, and text levels. Second, we wanted to suggest possible mechanisms, both cognitive and linguistic, underlying the disruption of discourse performance. Third, we wanted to compare discourse performance of subjects with different types of disorders and at different levels of severity. Since there is still relatively little known about discourse processing in impaired populations, most of our research has been exploratory in nature, with relatively small yet well-defined samples.

Although the focus of our studies has been on discourse, we have also examined sentential variables, including measures of syntactic complexity, use of modifiers, grammatical correctness, and so on. It is important to examine sentential variables in studies of discourse, because discourse-level structures are realized through sentence-level structures. While there is some degree of independence between the sentential and discourse levels of language, as our studies have indicated, sentence-level deficits do have an impact on the well-formedness of discourse.

In all of our studies, cognitive tests were administered to subjects to provide data on possible cognitive deficits that could contribute to discourse problems and to characterize subjects more completely. Additionally, standardized language tests were administered to provide information concerning possible deficits at the word or sentence level that might affect discourse performance.

Written Discourse in a Wernicke's Aphasic

The impetus for our studies of discourse in disordered populations was a single case study, reported in Ulatowska and Freedman-Stern (1978) and in Freedman-Stern, Ulatowska, Baker, and DeLacoste (1984). This patient was a Wernicke's aphasic who showed a marked dissociation in linguistic performance between the sentence level, which was severely disrupted, and the discourse level, which was relatively intact. This patient's ability to communicate effectively despite severe deficits in morphology and syntax provided empirical support for the existence of higher-level discourse structures that may be more important than morphosyntactic structures in mediating communication.

This study involved the analysis of written language, which was better preserved than oral language in this patient, who spent a great amount of time and effort in producing written discourse. From a linguistic perspective, written discourse may allow for a more sensitive analysis of certain text properties (e.g., cohesion) that are more fully realized in written than in oral discourse. The language samples in this study consisted of letters and extracts from a diary. Linguistic analysis revealed errors in morphology, including problems in verb tense and in pronoun gender and case; omission of articles and prepositions; and omission of derivational affixes. Problems at the syntactic level were also frequent, including a reduction of embedded clauses and reduction of clause length, errors in word order, and omission or misuse of conjunctions within the sentence. At the discourse level, however, the patient's language was more intact, as reflected by his control of narrative superstructure (i.e., use of narrative elements such as setting, complicating action, and resolution), his use of relatively sophisticated stylistic devices (e.g., foregrounding of important or unusual information), a skillful use of evaluation to indicate the significance of events, and marking of cohesive relations between sentences. (See sample 1 in Appendix 2 for an example of discourse produced by this patient.)

In addition to providing motivation for our later research in discourse, this single case study exemplified some of the advantages of a case study design, especially in the area of discourse. Careful analysis of a language sample, without reliance on a priori selection of a specific set of parameters, allows for a detailed exploration of the properties of disordered discourse and the relation between those properties and the communicative value of the discourse. However, group studies also have advantages, insofar as they allow for greater generalizability of findings and more powerful comparison of normal and disordered performance on specific parameters. It is to our group studies of discourse in aphasia that we will now turn.

Discourse in Mildly Impaired Aphasics

Our group studies of aphasic discourse were motivated by a desire to extend this case study to a larger population. Specifically, we were interested in using experimental discourse tasks to characterize at a linguistic level the nature of discourse produced by aphasics, to determine whether they would show a dissociation between sentence- and discourse-level structures, and to characterize the nature of that dissociation. The first group study (Ulatowska, North, and Macaluso-Haynes, 1981) examined discourse in a group of mildly impaired aphasics. Subjects were eight males and two females between the ages of 54 and 70 who had become aphasic following a single cerebrovascular accident to the left hemisphere. Two patients were classified as anterior, four as posterior, and four as mixed. A group of normal control subjects, matched by age, sex, and educational level, were also included to allow for direct comparison of normal and disordered discourse. The experimental discourse tasks were of two types, narrative and procedural. The narrative tasks included (1) telling about a "memorable experience" in the subject's life, (2) telling a story based on a sequence of pictures (see "Cat Story" in Appendix 1), (3) giving a summary for the "Cat Story," and (4) retelling a simple fable read by the examiner (see "Rooster Story" in Appendix 1). Procedural tasks involved explaining how to perform routine procedures (brushing teeth, combing hair, cutting bread, and making a sandwich) and more specialized procedures (bowling and changing a tire).

The language samples elicited by these tasks were analyzed at both the sentential and discourse levels. Sentential parameters included length of T-units, various measures of clausal embedding, and grammatical correctness. A T-unit was defined as one independent clause plus the dependent modifiers of that clause (Hunt, 1965). Measures of clausal embedding included number of clauses per T-unit and number of finite and nonfinite dependent clauses, expressed as percentages of total clauses. At the discourse level, narratives were analyzed with respect to the occurrence and length of superstructure elements such as setting, complicating action, and resolution. Procedures were analyzed in terms of number of steps produced and use of adverbial modification. Also, certain types of discourse errors were analyzed, including tense shifts, reference errors, incorrect use of connectives, and errors in sequencing events. A final stage of analysis involved having a group of raters score each text in terms of content and clarity.

Aphasic subjects were able to produce well-structured discourse although, compared to normals, they produced less complex language, more sentential errors, and more discourse errors. Their discourse was also rated lower on content and clarity. The most severe deficits were seen in the summarization task (see sample 2 in Appendix 2 for an example), which may place heavy cognitive as well as linguistic demands on subjects. However, the primary differences between normal and aphasic subjects were quantitative, not qualitative. These results confirm and extend some of the findings of the case study reported before, namely, that aphasic subjects could produce relatively well-structured discourse despite deficits at the sentence level. This is not to say that their discourse was "normal" but, instead, that a partial dissociation between the sentence level and discourse level was observed.

Discourse in Moderately Impaired Aphasics

The purpose of our second group study of discourse in aphasic subjects (Ulatowska, Doyel, Freedman-Stern, Macaluso-Haynes, and North, 1983; Ulatowska, Freedman-Stern, Doyel, Macaluso-Haynes, and North, 1983) was to extend the earlier study to moderately impaired subjects and to refine the methodology used to analyze disordered discourse. The subjects for this study were ten males and five females between the ages of 24 and 71. Thirteen subjects had become aphasic following a single cerebrovascular accident to the left hemisphere, while the remaining two subjects had suffered closed head injury. Eight subjects were classified as anterior, five as posterior, and two as mixed. Analysis of language samples from the discourse tasks was conducted at both the sentential and discourse levels, as in the first study. However, certain additions to the discourse-level analysis were made. The "Cat Story" and "Rooster Story" were analyzed for information content (i.e., how many propositions subjects included from the original stimulus). The "Memorable Experience" was analyzed for spectrum and profile (Longacre, 1976b). Spectrum analysis reveals a gradient of information contained in verb elements, ranging from the most dynamic elements of the story to the most static depictive elements. Profile analysis reveals the development of the plot of a story according to mounting and declining tension. At a more intuitive level, spectrum analysis examines types of verbs and use of verb tenses in terms of the amount of action conveyed and the importance or significance of those actions to the event line of the narrative. Profile analysis examines how a story builds up to a climax and then declines. Procedures were analyzed in terms of three types of steps: essential steps, optional steps, and target steps. Essential steps are defined as those that must be understood by the listener in order to know what actions are required to do the tasks, whereas optional steps are those that clarify or provide more detail about the essential steps. Target steps specify the goal or end-state of the procedure. Examples of these types of steps are provided in Appendix 2.

This study confirmed results of the first study, even though the subjects in the second study were more impaired. Several additional results were also obtained in the second study. In the "Memorable Experience," aphasic patients showed differences in profile, characterized by a more abrupt onset of the climax rather than a steady progression of events and by a reduction in linguistic devices used to mark the climax. Aphasic patients also showed differences in spectrum, characterized by a reduced range and structure of verbal elements. These differences in spectrum were associated with lower ratings of content and clarity for the aphasic subjects. In the procedures, aphasic subjects showed some reduction in the number of essential steps, although they were more likely to omit optional steps. Finally, these moderately impaired subjects produced a relatively large number of sentential errors and discourse errors, although discourse structure was preserved. (See samples 3 and 4 in Appendix 2 for examples of discourse produced by moderately impaired aphasics.)

Discourse in Severely Impaired Aphasics

In a third study, we examined discourse production in severely impaired aphasics (Bond, Ulatowska, Macaluso-Haynes, and May, 1983). Subjects were four males and one female ranging in age from 31 to 64 who had become aphasic following a single cerebrovascular accident to the left hemisphere. Four subjects were classified as anterior and one as posterior. Narrative discourse was elicited, using tasks similar to those described previously. Subjects showed a marked reduction in information content. Also, they showed a disruption in narrative superstructure, characterized primarily by errors in sequencing of events, and also by inadequate production of setting and resolution propositions. Thus, in the severely impaired group, there was evidence for a breakdown at the discourse level, as well as at the sentential level. (See samples 5 and 6 in Appendix 2 for examples.)

Discourse in Dementia

Although most of our research on discourse has been done with aphasic populations, we have used a similar line of research with other populations, including demented subjects and the normal elderly. These studies were conducted in part to investigate whether the patterns of linguistic performance in aphasic subjects would also be seen in other populations, or whether different patterns would emerge.

In a recent study (Ulatowska, Allard, Donnell, Bristow, Macaluso-Haynes, Flower, and North, in press), we examined narrative and procedural discourse in subjects with dementia of the Alzheimer's type (DAT) to specify the nature of linguistic deficits in this population and to compare the pattern of these deficits with the pattern seen in aphasia. Ten mildly to moderately impaired DAT subjects, six males and four females between the ages of 55 and 86, and ten matched controls were given discourse tasks similar to those in earlier studies. Subjects were diagnosed as having dementia of the Alzheimer's type on the basis of neurological, cognitive, and behavioral testing and exclusion of alternative diagnoses. Linguistic analysis was carried out at both the sentential and discourse levels and included measures of syntactic complexity, reference, information content, and superstructure. Results showed that the discourse of DAT subjects was characterized by (1) the relative preservation of sentence-level performance, (2) a reduction of essential information (i.e., information units that were determined a priori to be essential to each narrative or procedure), (3) an increase in tangential and irrelevant information, and (4) a disruption of reference, characterized especially by inappropriate use of pronouns in place of nouns. The production of summaries was markedly impaired in the DAT group. Overall, the pattern of deficits found in these DAT subjects differed from the pattern of deficits seen in aphasia in that the discourse of DAT subjects was relatively preserved at the sentence level but was characterized by intrusions of tangential and irrelevant information. (See sample 7 in Appendix 2 for an example of discourse produced by a DAT patient.)

Discourse in the Normal Elderly

Our studies of the normal elderly were motivated by a desire to extend the findings of our studies of aphasia and, since most of the subjects in our studies have been older, to investigate the possible contribution of normal aging to discourse problems. These studies of normal aging differed in a number of ways from our earlier studies of aphasia. First, a much more difficult task was added (the "O'Henry Story," described shortly), which allowed for a more sensitive investigation of subtle linguistic deficits, especially at the discourse level. Second, some new variables were added pertaining to reference. Our earlier studies of aphasia as well as work by other researchers had suggested that the reference system might be particularly susceptible to disruption, so we decided to study this system in more detail. Third, both production and comprehension of discourse were analyzed in contrast to our earlier studies of aphasia, which focused on production.

North, Ulatowska, Macaluso-Haynes, and Bell (1986), studied discourse performance in thirty-three elderly women between the ages of 64 and 92 and eighteen middle-aged women between the ages of 27 and 55. Subjects were given two narrative tasks, the "Cat Story" (described previously), and the "O'Henry Story," which involved retelling a complex story of about 600 words. Three procedural tasks were also used. The "Cat Story" was analyzed in terms of narrative superstructure and information content. The retellings of the "O'Henry Story" were analyzed in terms of information content (i.e., number of propositions recalled). Subjects' comprehension of the story was also tested. The procedures were analyzed in terms of number of essential steps. On the "Cat Story," older subjects, relative to middle-aged controls, produced fewer propositions, but superstructure was relatively intact. On the "O'Henry Story," older subjects produced fewer propositions in their retellings and showed poorer comprehension. On the procedures, older subjects produced fewer essential steps.

In an extension of this study using the same data base (Ulatowska, Hayashi, Cannito, and Fleming, 1986), a more detailed linguistic analysis was conducted focusing on disruption of reference. The following variables were measured: noun/pronoun ratio, number of reference ambiguities, noun phrase complexity, and specificity of nouns referring to characters in the narratives. Results showed that older subjects produced a higher proportion of pronouns, more reference ambiguities, and more general nouns.

Comprehension of Reference in Aphasia

While the major focus of our work has been directed toward discourse production, the recurring evidence of reference errors motivated studies of the comprehension of reference. Reference provides a structural framework, distinct from narrative superstructure, for organizing information. Resolving reference in discourse involves interpreting each noun or pronoun in relation to what is already known from textual or extratextual sources. We were interested in the differential contribution of textual and extratextual knowledge to discourse processing in general and reference processing in particular. Reference structure is concerned more with sequential organization, whereas narrative superstructure is concerned with the hierarchical nature of information.

We investigated comprehension of reference in discourse in two moderately impaired aphasic populations, one being moderately severe (Bond, 1986; Bond and Ulatowska, 1985; Chapman and Ulatowska, 1989). Subjects were seventeen aphasics between the ages of 28 and 65, of whom sixteen had suffered a cerebrovascular accident to the left hemisphere and one had suffered a closed head injury. A group of normal control subjects was also examined. The discourse tasks included six experimental narratives in which specificity and plausibility of reference were manipulated to control for textual and extratextual effects.

Results indicated that patients with both moderate and moderately severe levels of impairment had significant difficulty resolving referents whose identity depended on contextual linguistic cues. Both were more proficient at retrieving factual information from individual sentences comprising the narratives. It was hypothesized that both populations would have more difficulty when the linguistic information was counter to real-life expectations. The more severely impaired population performed more poorly when the textual information was not consistent with world knowledge. When the textual and world knowledge were equally plausible or neutral, the more severely impaired aphasics did somewhat better. For the less severely impaired population, however, little difference in performance was seen between the neutral and counterexpectation conditions. These findings support the belief that as language disruption increases, patients rely more heavily on world knowledge strategies even when the contextual linguistic information contradicts expectations. In addition, the more severely impaired subjects did not benefit as much as the moderately impaired aphasic subjects in the condition where the linguistic cues were consistent with world schemas. This finding suggests that even though the more severely impaired aphasics tended to rely on world knowledge, even this information may be impaired. In general, the aphasic patients had difficulty keeping track of reference identity that required bridging linguistic information across sentences. Their highest levels of performance were in retrieving explicitly stated noun referents or in recovering reference identity from world knowledge.

Interpretation of Results

In this section, we will interpret the most important findings from our research on discourse performance in disordered populations. The major issues to be discussed include (1) relations between levels of language, (2) manipulation of information structure, (3) disruption of reference, and (4) acceptability of discourse production in aphasic patients.

Relations Between Levels of Language

Our studies of aphasic subjects have indicated that there is some degree of dissociation between sentential and discourse levels of language; subjects with severe sentence-level deficits may still be able to produce discourse. This dissociation may result in part from the redundancy of language (i.e., subjects can use other linguistic and paralinguistic devices to compensate for syntactic deficits). Also, the relative preservation of discourse may result from the top-down nature of discourse production; i.e., the content and form of the discourse are planned before the individual sentences of the discourse are constructed. Furthermore, in the discourse types we have used (narratives and procedures), subjects' discourse production may be guided by relatively intact schemas or scripts that are more cognitive than linguistic in nature.

The dissociation of different levels of language underscores the need to analyze discourse at multiple levels (i.e., lexical-semantic, syntactic, pragmatic, and textual). Analysis of multiple linguistic levels can help to specify more precisely the nature of discourse problems experienced by a group of subjects. For example, in our study of dementia, some subjects showed relatively preserved syntax but disrupted discourse, suggesting that the source of the discourse problem involved higher linguistic levels (e.g., narrative superstructure). From a more theoretical perspective, analysis of multiple levels can help reveal what linguistic components are crucial to well-formed discourse and what components are optional or less important. For example, the fact that some of our aphasic subjects showed a reduced repertoire of syntactic structures, yet were able to produce well-formed narratives, suggests that complex syntax per se may be of limited importance in narrative discourse.

Manipulation of Information Structure

Aphasic subjects, compared to controls, produced a reduced amount of information, a finding supported by previous research (Berko-Gleason, Goodglass, Obler, Green, Hyde, and Weintraub, 1980). However, information structure was preserved for the mildly and moderately impaired aphasic populations, although for the severely impaired population structure was not preserved. Preservation of information structure was evidenced by the inclusion of the most essential information in both narrative and procedural discourse. For the narrative, this information included setting, complicating action, and resolution. For procedures this information was the necessary steps for completing a task. The severely impaired aphasic patients did not produce even the most basic information to the narrative task.

The preservation of discourse structure in mildly and moderately impaired aphasic individuals demonstrated that these patients were able to sort out the most important linguistic information, an important cognitive operation. Previous studies have postulated a number of processing strategies for aphasic patients (e.g., recency or primacy strategies). Using a recency strategy, subjects would tend to recall the most recently presented information, whereas using a primacy strategy they would be more likely to recall the first information heard. While many aphasic patients may use these processing strategies, our studies indicated that at least some aphasic patients could hierarchically organize information and that this organization could guide them during discourse production. This evidence of hierarchical organization of information by aphasic patients provided insights into cognitive operations used during discourse processing.

The fact that mildly and moderately impaired aphasic patients showed preservation of information structure indicates that information structure is more resistant to disruption than sentential structure, a finding supported by other research. Huber and Gleber (1982), for example, found that in processing narratives aphasic patients relied more on macrostructure information (i.e., global aspects of structure) than on microstructure information (i.e., particular details). One explanation for relative preservation of information structure is that both narratives and procedures are supported by cognitive schemas that are developed early in life and may be resistant to disruption. The results from our studies of severely impaired aphasics also provide evidence that these schemas may be resistant to disruption. Even though information structure was not preserved in these severely impaired patients, a "sense" of story was preserved, as evidenced by patients' ability to arrange a picture story (of up to five pictures) in correct sequence.

Our findings should not be interpreted as indicating that aphasic subjects show *no* decrements in manipulating information structure, since the stories and procedures used in our experiments were relatively simple. The stories had basically a single episodic structure, while the procedures involved simple action sequences. We suspect that given an unconventional sequence of events, the patients would have had more difficulty sequencing the events because their internal schemas could not adequately guide production. Some evidence of this was observed in patients' incorrect performance on unpredictable picture sequence tasks, which were administered as part of the nonverbal cognitive testing. In addition, the experimental stories were elicited by supporting stimuli, either visual or auditory. Such stimuli may have provided the patient with a needed source of information as well as shared context for the examiner. More difficult tasks may be necessary to tap subtle deficits in manipulating information structure.

Narrative superstructure operates at the macro-level of a text (i.e., it involves relations between large units of the text). Another aspect of information structure is chronological sequencing of events, which operates at a micro-level (i.e., between individual sentences of a text). The chronological sequence of events for both narratives and procedures was preserved in discourse production of mildly and moderately impaired aphasic individuals, perhaps because sequence of events is strongly supported by world knowledge scripts based on common, real-life occurrences of events and procedures. However, the sequence of events was not preserved in narrative discourse production of severely impaired aphasic patients.

Although mildly and moderately impaired aphasics showed an apparent preservation of superstructure in most of the tasks administered, these subjects did show marked deficits in the summarization task. This result is important because it suggests that subjects may, in fact, have subtle deficits in manipulating information structure, which may have been masked in easier tasks such as story retellings. Summarization is a cognitively demanding task that requires extraction of the most important information in a discourse. Subjects' deficits on this task could reflect a reduction in their ability to organize information in a hierarchical manner. Some of the normal subjects in our studies also showed deficits on the summarization task but, overall, the normal subjects performed substantially better.

Subjects with dementia of the Alzheimer's type did show some disruption of information structure, characterized particularly by intrusions of tangential and irrelevant information in their discourse. This disruption may reflect an inability to distinguish relevant from irrelevant information, or it could reflect a breakdown at the level of pragmatics, characterized by subjects' failure to monitor whether their discourse was clear to the listener. It could also reflect a deficit in using story schemas and script knowledge to guide production of narrative and procedural discourse. The fact that most of the essential components or steps were included in the discourse of these subjects suggests that the underlying schemas or scripts were relatively intact. The intrusion of irrelevant information may occur during the ongoing production of discourse, as a result of attention or memory problems.

Disruption of Reference

One of the more frequent findings in our studies was disruption of reference, both in comprehension and production tasks. Reference is a particularly important feature of discourse, because it connects lower and higher levels of language. For example, a disruption of function words such as pronouns, which reside at a lexical-semantic level, may lead to marked impairment at a discourse level. Deficits in manipulating reference were seen in all the populations we have studied and have also been documented in other studies of neurological populations (Hartley, 1984; Hier, Hagenlocker, and Shindler, 1985; Lovett, Dennis, and Newman, 1986; Nicholas, Obler, Albert, and Helm-Estabrooks, 1985). The system of reference may be particularly vulnerable to disruption because there are many points where a breakdown can occur. Because of the complexity of the reference system, different populations may show deficits in use of reference for different reasons, including word- and sentence-level deficits, as mentioned before. Disruptions in reference can also result from semantic, pragmatic, and/or cognitive deficits. At a semantic level, difficulties in building semantic networks of meaning across utterances can interfere with keeping referents distinguishable. At a pragmatic level, excessive use of pronouns may result from a failure to recognize the listener's needs for precision of reference. At a cognitive level, memory deficits can contribute to reference problems. Appropriate use of a pronoun as opposed to a noun requires that a speaker have some "trace" of previous discourse in memory.

Acceptability of Discourse

Our linguistic analyses of discourse of disordered subjects have revealed a variety of deficits. An important question is whether these specific deficits have an effect on the acceptability of discourse. Acceptability is a subjective but important text property that involves how a discourse is perceived by a hearer (i.e., whether the discourse is clear, well-formed, etc.). At a sentential level, acceptability corresponds to grammaticality (i.e., the well-formedness of individual sentences).

In some of our studies, acceptability was analyzed using ratings of discourse quality. Aphasic discourse even for the mildly impaired patients was inferior to that produced by normals, despite the evidence that discourse informativity was preserved in aphasic patients. Judges consistently rated aphasic narratives lower on clarity than narratives produced by normal subjects. Therefore, even at mild levels of linguistic impairment, the preservation of information structure is not sufficient for producing well-formed discourse. Objective measures of linguistic impairment provide some insight into contributing deficits. At a discourse level, the aphasic individuals produced more discourse errors, including errors of reference and verb tense and errors in use of prepositions and connectors. Aphasics also showed a reduction in syntactic structure, which could contribute to problems in marking given/new information or foregrounding important information, since syntax is one means of achieving these functions.

Narrative and Procedural Genre

Our studies of discourse in brain-damaged populations were not designed to compare performance across genres, but only to use both narrative and procedural genres to provide a more comprehensive picture of patients' discourse performance. However, a few tentative comments can be made concerning genre effects. Most important, brain-damaged patients seemed to show the same differences across genres as did normal subjects. For example, both normal and aphasic subjects showed a reduction in syntactic complexity in procedures relative to narratives. This finding suggests that brain-damaged patients retain knowledge concerning the demands of different discourse types, at least for the types we have studied.

Extensions of Discourse Studies

Most of our studies to date have been exploratory in nature, since relatively little was known about discourse performance in disordered populations when these studies were undertaken. The findings of these exploratory studies should now be examined in more experimentally rigorous, hypothesis-driven research. For example, one topic that warrants further investigation is disruption in the use of cohesive devices in discourse production. An unresolved question concerns the source of this disruption (i.e., whether it is cognitive or linguistic in nature, or a combination of both). In addition to investigating the nature and source of problems in manipulating cohesive devices, the communicative impact of these problems should be explored.

The performance of brain-damaged patients in manipulating information structure also needs to be explored more systematically. Certain populations (e.g., severely impaired aphasics and some dementia patients) show a disruption in information structure, although the nature of that disruption varies. The different manifestations of impaired information structure may have different sources and different communicative effects, which need to be more carefully investigated. The mildly and moderately impaired aphasics in our studies showed some evidence of subtle deficits in information structure on the summarization task, another finding that should be investigated in more detail, since it may reveal patients' strategies (and difficulties) in manipulating information in complex tasks.

Future studies of discourse performance in aphasia should consider differences between clinical subgroups (e.g., Broca's versus Wernicke's patients), since different patterns of deficits may be seen in various subgroups and different underlying mechanisms may contribute to similar problems in those subgroups. For example, Broca's aphasics often have difficulty producing function words, including pronouns and conjunctions, which could contribute to problems in achieving cohesion. In other subgroups, such as Wernicke's aphasia, problems in cohesion may result from an overuse of pronouns, which would contribute to a lack of specificity of reference.

In addition to comparing various subgroups within aphasia, future research should also directly compare discourse performance across different populations, including aphasia, dementia, right-hemisphere damage, and closed head injury. Aphasia is characterized by problems at the sentence level, which can contribute to discourse problems. Other neurological populations, however, do not have marked problems at the sentence level, although they may have marked problems at the discourse level. For example, Roman, Brownell, Potter, Seibold, and Gardner (1987) found that the discourse of right-hemisphere subjects, in a script-producing task, was characterized by intrusions of tangential information. Also, Joanette, Goulet, Ska, and Nespoulous (1986) found that the discourse of right-hemisphere subjects was characterized by reduced informativity. Comparison of different populations may therefore reveal different patterns of discourse disruption and different underlying mechanisms.

Certain methodological extensions may prove valuable in research on discourse performance. First, the cognitive demands of discourse tasks could be more systematically manipulated to help sort out the relative contributions of cognitive and linguistic deficits to discourse problems. Second, the effect of story schemas could be systematically manipulated (e.g., by using stories that conform to conventional schemas and stories that do not). Third, single case studies can allow for a micro-analysis of discourse, which may help to reveal features of disordered discourse and interactions among levels of language (e.g., word, sentence, and discourse levels), which might be overlooked in a group study. Fourth, studies of written discourse should be carried out, since there is a greater demand for use of certain linguistic devices (e.g., those marking cohesion) in written than in oral language.

Epilogue

Ten years have passed since the time of our first single case study, when an aphasic patient provided us with valuable insights into the nature of discourse and set us on the course of our subsequent studies. It was this patient who taught us, through his painstaking efforts in writing his diary, that storytelling is one of the most compelling and rewarding experiences of human existence. Just recently, another aphasic patient, also involved in a single case study of discourse, turned in a written assignment with the comment: "It took me four hours to produce this page and a half, but it is not a composition, just a collection of individual sentences." We acknowledge our debt to these aphasic patients in the work described in this chapter.

Appendix 1 Stimulus Materials

Original text for the "Rooster Story"

Two roosters were fighting over the chicken yard. The one who was defeated hid himself in the corner. The other rooster flew to the top of the roost and began crowing and flapping his wings to boast of his victory. Suddenly, an eagle swooped down, grabbed the rooster and carried him away. This was good luck for the defeated rooster. Now he could rule over the roost and have all the hens that he desired.

"Cat Story"
The content of the story depicted in the "Cat Story" picture sequence is presented here.

The little girl is crying because her cat is in the tree. She tells her father, who decides to help. The father climbs the tree, but as he approaches the cat it begins hissing at him. When the father reaches for the cat, it jumps down. The little girl holds out her arms to catch the cat. Then the father slips and gets hung up on the tree. The little girl begins crying. The fire department has to come and rescue the father, while the cat sits on the ground licking itself.

Appendix 2 Discourse Samples

1. *Written narrative: moderately impaired posterior aphasic*
This sample shows preservation of narrative superstructure despite sentence-level deficits.

Setting	No man for island, animals have 6 apes, female.
	We had lots of fruit of different kinds.
	The apes gave my cook, wash the clothes, hunt me
	for dr. the headache, etc.
	I lived for 2 years, no seen a man....
Evaluation	I was sure need some friends.
Action	One morning I could see the horizon on a raft. I
	could see 3 people....
	They were three women.
	Hot dam, they were 3 girls of prettiest I ever
	saw....
	They introduce each.
	She said E., B., C.!
	They wanted me, how long I was here!
	I told them that *first* we need the business first.
	Then we can talk later.
	One was going ready to Amen.
Resolution	Damn, I woke.
Coda	I take all last night and couldn't get me again, again.
	Sept. 5, 1976, I have been looking for re-dream that
	dream and trip back to M. A. Island Eden.

2. Summarization task: mildly impaired aphasic
This sample shows inclusion of unimportant information in a summary.

	Two roosters were fighting.
	One whipped the other.
Unimportant detail	The one that whipped the other got up on the roof
	and was crowing and shouting.
	And a hawk came down and carried him off.
Unimportant detail	Which in turn was very enchanting to the rooster
	that was left.

3. Memorable experience: moderately impaired aphasic
This sample shows preservation of narrative superstructure, despite deficits at the sentence level.

Setting	Going to Possum Kingdom
	Almost there
	Other guy was drunk
	Head on collision
	And Mike S. he was driving
	And me passenger
	Head on collision
	And would've died
Action	Some guy stopped along the road
Resolution	And put a snorkel in my throat

	And would've died
	And other guy went insane
Coda	And that's it

4. *Sandwich procedure: moderately impaired aphasic*
This example shows a preservation of discourse structure in a procedure, despite problems at the sentential level.

Essential step	Two slices of bread
Essential step	Open the peanut butter jar
Optional step	And get the knife
Essential step	And dip the spread it on the slices
Target step	And fold it
Coda	And sandwiches

5. *"Cat Story": severely impaired posterior aphasic*
The following narrative shows a disruption in narrative superstructure, problems in reference, and reduced verb specificity.

Incomplete setting	Little girl—she is a hurting
	She's holler—hoow-haa-haa
	So maybe somebody'd hear
Ambiguous reference	So *he* look each other
	So he turn away
	She look at
	So he gonna turn around
Reduced specificity	He started *working*
Ambiguous reference	*it*
	So he gonna turn around
Ambiguous reference	Work inside each *other*
	He kinda got a little bit back there
	He's gonna watch out
	But he could see it
Reduced specificity	Really didn't *do* anything
	But it jumped off right quick
	Ahh—beautiful
	Ahh-I love it
Unclear resolution	Oh—fellow right there trying to tell the police
	"Throw that back there"

6. *"Rooster Story": severely impaired anterior aphasic*
The following narrative also shows a disruption of narrative superstructure and a marked reduction in information content.

Omitted setting	Cock-a-doodle-doo
Disrupted sequence	Fighting and fighting—rooster and rooster
Ambiguous reference	*Rooster*—King Kong
Ambiguous reference	*Rooster* is gone
Unclear resolution	But this one—King Kong—myself

7. *Light procedure: moderately impaired dementia subject*
This sample shows marked impairment of reference and intrusion of irrelevant information.

Indefinite reference	Well, first thing, *it's*—it's high enough that—that I couldn't reach it from the floor,
	but I do have a beautiful stand at the end of the bed and—
Digression	and I have on this stand—
	I have a red velvet that I—
	My wife loves me to put it on the bed,
	and so we put that—
	It's folded up
	so I have to take this red velvet off of the bed—off of the stand
	and put it on the bed.
	Then I step on that stand
	and then I can reach up and—
Indefinite reference	and unscrew the *thing* from the glass.
Digression	Now I did one in the kitchen
Indefinite reference	and *it* had a *thing* that long.
Indefinite reference	*It* was in a case like,
Indefinite reference	so I don't know whether *this* would be the same or not.

References

Berko-Gleason, J., Goodglass, H., Obler, L., Green, E., Hyde, M.R., & Weintraub, S. (1980). Narrative strategies of aphasic and normal-speaking subjects. *Journal of Speech and Hearing Research, 23*, 370–382.

Bond, S.A. (1986). *Reference in aphasia: Processing of nouns and pronouns in narrative discourse.* Unpublished Ph.D. dissertation, University of Texas at Dallas.

Bond, S.L., & Ulatowska, H.K. (1985). Methodology for assessing auditory comprehension of discourse in aphasia. In R.H. Brookshire (Ed.), *Proceedings of the clinical aphasiology conference.* Minneapolis: BRK Publishers.

Bond, S.L., Ulatowska, H.K., Macaluso-Haynes, S., & May, E.B. (1983). Discourse production in aphasia: Relationship to severity of impairment. In R.H. Brookshire (Ed.), *Proceedings of the clinical aphasiology conference.* Minneapolis: BRK Publishers.

Chapman, S.B., & Ulatowska, H.K. (1989). Discourse in aphasia: Integration deficits in processing referents. *Brain and Language, 36*, 651–668.

Freedman-Stern, R., Ulatowska, H.K., Baker, T., & DeLacoste, C. (1984). Disruption of written language in aphasia: A case study. *Brain and Language, 21*, 181–205.

Hartley, L. (1984). *Narrative and procedural discourse following closed head injury.* Unpublished Ph.D. dissertation, University of Florida.

Hier, D.B., Hagenlocker, K., & Shindler, A.G. (1985). Language disintegration in dementia: Effects of etiology and severity. *Brain and Language, 25*, 117–133.

Huber, W., & Gleber, J. (1982). Linguistic and nonlinguistic processing of narratives in aphasia. *Brain and Language, 16*, 1–18.

Hunt, K.W. (1965). Grammatical structures written at three grade levels. Research Report No. 3. Champaign, Ill: National Council of Teachers of English.

Joanette, J., Goulet, P., Ska, B., & Nespoulous, J.-L. (1986). Informative content of narrative discourse in right-brain-damaged right-handers. *Brain and Language, 29*, 81–105.

Longacre, R. (1976a). *An anatomy of speech notions.* Lisse: The Peter de Ridder Press.

Longacre, R. (1976b). A spectrum and profile approach to discourse analysis. *Text, 1*, 338–359.

Lovett, M.W., Dennis, M., & Newman, J.E. (1986). Making reference: The cohesive use of pronouns in the narrative discourse of hemidecorticate adolescents. *Brain and Language, 29*, 224–251.

Nicholas, M., Obler, L.K., Albert, M.L., & Helm-Estabrooks, N. (1985). Empty speech in Alzheimer's disease and fluent aphasia. *Journal of Speech and Hearing Research, 28*, 405–410.

North, A.J., Ulatowska, H.K., Macaluso-Haynes, S., & Bell, H. (1986). Discourse performance in older adults. *International Journal of Aging and Human Development, 23*, 267–283.

Roman, M., Brownell, H.H., Potter, H.H., Seibold, M.S., & Gardner, H. (1987). Script knowledge in right hemisphere-damaged and in normal elderly adults. *Brain and Language, 31*, 151–170.

Ulatowska, H.K., Allard, L., Donnell, A., Bristow, J., Haynes, S.M., Flower, A., & North, A.J. (1988). Discourse performance in subjects with dementia of the Alzheimer type. In H.A. Whitaker (Ed.), *Neuropsychological studies of non-focal brain damage: Trauma and dementia.* New York: Springer-Verlag.

Ulatowska, H.K., Doyel, A.W., Freedman-Stern, R., Macaluso-Haynes, S., & North, A.J. (1983). Production of procedural discourse in aphasia. *Brain and Language, 18*, 315–341.

Ulatowska, H.K., & Freedman-Stern, R. (1978). Analysis of aphasic writing. Paper delivered at the Aphasia Research Group, World Federation of Neurologists, University of Iowa, Iowa City.

Ulatowska, H.K., Freedman-Stern, R., Doyel, A.W., Macaluso-Haynes, S., & North, A.J. (1983). Production of narrative discourse in aphasia. *Brain and Language, 19*, 317–334.

Ulatowska, H.K., Hayashi, M.M., Cannito, M.P., & Fleming, S.G. (1986). Disruption of reference in aging. *Brain and Language, 28*, 24–41.

Ulatowska, H.K., North, A.J., & Macaluso-Haynes, S. (1981). Production of narrative and procedural discourse in aphasia. *Brain and Language, 13*, 345–371.

9
Discourse Ability in Children After Brain Damage

Maureen Dennis and Maureen W. Lovett

The Study of Discourse

Discourse is language in the contextual, narrative, and conversational settings in which it is daily used and understood. The study of discourse is the study of communicative language in context, in contrast to other types of language analysis at the level of closed, formal, linguistic systems.

For both speaker and listener, the communicative success of connected language, or language operating in some of its naturally occurring environmental contexts, depends first on the intactness of lexicon and grammar, which is typically assessed in a formal language assessment. The production and comprehension of connected language, however, also rely on an *interface* of lexicon and grammar with functions that are less well understood and far less commonly studied: pragmatic competence involving aspects of social perception and cognition; and aspects of cognitive function and learning such as how events are represented in memory, the integration of new and existing knowledge, and ease of access to specific types of knowledge representation. Successful production and comprehension of discourse depend, therefore, on establishing interconnections among the formally specified aspect of language, or grammar, its content domain, or lexicon, and the pragmatic, cognitive, and information bases relevant to a particular social linguistic context.

The connectedness of discourse comes from a variety of sources. Local connections may be established between elements in adjacent parts of a text as, for example, when a cohesive, anaphoric relationship exists between a noun in one sentence and a pronoun in a later sentence. Prior world knowledge may be integrated with textual information to form a script, a conceptual representation of stereotyped, real-world events. The social and interpersonal context is woven into a text to produce narratives and conversations.

This central feature of discourse — its connectedness — has recently become the focus of research with a variety of populations, normal and pathological, young and old. One by-product of this research into just what makes discourse connected has been the development of new methods of discourse assessment.

Our purposes in this chapter are three. We discuss some of the procedures available for, and appropriate to, the study of connectedness in texts, folk tale narratives, and conversations, and we suggest new procedures that might be applied profitably to the analysis of previously unstudied aspects of discourse competence. We describe some of the procedures that have already been used to analyze discourse in brain-damaged children. And we explore how discourse data from brain-damaged children can be brought to bear on a particular set of theoretical issues.

Why Study Discourse in Brain-Damaged Children?

The discourse skills of brain-damaged children are poorly understood, although this aspect of their pragmatic language competence is critical to successful academic functioning and crucial to understanding some of the recently described effects of early brain damage on language. After some forms of early brain damage, the rate at which some language skills are acquired is slowed with increasing age, so that the brain-damaged group are progressively less able than their peers to maintain age-appropriate increments in language performance (Dennis, Hendrick, Hoffman, and Humphreys, 1987).

Such interactions between age and early brain damage have increasingly important implications for cognitive and social development. Some effects of early brain damage on later language or cognitive functioning may become more, rather than less, apparent as the child develops. The consequence of this may be that early brain-damaged children and adolescents experience particular difficulty with later-developing skills, such as the use and understanding of language in expository, narrative, and conversational contexts. And the further the child moves into his developmental course, the more critical becomes the effective use of language in its social and interpersonal contexts. The ability to access and to integrate representations of existing knowledge (i.e., the ability to apply old knowledge to new problems), the need to see parallels between old and new problems, and the ability to integrate new knowledge with prior networks all become increasingly important to the child's mastery of language.

Representing Discourse Information

The discourse literature has provided us with some insight into the various levels and types of information contained within any segment of connected discourse and has provided an assortment of different formalisms with which to represent this information on a theoretical level. One purpose of this chapter is to demonstrate how this theoretical information from the study of discourse can be shaped to study performance; specifically, how it can be adapted to analyze the discourse production and discourse comprehension of individuals.

The following discussion outlines some domains of interest in the study of discourse, with special reference to different ways to represent the information contained in connected discourse. With an appreciation of these possible representational structures, it will be possible to explore their potential applications to the task of assessing linguistic functions in brain-damaged and other language-disordered populations, child and adult.

Two broad classes of concepts will be introduced. One stems from ongoing work on the formal representation of textual information; the other arises from attempts to characterize the cognitive processes involved in discourse production and discourse comprehension.

Textual information can be represented on several different levels. The text-grammar approach attempts to account for linguistic and conceptual systematicity at the whole text level; *text* is understood to be the abstract underlying structure of *discourse*, with discourse considered an observational, more empirical, construct and text a theoretical notion (van Dijk, 1980; van Dijk and Kintsch, 1983). The concept of macrostructures is part of the text-grammar tradition, macrostructures being defined as theoretical representations of a text's conceptual content, accounting for what is usually called the gist, the upshot, the theme, or the topic, of a text (van Dijk and Kintsch, 1983). An example of a text-grammar application is the story grammar, a rule system describing story constituents and their conceptual and structural interrelationships in narratives. At more local levels, the continuity or essential connectedness of discourse is represented by the referential relationships that maintain text cohesion and coherence. It should be noted that, as they find application by different authors, these categories of formal representation show partially overlapping boundaries.

The basic ideas communicated in a text are characteristically described in terms of propositional units. The term "proposition" is used to describe units at both a macro- and a microlevel of text analysis. For the former, a proposition is simply considered as a single idea unit, sometimes corresponding to the independent clausal units of a text; for the latter, a proposition is an underlying semantic structure consisting of a predicate and its arguments.

Although the cognitive, memory, and general neuropsychological processes necessary for successful discourse processing have yet to be fully defined, there have been some advances in characterizing the cognitive structures and related processes involved. Skilled comprehenders are thought to approach texts with a story schema, a cognitive representation of "story-ness" based on previous discourse experiences, which generates expectations about the way in which a story might progress. An individual's story schema is critical to her ability to generate and comprehend a text macrostructure. A related concept is that of a script, also a cognitive structure that, when activated, organizes the understanding of real-world events and their sequelae. Both scripts and story schemas are attempts to characterize prerequisite memory representations of the contextual information and metacognitive knowledge involved in discourse processing. All of the processes inherent to knowledge acquisition and the integration of old and new knowledge are also relevant to the study of discourse processing, because the interface of real-world knowledge with formal discourse information defines the act of discourse processing.

Formal Representations of Textual Information

Story Grammars

Macrostructures attempt to represent formally the conceptual content of discourse and contextual and abstract discourse structures. The study of macrostructures is important for their potential in showing how ideas are interrelated and structured in a person's discourse comprehension and production as well as for specifying the structuring of ideas in conversations and narratives.

A story grammar, one type of macrostructure, is a rule system outlined for the purpose of describing regularities in one particular kind of text, a folk tale or story (Mandler, 1984). The rules describe story constituents and their conceptual and structural interrelationships in the story structure. As Mandler (1984) has noted, the term "grammar" does not necessarily connote built-in or native linguistic attributes; a grammar is merely a rule system that describes language in terms of a set of units and the ways in which these units are sequenced. Although story grammars are predicated on the idea that the abstract form of stories can be studied without reference to their specific content, it is obviously the case that any story form is always instantiated with some type of story content.

The core of the story grammar is the idea that stories have a base structure that is quite invariant over different story contents (Johnson and Mandler, 1980; Mandler, 1978, 1984; Mandler and Johnson, 1977). The base structure consists of a number of ordered constituents. Traditional stories begin with a setting, which introduces the protagonist(s), as well as the time and story locale. The overall plot structure of the story consists of one or more episodes, each of which has a beginning, a development, and an ending. Each constituent in the story has a specific type of connection to the ones that follow. The base story structure can be generated by the set of rewrite rules describing how the story constituents are interrelated.

Cohesion and Coherence

The cohesiveness of a text refers to the clarity with which its elements are connected to one another. *Cohesion* is a semantic relation between an element in the text and some other element that is crucial to its interpretation; it refers to the range of possibilities that exist for linking something with what has gone before. This linking does not depend on structural characteristics of the text, but is content based (Mandler, 1984), and so it is achieved through relations in meaning (Halliday and Hasan, 1976). Because cohesive relations are not primarily concerned with text structure, they may occur just as well within a sentence as between sentences.

The simplest and most general forms of the cohesive relationship are "equals" and "and": identity of reference and conjoining. Another simple form of cohesion is one in which the presupposed element is verbally explicit and is found in the immediately preceding sentence. [See, e.g., Halliday and Hasan (1976): "Did the gardener water my hydrangeas? He said so."] In more complex cohesive forms, the presupposed element is located elsewhere (in a preceding or following sentence), or is even missing from the text.

Textual semantics has also defined the notion of local and global *coherence*. Local coherence refers to various relationships between propositions and the facts they denote (van Dijk and Kintsch, 1983). In order for a text to maintain global coherence, which is a general constraint that monitors the production or comprehension of the discourse, some form of organizing topic is required (van Dijk, 1980).

There are a variety of conventions for representing texts. Most of the representational conventions just outlined are discussed in more detail elsewhere in this book (see Mross, Chapter 3).

Discourse Processing

Story Schemas and Scripts

A story schema is a cognitive representation of "story-ness" that generates expectations about the way in which stories progress; it is what readers and listeners have extracted from their experience with stories. The story schema guides the formation of a text macrostructure; that is, the main events of the story are assigned to schematic categories (Kintsch and van Dijk, 1978; van Dijk and Kintsch, 1977). To form a story macrostructure, knowledge about goals and actions is also necessary, and story grammars are an attempt at accounting for how these factors operate together. What is in dispute is whether narrative structures have processing reality—that is, whether people actually process discourse in units or domains that correspond to these ideational structures—and whether there is any theoretically motivated way of formulating grammars for text structures (Black and Wilensky, 1979).

A script is a hypothesized cognitive structure that, as it is activated, organizes the understanding of event-based situations (Abelson, 1981; Schank and Abelson, 1977). Scripts represent stereotyped event sequences, and they are activated when the listener expects events in the sequence to occur in the text. A script is a type of event schema, one that includes knowledge about what will happen in a given situation and, often, the order in which the individual events will take place (Mandler, 1984). Scripts involve various inferential processes (Clark and Clark, 1977; den Uyl and van Oostendorp, 1980). The value of scripts for maintaining the connectedness of discourse is that they allow narrated events to be seen in relation to familiar contexts rather than in isolation.

Knowledge and Discourse

The domain of textlinguistics ultimately is dependent on topics central to the study of cognition—how knowledge is represented and accessed in memory. Models of discourse processing assume certain amounts of real-world knowledge, both episodic and more abstract semantic knowledge. For instance, van Dijk and Kintsch (1983) assume that, in the understanding of a text, the application of prior knowledge involves a flow of information between long-term and short-term memory in order to support specific comprehension strategies and, further, that such strategies will vary with the goals of the language user, the context in which elaborative inferences are made, the knowledge available from a text and a specific context, and the degree of coherence needed for comprehension (Mandler, 1984; Reder, 1980; Sanford and Garrod, 1981; Whitney, 1987).

An important aspect of discourse production and comprehension is the ability to integrate prior real-world knowledge to facilitate interpretation of ongoing discourse. A failure to understand discourse may be due to inadequate integration and use of world knowledge during listening (Royer and Cunningham, 1981); it is known, for example, that failure to use real-world knowledge leads to problems in understanding figurative language and in drawing correct contextual inferences. Issues of interest here concern how real-world knowledge is represented, how well such knowledge can be accessed, how old knowledge is applied to new contexts, how old and new information about a topic are integrated, and how links are established to knowledge on related topics.

Discourse Analysis Methods and Applications

A variety of methods emerged from basic discourse analysis research in the 1970s conducted both with normal developmental populations (for example, Meyer 1975; and Meyer and Freedle 1984) and with adults (Mandler and Johnson, 1977; Thorndyke, 1977). These studies were concerned with the structure of discourse, with the organization that binds it together and specifies the logical connections among ideas as well as the subordination of some ideas to others. Most of these studies addressed the memorability of different levels and types of text structure. The goals of this line of research were both to assess efforts to approximate the representation of text structures in memory and to evaluate the priority given different types of text information during discourse processing by normal samples.

Our interests in, and use of, discourse analysis are different. Our goal is to analyze individuals' ability to produce and comprehend extended units of discourse, such as those found in texts, narratives, and conversations. We are concerned, not with the prediction of text recall, but with the description of how individual subjects, and selected samples of subjects, produce and understand connected discourse. Our particular interests are in the development and application of new discourse-analysis procedures to the study of language development in brain-damaged children. These procedures and new directions are also relevant, however, to the study of functional language in normally developing and language-disordered samples.

Discourse Competence

Language competence requires appropriateness both in the use and understanding of language content and in the responsiveness to communicative demands. An example of one standardized test that attempts to assess both domains is The *Test of Language Competence* (Wiig and Secord, 1989). This test was designed to evaluate delays in the emergence of linguistic competence and problems in the use of semantic, syntactic, and pragmatic language strategies.

The test consists of four subtests. The first—Understanding Ambiguous Sentences—evaluates the ability to recognize and interpret the alternative meanings of selected lexical and structural ambiguities (e.g., "The elephant was ready to lift." What might this mean? What else might it mean?). The second subtest—Making Inferences—requires the child to make plausible inferences from the lead-in and lead-out sentences of causal event chains that constitute situational and instrumental scripts (e.g., "Mother wanted to have the turkey at home. The family was disappointed to eat Thanksgiving dinner in a restaurant." What happened?) The third subtest—Recreating Sentences—requires the child to formulate propositions in grammatically complete sentences with the incorporation of key words related to the context of a given situation; the child recreates a sentence that could have been produced by one of the speakers in an illustrated situation, using key words provided by the experimenter (e.g., "Here are people in a park. Tell me a sentence one of them said that contains these words: sit . . . painted . . . because."). The fourth subtest—Understanding Metaphoric Expressions—requires the ability to interpret metaphoric expressions and to match structurally related metaphoric expressions by shared meaning (e.g., "I just can't swallow that.").

The *Test of Language Competence* might more properly be regarded as a survey of four discourse-related skills than as a technique primarily designed for a systematic analysis of the linguistic and pragmatic structures underlying discourse. Nevertheless, it is worth noting that each subtest in the test taps a particular domain of discourse study. The first subtest—Understanding Ambiguous Sentences—involves the identification of sentence ambiguity that could have been encountered in a specific topical-situational context; data from this subtest bear on questions about how contextual ambiguity (lexical, surface, or deep structure) is perceived and resolved (e.g., Carey, Mehler, and Bever, 1970; Fodor and Garrett, 1967). The second subtest—Making Inferences—elicits memory for one or more intervening event chains or scripts. It is based on a model of episodic memory and inferential knowledge described by Schank and Abelson (1977) in which concepts and lexical items are organized around propositions that, in turn, are connected by their co-occurrence in the same event or time span. Within a framework of speech act theory (Searle, 1969), the items of the third subtest — Recreating Sentences — were designed to elicit speech acts (illocutions) that express the speaker's intent or complex sentences (locutions) to carry the communication. The fourth subtest — Understanding Metaphoric Expressions — exploits the Lakoff and Johnson (1980) model for categorizing and systematizing metaphorical concepts; within this model, metaphorical expressions used in discourse and conversations are considered to be tied to metaphorical concepts in a systematic and structured manner.

The *Test of Language Competence* broadens the range of tested language skills from clinical signs to contextual and discourse functions, thereby providing a component to the neuropsychological assessment of language that approximates how language is used and understood on a day-to-day basis. It evaluates the acquisition of cognitive strategies related to conversational and discourse functions.

The technical manual for the *Test of Language Competence* provides information about test development, standardization, the derivation of standard scores and confidence intervals, as well as validity and reliability data. At present, the test is the only commercially available discourse evaluation tool; standardized scores allow children's test performances to be compared with those of normally achieving students in public school classes.

Current Applications of Discourse Procedures to Brain-Damaged Children

Discourse procedures have not been widely used in the study of brain-damaged children. One reason for this may be their relative novelty. Perhaps another is the tendency, in the study of both child and adult language, to assume that higher-level or contextual language does not warrant investigation in individuals with impairments in lexicon or grammar. Nonetheless, some applications to brain-damaged children and adolescents have been made, and three of these applications will be discussed that have provided information about how closed head injury affects a variety of discourse-related functions, about the clarity with which the content elements in a story text are connected to each other, and about the structural basis of folk and fairy tales.

Language Competence and Closed Head Injury

The application of tests of language competence to individuals after clinical recovery from closed head injury has revealed that this type of brain injury has consequences for certain aspects of discourse use and understanding. This seems true in children, adolescents, and adults.

After traumatic head injury, pragmatic language may continue to be impaired, sometimes even when no clinical language deficits are apparent: Milton, Prutting, and Binder (1984) described inappropriate regulation of discourse between speakers and listeners in some head-injured adults, and Holland (1982) has observed that such adults talk better than they communicate. In a study of the performance of head-injured adolescents and young adults on the Test of Language Competence, Wiig, Alexander, and Secord (1988) found that, controlling for the duration of post-traumatic coma and post-traumatic amnesia, individuals with lower levels of cognitive functioning had poorer levels of language competence. In particular, they had lower scores on the test of comprehension for metaphoric expressions, although they did not differ from norms on tests of paired associate word recall. These data show that lower levels of rated cognitive function at the time of closed head injury are indicative of a loss of language competence and discourse-related skills. The *Test of Language Competence* has also identified impairments in the pragmatic structures underlying discourse in children and adolescents after closed head injury; the magnitude of such discourse impairment does not seem well correlated with extent of clinical language deficit as assessed by standard tests of naming, fluency, and comprehension (Dennis and Barnes, 1988). Such data highlight the importance of a post-trauma language assessment that includes a specific evaluation of discourse functions.

Pronoun Use and Text Cohesion in the Discourse of Hemidecorticate Adolescents

The analysis of one level of text cohesion in individuals' narrative productions has been used to study the discourse strategies of adolescents who had undergone left or right hemidecortication in infancy (Lovett, Dennis, and Newman, 1986; Newman, Lovett, and Dennis, 1986). A formalism was developed to analyze the cohesive use of referential language, specifically pronouns, in the narrative discourse of three hemidecorticate adolescents.

In these studies, transcriptions of the subjects' retelling of four fairy tales were analyzed with respect to pronoun distribution; pronoun:referent distribution patterns; types of cohesive links both within and across propositional boundaries; and classes of text cohesion used, such as anaphora, cataphora, and exophora. In addition, sections of each subject's narratives were illustrated in a rebus format to demonstrate graphically the intra- and intersubject differences in the complexity of cohesive relationships embedded within a continuous story line (see Lovett, Dennis, and Newman, 1986, pp. 237–245, for examples).

Over all stories, the pattern of results revealed in these analyses was one of some shared competencies and some distinctive differences in the subject's narrative strategies. Each of the subjects used text cohesion effectively and correctly in their retelling of the fairy tales. Both left and right hemidecorticates demonstrate the basic comprehension, memory, and speech production processes required for the production and understanding of cohesive text.

Marked individual differences emerged, however, in patterns of pronoun use, and these suggested more basic differences in these subjects' narrative strategies. Neither left hemidecorticate seemed to plan a narrative in extended units. The two left hemidecorticates were different from each other. One adopted a linear, very explicit narrative style characterized by a highly redundant overstatement of referent nouns, while the other demonstrated a cluttered style, producing narratives with ambiguous as well as correct reference, and relying on nonpersonal pronouns at the cost of narrative specificity.

The right hemidecorticate's narrative style was clearly different. The stories he retold were rich in pronoun use and both economical and cohesive in their referential structure. His narratives included well-maintained, intersecting chains of referential relationships, and he was the only one of the three subjects to succeed in maintaining simultaneous story lines with multiple pronouns and referential relationships cohesively embedded. As a result, his discourse was both more economical in form and far richer in ideational content.

This pattern of results is illustrated in a rebus representation of the same story segment as retold by each of the subjects. The rebuses are shown in Figure 9.1, where part of *The Practical Princess* story is retold.

In this section of the story, the characters are discussing a course of action in response to a dragon's threat to devour either the kingdom or the princess, Bedelia. The canonical text reads as follows:

Sadly, King Ludwig called together his councilors and read them the message. "Perhaps," said the Prime Minister, "we had better advertise for a knight to slay the dragon. That is what is generally done in these cases." "I'm afraid we haven't time," answered the King. "The dragon has only given us until tomorrow morning. There is no help for it. We shall have to send him the princess." Princess Bedelia had come to the meeting because, as she said, she liked to mind her own business and this was certainly her business. "Rubbish!" she said, "Dragons can't tell the difference between princesses and anyone else. Use your common sense. He's just asking for me because he's a snob." "That may be so," said her father, "but if we don't send you along, he'll destroy the kingdom." Bedelia said, "I see I'll have to deal with this myself!"

In his rebus representation, the right hemidecorticate, M.W., was found to use direct referents sparingly, successfully maintaining extended cohesive chains while also preserving multiple simultaneous chains of reference. His story segment was rich in appropriate pronoun use and economical and highly cohesive in its referential structure. The same narrative segment of the left hemidecorticate, S.M., was impoverished in pronoun use and dominated by redundant overstatement of explicit referent nouns. He tended to use pronouns redundantly rather than as cohesive text elements and occasionally required successive approximations to achieve the correct pronoun case. The second left hemidecorticate, C.A., was less adept at using mediated chains, and she did not produce any overlapping or intersecting cohesive relationships. She flavored her narrative segment with the nonpersonal "it" pronoun (sometimes related to an appropriate contextual referent but, in other instances, referentially ambiguous), which reduced the specificity of her narration.

This application of a formalism to examine individual speakers' use of text cohesion devices has suggested hemisphere-specific differences in overall dis-

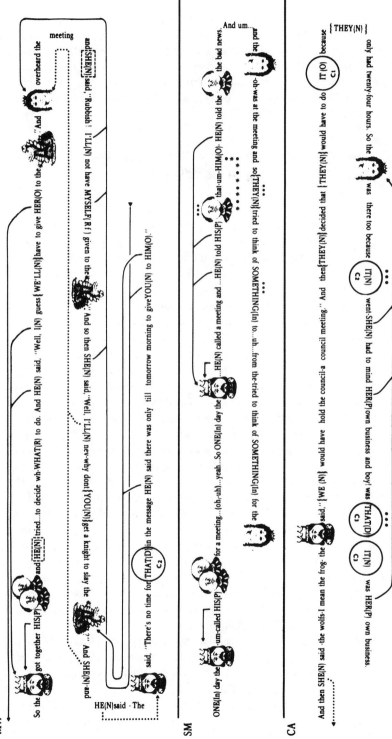

FIGURE 9.1. Rebus representations of a segment of *The Practical Princess* as retold by three hemidecorticate adolescents.

course skill and has provided a means of examining individual differences in narrative strategy. The formalism developed in Lovett, Dennis, and Newman (1986) has been illustrated here in its application to hemidecorticate language, but it has the potential to provide an assessment of discourse competence in a number of different language-disordered groups, thereby yielding a perspective on higher-level language functions that is not available from standardized tests of language use.

Story Grammars After Acquired and Congenital Left-Hemisphere Lesions in Childhood

Acquired Left-Hemisphere Arteriopathy

Children do suffer cerebrovascular accidents or strokes, less commonly than adults but occasionally from the same pathological mechanisms. When such strokes occur in the language areas of the left hemisphere, the production and comprehension of speech and language is disrupted (Dennis, 1980) and recovery is relatively poorer than in those instances where childhood language disorders arise from trauma (van Dongen and Loonen, 1977).

Language disruption after strokes in childhood has been rarely studied, and many important questions about language remain unanswered. One question of significance for the study of discourse is whether intact schemata for stories can coexist with impoverished and agrammatic expressive language. In a childhood stroke case, Dennis (1980) applied story grammar rewrite rules to the analysis of a child's retelling of the classic fairy tale, *Little Red Riding Hood*.

The Mandler and Johnson (1977) rewrite rules were applied to the series of propositions in the canonical *Little Red Riding Hood* text and a tree structure drawn to represent visually the hierarchical and sequential interrelationships of the story constituents. As with most classic folk and fairy tales, the story is well structured. The setting of the story introduces the Little Red Riding Hood character and explains how she got her name. The supraordinate or Story episode begins with the mother's request that Little Red Riding Hood visit Grandmother, is developed throughout the events of the visit, and ends with retribution for the wolf. The development of the overall Story episode involves Little Red Riding Hood setting off for her grandmother's house. The outcome is the Wolf subepisode, beginning with Little Red Riding Hood meeting the Wolf, developing with the wolf's nefarious plan, and ending with a Grandmother's House subepisode covering Little Red Riding Hood's adventures at Grandmother's house, the ending of which reveals the Wolf's identity and bad character.

The childhood stroke case, a girl with normal language development preceding a cerebrovascular accident at age 9, was asked to retell the *Little Red Riding Hood* story, and a tree structure was drawn for her retelling, according to the same rewrite rules used to analyze the canonical text. Application of the Mandler and Johnson (1977) rewrite rules to the child's retold *Little Red Riding Hood* story (the proposition list is shown in Table 9.1) resulted in the generation of the tree structure shown in Figure 9.2.

TABLE 9.1. Proposition list for *Little Red Riding Hood* retold by a childhood stroke case. Prompted propositions (those produced in response to examiner queries ("What happened"?) are in italics; propositions supplied by the examiner are in boldface; all others are spontaneously produced by the subject. Numbers refer to propositions in the tree structure in Figure 9.2.

 1. The wolf comes
 2. *Look at my little basket*
 3. *my mom made this, and this, and this, and my ribbon*
 4. And say something, "Hi, Little Red'n Hood, where you going?"
 5. "To Grandma's"
 6. "Well, I'm going too"
 7. "You go this way
 8. and I'll go that way"
 9. Come
10. Knock
11. "Come in"
12. *And then he goes to bed and then Little Red*
13. *He's puttin' on the tat*
12. *He goes to bed*
14. SOUND EFFECT: KNOCKING
15. "Oh grandma, you, you have big eyes!"
16. **"Oh grandma, what big arms you've got!"**
17. *"To hug you with!"*
18. "Oh grandma, you have big eyes, eyes, eyes, eyes!"
19. *He says, "Shut up!"*
20. *"To see you with!"*
21. "Oh grandma, big ears you have!"
22. "To, uh, hear you with!"
23. "Oh grandma, how big is your mouth!"
24. *"To somethin' eat you with!"*
25. Um, somethin' ate 'im. Her . . A wolf. No she didn't.
26. The, the somethin' come, the woodcutter come
27. *He shoot him*
28. And then he'll never come again
29. *Granny came out. The clothes hozen, the closet . . the closet!*
30. **Boy, it's a good thing that guy comes along and shot that wolf, eh? My goodness, he would've eaten both of them up, I think!"**
31. Yes, all bastard!

The rewrite rules parse each story into a series of episodes with a beginning (BEGIN), a development (DEVELOP), and an ending (END). In illustrating how episodes are sequenced and embedded and in specifying the intermediate-level structures into which they rewrite, the tree structures document the extent to which a given text or protocol is internally structured and the constituent ideas are well organized. At the local level of single propositional statements, the tree structure graphs the specific connection between and among individual ideas, illustrating how well story components are elaborated and how systematically they are sequenced.

In relation to those in the canonical story, the childhood stroke case's propositions were semantically impoverished, reduced, or overgeneralized. Unless the

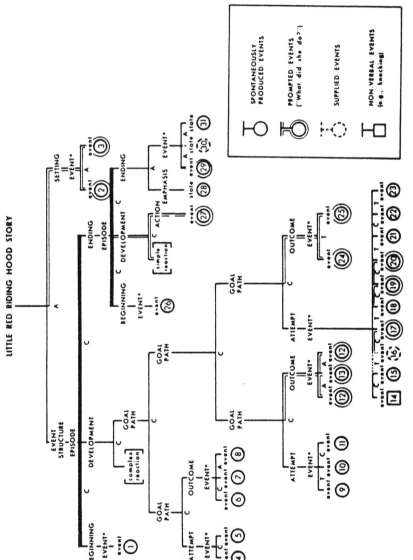

FIGURE 9.2. Story grammar representation of the retelling of *Little Red Riding Hood* by a childhood stroke case.

examiner provided a prompt for the outcome, she tended simply to concatenate events. Her story was simplified, with its internal structure disordered in several ways. She omitted outcomes, ignored settings, and produced no internal states. She could not produce a story setting without prompting. Her story had no true structure involving embedded episodes, and she produced only one episode spontaneously, the others being replaced by middle-level structures in the story grammar hierarchy. She seemed to have produced the story without reference to its embedded episodic structure.

Strokes to language areas of the left hemisphere in middle childhood may produce agrammatic speech and language as well as agrammatic comprehension. In addition, they may disrupt the ability to produce discourse that effectively conveys the structures involved in a simple and overlearned fairy tale. More generally, the story grammar procedures developed in this study provide a technique for evaluating the intactness of the structures underlying narrative discourse in individuals with varying levels of functioning oral language.

Story Structure in Adolescence After Early Left Hemidecortication

Currently, we are using story grammar formalisms to analyze the story retelling of the hemidecorticate adolescents who participated in the cohesion study described earlier. Each hemidecorticate subject retold four fairy tales, allowing a comparison of performance on familiar and unfamiliar narrative materials. The three hemidecorticates succeeded in understanding the plots of these fairy tales and, in most cases, in retelling a majority of their main ideas in a multiepisodic story. The subjects differed substantially in the ease with which they retold their stories and in the extent to which they integrated and interrelated individual ideas.

Consistent with what was demonstrated in the cohesion analyses, the stories of the right hemidecorticate, M.W., reflected an economical and effective narrative style. His episodic structures were closely interdependent in their embeddings and his expression of individual propositions was simultaneously rich in ideational content and free of jargon, colloquialisms, and lexical clutter. In contrast, the two left hemidecorticates demonstrated less efficient narrative strategies, although the problems illustrated in of one of their tales, *The Frog Prince*, seemed to involve different levels of story structure. S.M.'s individual ideas seemed more precisely articulated, but were overall more loosely structured, while C.A.'s overall structure contained more embedded constituents, with the expression of individual constituents occasionally imprecise, inaccurately described, or simply misspoken.

Narrative Production (NaP) Grammar

Story grammars such as Mandler and Johnson's capture important information about the episodic structure of folk and fairy tales. At the same time, there are other aspects of productive language competence involved in relling these stories that these grammars do not address. Recently, we have developed the Narrative Production (NaP) story grammar for use with brain-damaged children, a grammar that attempts to characterize some of these other features of story retelling, such as conversational exchanges; the sequential and nonsequential progress of the events in a story; and aspects of internal state and motivation (Dennis and Lovett, in preparation).

Like the Mandler and Johnson (1977) and other story grammars, our NaP grammar parses stories into a series of episodes, each with beginning, development, and ending rewriting into intermediate-level structures and ultimately into single propositions or idea units. The NaP grammar differs from earlier grammars at both intermediate and terminal propositional levels of the tree structure used to characterize story organization. At both levels, the differences involve more detailed specification or elaboration of story content.

When independent ideas or propositions are classified in the NaP grammar, the distinction between different types of ideas is refined. In the Mandler and Johnson grammar, propositions are represented as events or states. In the NaP grammar, nine types of propositions are represented, distinguishing action, situation, and state from different elements of dialogue (e.g., queries, commands, and statements) and psychological perspective (e.g., thought, emotion, and aspiration). The relationship between and among individual propositions also is elaborated in the NaP rewrite rules. The range of possible connectors between individual ideas is extended to include conditional and specific semantic connections (e.g., comparative and appositional), in addition to the traditional additive (neutral), sequential (temporal), and causal relationships.

The NaP grammar also allows further specification of story content at the level of intermediate story structures—as when an episode develops through a directed sequence of events that may be characterized as an attempt to realize a goal, and the outcome of that attempt. Episodic development in the NaP grammar allows the plot to advance through the movement of conversation or dialogue, a central feature of fairy tales such as *Little Red Riding Hood* and many other types of stories. In previous story grammar systems, events and dialogue have been forced to rewrite into traditional "goal paths"–that is, as some attempt and its designated outcome; the NaP grammar extends the options for episodic development to include topic-comment and even looser recursive conversational structures.

The ability of the NaP grammar to characterize dialogue and motivational information allowed an important difference between two individual right- and left-hemidecorticate storytellers to be revealed. In their retelling of *The Frog Prince*, for example, the two subjects, M.W. and C.A., differed in their ability to convey the protagonist's emotions. At the point in the story when the princess loses her treasured golden ball, M.W. states very simply, "she was sorry because her ball fell in" and later, when the frog retrieves it from the pond, "she was so happy that she ran off. . . ." C.A., in her retelling of the same story segments, used four propositions to convey what could have been conveyed in one: "Then she started to cry and boo-hooing and she was so unhappy that she just fell on the ground and started crying like crazy." C.A. tended to externalize the princess's emotion and describe it as physical behavior. At a later point in the story, when the princess's ball had been successfully retrieved, C.A. describes her, not as happy, but in action: "She was jumping like crazy because she-she got it back and everything." In this instance, left-hemidecorticate S.M. more resembled right-hemidecorticate M.W. in his ability to attribute appropriate emotion succinctly (S.M.: "And the princess was so happy that she forgot all about the frog."). C.A.'s quote describing the princess's distress illustrates not only her difficulties in conveying thought and emotion in the story's characters, but also the uneconomical and superfluous nature of her narration.

Story grammar applications describing the narrative productions of brain-injured subjects have highlighted the usefulness of formalisms such as the NaP grammar that can capture both the explicit and implicit ideational and structural content of stories. Story grammars that allow a fuller account of dialogue, as well as greater elaboration of internal states that signal motivational and psychological information, will be more successful in assessing real-life pragmatic functions.

Potential Applications of Discourse Procedures

Individual Differences

The formalisms just described are well suited to the study of individual differences in the competence and strategies of both speaker and listener. Data of this kind could answer questions about the internal organization of discourse systems at different developmental stages, at different levels of language skill, and with different forms of language disorder. Analyses of individual differences in discourse processing may be equally valuable in the study of normal and aberrant language development and in the study of developmental and acquired language disorders.

Brain-Injured Children

The discourse procedures discussed have many other potential applications. Three of these will be outlined.

Epileptic Aphasias

Certain epileptic conditions in childhood and adolescence are accompanied by language disturbances (Cooper and Ferry, 1978; Gascon, Victor, Lombroso, and Goodglass, 1973; Lou, Brandt, and Bruhn, 1977; Mantovani and Landau, 1980; Msall, Shapiro, Balfour, Niedermeyer, and Capute, 1986). Speech and language disturbances may fluctuate in and around the clinical seizures and vary throughout the course of treatment regimes. In adults, the speech and language disturbances have been directly related to ictal EEG seizure abnormalities

(Rosenbaum, Siegel, Barr, and Rowan, 1986) and there has been some suggestion that a similar relationship may exist in children (Razdan and Koul, 1987).

Discourse analyses of the language of such childhood cases would be highly informative. In particular, the ability to monitor the cohesiveness and the structure of extended discourse throughout the course of treatment regimes or epileptic conditions that involve ictal changes in speech would likely reveal important information relevant to the nature of language and cognitive disturbances in such children.

Acquired Aphasias of Childhood

The course of recovery from sudden-onset aphasias of childhood, such as those produced by stroke or trauma, is largely unknown. With children, as with adults, any improvement of language is usually studied with reference to particular tests or clinical measures that sample selected aspects of lexicon and grammar. It is not known how fully discourse production and discourse comprehension recover after injury to the child's brain. Nor is it known whether any recovery of discourse function proceeds in full or partial parallel with recovery of lexicon or grammar or whether it is asynchronous with these features of language. Application of currently available discourse-analysis procedures to childhood aphasia cases at various intervals after the onset of stroke or trauma would provide a means of addressing these important and understudied questions.

Childhood Hydrocephalus

Childhood hydrocephalus is often characterized by some degree of disorganization in extended, propositional speech. This disorganization is especially evident with fluctuations in the level of intracranial pressure. Discourse-analysis procedures could be usefully applied to hydrocephalic children in order to establish language markers for the presence of clinical increased intracranial pressure and also to establish correlations between any such language markers and more direct indices of intracranial pressure disturbances such as papilledema.

Issues on Which Early Brain-Damaged Discourse Processing Data Bear

Theoretical Issues in the Analysis of Discourse Processing

Data from brain-damaged children, of the type described in this chapter, bear on some theoretical issues in the analysis of discourse processing. Two of these will be outlined.

Cohesion

Appropriate use of the referential system provides cohesion and indicates topical links across utterances. Texts that lack cohesion are disjointed, seemingly dysfluent, and are difficult to understand. What is not clear is whether the various ways in which texts can lack cohesion are as separate in language performance as they are in linguistic theory. A text may lack cohesion because speakers violate the Given-New Contract (Clark and Haviland, 1977), that is, they fail to introduce a referent before using a pronoun to refer to it, and a text may lack cohesion because referents are reintroduced unnecessarily, leading the listener to wonder whether the speaker has introduced a new person with the same name.

In the study of pronoun-referential text cohesion outlined previously (Lovett, Dennis, and Newman, 1986), each of these two cohesion violations was typical of the narrative story productions of the isolated left hemisphere, but they occurred in separate individuals (violation of the Given-New Contract in subject C.A., and violation of cognitive economy in subject S.M.). Such breakdowns in text cohesion may be used to study the interrelationship of cohesive narrative production with other aspects of language use and understanding, for example, the ability to understand sentential information about topic and comment. And by studying how successful pronominal reference in narrative texts relates to measures of oral and written syntax in the same subjects, the question of how anaphoric reference depends on mastery of the syntactic system may be addressed.

Story Grammars

There is ample evidence from the experimental literature on story recall to support the psychological validity of episodic and story constituent constructs in story schemas (Mandler, 1978; Mandler and DeForest, 1979; Stein and Glenn, 1979; Thorndyke, 1977). Similarly, multiple regression analyses of text constituent reading times (Haberlandt, 1980; Haberlandt, Berian, and Sandson, 1980; Mandler and Goodman, 1982) have suggested that story schemas influence the way individuals understand stories as well as the way they remember them. Mandler (1984) concludes that our understanding of story organization and its regularities, and of their mental schematic representation, at this point probably surpass our understanding of real-world events and of their representative schemas.

It is in the latter domain that some of the discourse-processing data described previously may prove particularly interesting. By applying a text grammar formalism to the discourse productions of brain-damaged and normally developing children, new information about perceived invariance in real-world events and settings may be provided. In subjects' telling or retelling of an event sequence—whether it is spontaneously recounted or recalled following specific narration—perceived organization in individually experienced event sequences and their corresponding expectations and representative mental structures may be revealed.

Application of story grammar formalisms to the retold stories of individual brain-damaged children has also identified two developmental brain perturbations—loss of the left hemisphere at birth and focal damage to the left hemisphere in middle childhood—that are subsequently associated with a less than complete mental representation of text structures. In our studies of narrated discourse in hemidecorticate subjects, both left and right hemidecorticates were able to produce a multiepisodic discourse structure that represented a story's main ideas; but only the isolated left hemisphere articulated a fully elaborated embedded episodic structure, rich in ideational content while economical in form and organization. In contrast, the child with left-hemisphere stroke (Dennis, 1980) seemed to encode an overlearned fairy tale largely without reference to, or understanding of, its embedded episodic structure: she failed to represent even the story gist. From these initial applications, some aspects of left-hemisphere functioning in childhood and adolescence would seem to be a prerequisite for complete processing of some of the hierarchical features of certain tightly constructed (i.e., episodically embedded) texts.

Discourse ability has not thus far been studied in many of the forms of childhood brain damage, and our understanding of what is required in terms of a brain substrate for successful discourse processing is far from complete. Nevertheless, data of the kind outlined here are important, not only because they begin to provide such a data base, but also because they may bear on the functional reality of dissociations made in the discourse-processing literature.

Theoretical Issues in Early Brain Damage

It was proposed long ago that the brain systems required to acquire a behavior might differ from those needed to sustain the behavior, once acquired (e.g., Hebb, 1942). Later research has supported this principle. In nonhuman primates, damage to one part of the prefrontal cortex produces a behavioral deficit that later resolves, whereas damage to a different prefrontal region delays or prevents the future acquisition of another behavior (Goldman, 1972). In humans, Rourke (1987) has suggested that what the brain's subcortex and white matter contribute to the acquisition of functional systems within the cortex is different from what they add to the maintenance of these systems once they are acquired. And recent research with brain-damaged children suggests that skill acquisition and skill maintenance may call on different localizations within each hemisphere of the brain, or even on different hemispheres.

Within the right hemisphere, there seems to be a depth shift during development, such that the functions underlying non-verbal intelligence become progressively more encephalized. Non-verbal intelligence is most disrupted by subcortical lesions in childhood (Dennis, 1985a, 1985b) but by acute cortical lesions in adulthood (e.g., Fitzhugh, Fitzhugh, and Reitan, 1962). Within the left hemisphere, also, there are suggestions of a functional depth shift in certain language skills. Access to the lexicon through the sound structure of words is typically impaired by left cortical lesions in adulthood (Lecours, Lhermitte, and Bryans, 1983); but, while left cortical lesions also impair this skill in early-damaged individuals, left subcortical lesions are relatively more disruptive (Dennis, 1987).

And perhaps one aspect of these developmental shifts in brain localization involves a switch in functional control from one hemisphere to the other. The development of non-verbal skills after early brain injury possibly may involve a left hemisphere mediation of skills that are characteristically maintained by a right hemisphere in adulthood (Kohn and Dennis, 1974). Pragmatic discourse competence is usually held to be impaired by right hemisphere lesions in adulthood (Weylman, Brownell, and Gardner, 1988; Joanette, Goulet, Ska, and Nespoulous, 1986), but the evidence thus far suggests that early left hemisphere damage and removal seems to impair these functions in children and adolescents (Newman, Lovett, and Dennis, 1986).

This issue of possible developmental shifts in the brain mechanisms of pragmatics, of course, is far from understood. For one thing, left hemisphere adult lesions must have some effect on the pragmatics of language. [Otherwise, as Newman, Lovett, and Dennis (1986) point out, the differences reported to exist between Broca's and Wernicke's aphasics, both with left hemisphere damage, could not have been obtained.] For another, the comparison of child and adult may possibly be confounded by differences between tissue atrophy or loss, in the child, and tissue damage, in the adult. And the important comparisons – those between left- and right-lateralized lesioned children and adults on the same pragmatic language tests – have not yet been conducted.

Practical Issues

In adults, the most dramatic loss of cognitive function follows closely in time the cerebral insult that caused it as, for example, when an aphasic language loss accompanies a stroke. When the brain injury is a developmental one, in contrast, some of its most substantial impacts on language capacities may be apparent at a developmental stage far removed from the one during which it was sustained (Dennis, 1988). In consequence, different types of later-developing language disorders may require remedial intervention at different points during the time span of educational acquisition (Rourke, 1987). If remedial efforts for language and educational skills are to be optimally geared to the developmental time scale imposed by early brain damage, we need to understand how early brain damage influences the emergence and evolution of discourse competence.

Recent explorations of discourse in brain-damaged children and adolescents have contributed to the establishment of formalized and operationalized procedures for studying language, not through the rather artificial medium of a conventional psychometric test, nor through the assessment of formal systems and structures of lexicon and grammar, but through some of the contextual and conversational settings in which language is daily used and understood. The particular results described here may prove to be specific to children and adolescents with early brain injury; the contextual and conversational language procedures that are emerging, however, are likely to prove applicable to a much broader range of communication disorders during development – and they will probably also provide insights into how discourse develops under more typical conditions, that is, without overt or demonstrable brain damage.

Acknowledgment. Preparation of this chapter was supported by personal awards to each author from The Ontario Mental Health Foundation; and by project awards, to the first author, from The Ontario Mental Health Foundation and, to the second author, from the Medical Research Council of Canada. We thank Dr. Marcia Barnes for her comments on the manuscript.

References

Abelson, R.P. (1981). Psychological status of the script concept. *American Psychologist*, *36*, 715–729.

Black, J.B., & Wilensky, R. (1979). An evaluation of story grammars. *Cognitive Science*, *3*, 213–230.

Carey, P., Mehler, J., & Bever, T. (1970). Judging the veracity of ambiguous sentences. *Journal of Verbal Learning and Verbal Behaviour*, *9*, 243–254.

Clark, H.H., & Clark, E.V. (1977). *Psychology and language*. New York: Harcourt Brace Jovanovitch.

Clark, H.H., & Haviland, S.E. (1977). Comprehension and the given-new contract. In R.O. Freedle (Ed.), *Discourse production and comprehension* (pp. 1–40). Norwood, N.J.: Ablex.

Cooper, J.A., & Ferry, P.C. (1978). Acquired auditory verbal agnosia and seizures in childhood. *Journal of Speech and Hearing Disorders*, *43*, 176–184.

Dennis, M. (1980). Strokes in childhood I: Communicative intent, expression, and comprehension after left hemisphere arteriopathy in a right-handed 9-year-old. In R. Rieber (Ed.), *Language development and aphasia in children* (pp. 45–67). New York: Academic Press.

Dennis, M. (1985a). Intelligence after early brain injury I: Predicting IQ scores from medical variables. *Journal of Clinical and Experimental Neuropsychology*, *7*, 526–554.

Dennis, M. (1985b). Intelligence after early brain injury II: IQ scores of subjects classified on the basis of medical history variables. *Journal of Clinical and Experimental Neuropsychology*, *7*, 555–576.

Dennis, M. (1987). Using language to parse the young damaged brain. *Journal of Clinical and Experimental Neuropsychology*, *9*, 723–753.

Dennis, M. (1988). Language and the young damaged brain. In T. Boll & G. VandenBos (Eds.), *The master lecture series: Neuropsychology* (pp. 89–123). Washington, D.C.: American Psychological Association.

Dennis, M., & Barnes, M.A. (1988). Clinical and social-pragmatic language in children and adolescents after closed head injury. Conference presentation. *Challenge and change in childhood psychopathology*, Clarke Institute of Psychiatry, Toronto, November 17–18, 1988.

Dennis, M., Hendrick, E.B., Hoffman, H.J., & Humphreys, R.P. (1987). Language of hydrocephalic children and adolescents. *Journal of Clinical and Experimental Neuropsychology*, *9*, 593–621.

Dennis, M., & Lovett, M.W. (in preparation). Storied syntax: The architecture of grammatical elements in the narrative discourse of hemidecorticate adolescents.

den Uyl, M., & van Oostendorp, H. (1980). The use of scripts in text comprehension. *Poetics*, *9*, 275–294.

Fitzhugh, K.B., Fitzhugh, L.C., & Reitan, R.M. (1962). Wechsler-Bellevue comparisons in groups with "chronic" and "current" lateralized and diffuse brain lesions. *Journal of Consulting Psychology*, *26*, 306–310.

Fodor, J.A., & Garrett, M.F. (1967). Some syntactic determinants of sentential complexity. *Perception and Psychophysics*, *2*, 289–296.

Gascon, G., Victor, D., Lombroso, C.T., & Goodglass, H. (1973). Language disorder, convulsive disorder, and electroencephalographic abnormalities. *Archives of Neurology*, *28*, 156–162.

Goldman, P.S. (1972). Developmental determinants of cortical plasticity. *Acta Neurobiologica Experimentalis*, *32*, 495–511.

Haberlandt, K. (1980). Story grammar and reading time of story constituents. *Poetics*, *9*, 99–118.

Haberlandt, K., Berian, C., & Sandson, J. (1980). The episode schema in story processing. *Journal of Verbal Learning and Verbal Behavior*, *19*, 635–650.

Halliday, M.A.K., & Hasan, R. (1976). *Cohesion in English*. London: Longman.

Hebb, D.O. (1942). The effect of early and late brain injury upon test scores, and the nature of normal adult intelligence. *Proceedings of the American Philosophical Society*, *85*, 275–292.

Holland, A.L. (1980). When is aphasia aphasia? The problem of closed head injury. In R.H. Brookshire (Ed.), *Clinical aphasiology. Conference Proceedings* (pp. 345–349). Minneapolis: BRK Publishers.

Joanette, Y., Goulet, P., Ska, B., & Nespoulous, J-L. (1986). Informative content of narrative discourse in right-brain-damaged right-handers. *Brain and Language*, *29*, 81–105.

Johnson, N.S., & Mandler, J.M. (1980). A tale of two structures: Underlying and surface forms in stories. *Poetics*, *9*, 51–86.

Kintsch, W., & van Dijk, T.A. (1978) Toward a model of text comprehension and production. *Psychological Review*, *85*, 363–394.

Kohn, B., & Dennis, M. (1974). Patterns of hemispheric specialization after hemidecortication for infantile hemiplegia. In M. Kinsbourne & W.L. Smith (Eds.), *Hemispheric disconnection and cerebral function* (pp. 34–47). Springfield, Ill.: Charles C. Thomas.

Lakoff, G., & Johnson, M. (1980). *Metaphors we live by*. Chicago: Chicago University Press.

Lecours, A-R., Lhermitte, F., & Bryans, B. (1983). *Aphasiology*. London: Bailliere Tindall.

Lou, H.C., Brandt, S., & Bruhn, P. (1977). Aphasia and epilepsy in childhood. *Acta Neurologica Scandinavia*, *56*, 46–54.

Lovett, M.W., Dennis, M., & Newman, J.E. (1986). Making reference: The cohesive use of pronouns in the narrative discourse of hemidecorticate adolescents. *Brain and Language*, *29*, 1986, 224–251.

Mandler, J.M. (1978). A code in the node: The use of a story schema in retrieval. *Discourse Processes*, *1*, 14–35.

Mandler, J.M. (1984). *Stories, scripts, and scenes: Aspects of schema theory*. Hillsdale, N.J.: Erlbaum.

Mandler, J.M., & DeForest, M. (1979). Is there more than one way to recall a story? *Child Development*, *50*, 886–889.

Mandler, J.M., & Goodman, M.S. (1982). On the psychological validity of story structure. *Journal of Verbal Learning and Verbal Behavior*, *21*, 507–523.

Mandler, J.M., & Johnson, N.S. (1977). Remembrance of things parsed: Story structure and recall. *Cognitive Psychology, 9*, 111–151.

Mantovani, J.F., & Landau, W.M. (1980). Acquired aphasia with convulsive disorder: Course and prognosis. *Neurology, 30*, 524–529.

Meyer, B.J.F. (1975). *The organization of prose and its effects on memory.* Amsterdam: North Holland.

Meyer, B.J.F., & Freedle, R.O. (1984). The effects of different discourse types on recall. *American Educational Research Journal, 21*, 121–143.

Milton, S.B., Prutting, C.A., & Binder, G.M. (1984). Appraisal of communicative competence in head injured adults. In R.H. Brookshire (Ed.), *Clinical aphasiology. Conference Proceedings* (pp. 114–123). Minneapolis: BRK Publishers.

Mross, E.F. (1989). Text analysis: Macro- and microstructural aspects of discourse processing. In Y. Joanette & H.H. Brownell (Eds.), *Discourse ability and brain damage: Theoretical and empirical perspectives* (pp. 50–68). New York: Springer-Verlag.

Msall, M., Shapiro, B. Balfour, P.B., Niedermeyer, E., & Capute, A. (1986). Acquired epileptic aphasia. *Clinical Pediatrics, 25*, 248–251.

Newman, J.E., Lovett, M.W., & Dennis, M. (1986). The use of discourse analysis in neurolinguistics: Some findings from the narratives of hemidecorticate adolescents. *Topics in Language Disorders 7*, 31–44.

Razdan, S., & Koul, R.L. (1987). Epileptic aphasia. *Neurology, 37*, 1571.

Reder, L.M. (1980). The role of elaboration in the comprehension and retention of prose: A critical review. *Review of Education Research, 50*, 5–53.

Rosenbaum, D.H., Siegel, M., Barr, W.B., & Rowan, A.J. (1986). Epileptic aphasia. *Neurology, 36*, 822–825.

Rourke, B.P. (1987). Syndrome of nonverbal learning disabilities: The final common pathway of white matter disease/dysfunction? *The Clinical Neuropsychologist, 1*, 209–234.

Royer, J.M., & Cunningham, D.J. (1981). On the theory and measurement of reading comprehension. *Contemporary Educational Psychology, 6*, 187–216.

Sanford, A.J., & Garrod, S.C. (1981). *Understanding written language.* New York: Wiley.

Schank, R., & Abelson, R. (1977). *Scripts, plans, goals, and understanding.* Hillsdale, N.J.: Erlbaum.

Searle, T.R. (1969). *Speech acts: An essay in the philosophy of language.* Cambridge: Cambridge University Press.

Stein, N.L., & Glenn, C.G., (1979). An analysis of story comprehension in elementary school children. In R. Freedle (Ed.), *New directions in discourse processing*, Vol. 11 (pp. 53–120). Norwood, N.J.: Ablex.

Thorndyke, P.W. (1977). Cognitive structures in comprehension and memory of narrative discourse. *Cognitive Psychology, 9*, 77–110.

van Dijk, T.A. (1980). *Macrostructures.* Hillsdale, N.J.: Erlbaum.

van Dijk, T.A., & Kintsch, W. (1977). Cognitive psychology and discourse: Recalling and summarizing stories. In W.U. Dressler (Ed.), *Current trends in text linguistics.* Berlin/New York: de Gruyter.

van Dijk, T.A., & Kintsch, W. (1983). *Strategies of discourse comprehension.* New York: Academic Press.

van Dongen, H.R., & Loonen, M.C.B. (1977). Factors related to prognosis of acquired aphasia in children. *Cortex, 13*, 131–136.

Weylman, S.T., Brownell, H.H., & Gardner, H. (1988). "It's what you mean, not what you say": Pragmatic language use in brain-damaged patients. In F. Plum (Ed.), *Language, communication, and the brain* (pp. 229–243). New York: Raven Press.

Whitney, P. (1987). Psychological theories of elaborative inferences: Implications for schema-theoretic views of comprehension. *Reading Research Quarterly, 22*, 299–310.

Wiig, E.H., Alexander, E.W., & Secord, W. (1988). Linguistic competence and level of cognitive functioning in adults with traumatic closed head injury. In H.A. Whitaker (Ed.), *Neuropsychological studies of non-focal brain damage: Dementia and trauma* (pp. 186–201). New York: Springer-Verlag.

Wiig, E.H., & Secord, W. (1989). *Test of language competence. Expanded Edition.* San Antonio, Texas: Psychological Corporation.

10
Discourse Abilities and Deficits in Multilingual Dementia

Susan de Santi, Loraine K. Obler, Helene Sabo-Abramson, and Joan Goldberger

Introduction

Multilinguals have more than twice as many linguistic options as monolinguals. They can choose to speak any one of their languages—"language choice"—but they can also choose to code-switch (i.e., to mix words or phrases of one language into the other). For the healthy bilingual or multilingual speaker (hereafter we will use the term "bilingual" to encompass multilingual as well), decisions concerning language choice or code-switching are based on sophisticated linguistic and social rules (Grosjean, 1982). In dementia, a few studies have reported, these rules seem to break down.

This chapter will illustrate the extent to which factors that determine code-switching and language choice in healthy bilinguals remain active in bilingual demented patients. To do this, we undertake analysis of the discourse produced by four bilingual patients with senile dementia of the Alzheimer's type (SDAT). Through study of discourse inappropriateness and incoherence in these patients, we may identify pragmatic rules of conversational and test-taking discourse in normal bilinguals. To the extent that normal rules are violated in the patients we studied, we must consider their errors in the context of the general discourse phenomena previously described in demented monolingual individuals. Among the unique discourse features present in the language of our bilingual or multilingual demented patients, we describe the nature of these patients' language interaction in conversational and test-taking discourse, including examples of appropriate and inappropriate code-switching, appropriate and innapropriate language choice, spontaneous and elicited translation, use of neologisms, and language correction.

Our specific research questions were as follows:

1. Are the language problems present in the language of monolingual demented subjects also present in each of the languages of a bilingual demented patient?
2. Do problems with language choice and code-switching occur in all bilingual demented subjects?
3. If a bilingual demented subject makes code-switching and language-choice errors, does this relate to the severity of the dementia?

4. How can we characterize the nature of the code-switching and language-choice errors of the bilingual demented subject, and what do we learn about the normal's abilities from such qualitative analysis?

Literature Review

Language choice is the selection by the bilingual of a base language for communication. Pragmatic and sociolinguistic cues, primary among these the monolingual or bilingual status of the interlocutor, determine the choice of a base language. Thus, when a healthy bilingual speaks to a monolingual, code-switching does not occur. According to Grosjean (1982), when a bilingual speaks to another bilingual, the choice of a base language is determined by a number of factors, including interlocutor characteristics, situation, topic, and purpose of discourse.

Moreover, code-switching may occur appropriately with any bilingual interlocutor. Grosjean (1982) defines code-switching as the rule-governed "mixing" of two languages when speaking with another bilingual. Code-switching may serve numerous functions depending, for example, on the proficiency of a speaker in each of the languages, the specificity of the meaning of a word in one language, or one language not containing a lexical item that another language contains (Grosjean, 1982). Clearly, the nature of code-switching is more strictly linguistically determined, whereas language choice is more pragmatically determined.

Poplack (1979) formulated two rules that describe when code-switching occurs. The smallest unit that may be involved in a switch is the free morpheme or its equivalent. Therefore, according to the first rule, switching languages between a word's stem and its inflection is precluded by this constraint. Furthermore, there are word-order constraints: the word order on either side of the code-switch must be the same in both languages (Poplack, 1978). Poplack called this second rule the equivalence constraint. Thus the sentence "*Mangiamo* [we are eating] chicken for dinner" conforms to the free morpheme constraint, whereas "*Eatiamo*" [we are eating] does not.

Similarly, Lipski's (1978) example "*No se, porque* I never used it" is a legitimate code-switch, following the word-order-equivalence constraint, because the word order on either side of the switch is the same in both Spanish (*no se /porque/ nunca lo use.*) and in English (I didn't know because I never used it.). By contrast, Poplack cites an illegal code-switch that does not follow the word-order constraint: "*J'ai acheté* /an American / *voiture*," since the French structure is "*J'ai acheté / une voiture Americaine*," whereas the English is "I bought /an American car." The object noun phrases are not similar in the two languages.

The issue of word-order equivalence between languages has caused some debate. Nishimura (1986), for example, reports that code-switching does occur between languages at points where word order is not equivalent in language pairs which are structurally quite different. In a study that examined the code-switches between English and Japanese, Nishimura found a large number of sentences in her corpora where code-switching occurred between constituents whose order was not shared by the two languages. For example, a healthy subject might say "Only small prizes / *moratta ne*," where "*moratta ne*" means got. The translation equivalent in English is "(We) got only small prizes, you know," where the verb "got" has a different position.

Code-switching and language choice in two bilingual demented patients (one Swedish-Finnish, one Swedish-German) were investigated by Hyltenstam and Stroud (in press). These researchers found that their subjects had difficulties in choosing the appropriate language and in keeping the two languages separate when speaking to a monolingual. In addition, they reported that mixing of the two languages (i.e., code-switching) did, in fact, occur when speaking to a monolingual but was not haphazard; instead, it conformed, for the most part, to the grammatical constraints that govern healthy code-switching behavior.

Analysis of pragmatic skills in their patients revealed differential abilities in each language. Included in their evaluation were topic treatment, turn structure, lexical search problems, and automatic speech abilities. The results suggested that one subject's first learned language was less impaired on these aspects of language than the second learned language. The other subject showed a smaller advantage in the first learned language.

Dronkers et al. (1986) described a multilingual demented subject who progressively reduced her use of English and spoke primarily Dutch to non-Dutch speakers. The researchers evaluated the subject's linguistic abilities in both languages and noted that each language (English and Dutch) was equally affected. They concluded that the subject's tendency to employ Dutch more frequently than English reflected the memory deficit typically seen in Alzheimer's dementia rather than differential impairment to one or the other language.

Two other sets of bilingual phenomena we observed in our patients have not been described, to our knowledge, in the small literature on discourse in demented bilingual subjects. They are translation to help the interlocutor and correcting the speech used by the interlocutor. Both phenomena may occur in normal interactions where a bilingual is speaking with an interlocutor who has not fully mastered the language being spoken. To use them appropriately requires careful monitoring of the interlocutor's speech (in the case of correction) and comprehension (in the case of translation), as well as thoughtful consideration of the relative status of the subject and the interlocutor (i.e., it is appropriate to correct a junior person, but not a superior).

Description of Cases

Four female Yiddish-English-speaking patients with the diagnosis of probable SDAT were studied. The patients ranged in age from 87 to 96 years ($\bar{X} = 92$). The diagnosis of probable SDAT was determined by a physician on the basis of progression of the symptoms, memory, behavioral and other cognitive abilities, and possible causes of pseudo-dementia. All patients were residents of The Parker Jewish Geriatric Institute in New Hyde Park, New York. For demographic data see Table 10.1. One patient was born in the United States and learned how

TABLE 10.1. Demographic data on patients.

Patient	Age	Country born	L1[a]	L2[b]	Age L2 acquisition	Other language
B	96	Russia	Yiddish	English	18	Russian
C	96	Russia	Yiddish	English	16	Russian
D	89	United States	English	Yiddish	0	None
E	87	Poland	Yiddish	English	19	Polish

[a] L1 = first learned language.
[b] L2 = second learned language.

to speak Yiddish at home. The remaining three patients were born in Eastern Europe and immigrated to the United States during their childhood or teens. All spoke Yiddish at home initially. Three of the patients had elementary-school educations, and one was a graduate of a secretarial school. All four patients worked outside the home for a time, using English at work. Three worked until they had children; one continued to work until retirement. Three of the four patients knew languages other than English and Yiddish, but our testing was conducted only in these languages.

Procedure

Patients were interviewed by two different examiners on separate occasions: by a monolingual English-speaking examiner and by a bilingual English-Yiddish-speaking examiner. When the monolingual examiner interviewed the patients, the interaction was intended to be in English. When the bilingual examiner interviewed the patients, the interaction was intended to be in Yiddish. The bilingual examiner did not, however, feign ignorance of English. When a patient spoke to the bilingual examiner in English, the examiner reiterated in Yiddish what the patient said and continued the conversation in Yiddish.

The English and Yiddish sessions were conducted on different days. The interview and test sessions extended for four to eight sessions so that all interviews and testing in both languages could be completed. This was necessary because the patients had difficulties sustaining attention during formal testing for long periods of time.

All interviews were tape-recorded for later transcription and analysis. When the transcribed tapes were scored, all instances of non-English productions occurring with the monolingual examiner were reviewed by the bilingual examiner in order to differentiate between code-switches into Yiddish and neologisms.

Methods

Language abilities of the subjects were assessed by the monolingual examiner through spontaneous speech samples and through administration of specific

TABLE 10.2. Test scores (English)

	Patient C	Patient E	Patient B	Patient D
BNT[a]	7/60	7/60	14/60	30/60
ANT[b]	11/55	6/28	16/55	29/55
BDAE[c]				
Automatic speech	Refused	8/19	15/19	19/19
Oral reading	6/10	3/10	N/A[d]	10/10
Reading comprehension	Refused	5/18	N/A	11/18
Writing	Refused	8/15	N/A	13/15

[a] BNT = Boston Naming Test.
[b] ANT = Action Naming Test.
[c] BDAE = Boston Diagnostic Aphasia Examination.
[d] N/A = Not Applicable because patient was illiterate.

sections of the Boston Diagnostic Aphasia Exam (Goodglass and Kaplan, 1972), including:

Conversation and expository speech
Automatic speech
Repetition
Oral reading and reading comprehension
Writing

Additionally, the Boston Naming Test (Kaplan, Goodglass, and Weintraub, 1983) and the Action Naming Test (Obler and Albert, 1986) were administered. All sections of these tests were administered in English by the monolingual examiner, and pertinent sections were translated into Yiddish and administered by the bilingual examiner. The subjects' scores in English are noted in Table 10.2.

The general language behavior that characterized these patients include word-finding problems, verbal paraphasias, literal paraphasias, neologisms,[1] perseveration of an idea, perseveration of a word, repetition, unreferenced pronouns, pronoun confusion, and incorrect use of prepositions.

The degree of language impairment and hence the stage of dementia, as described by Obler and Albert (1984), for each patient was determined; patient B was at stage II, patient D at stage III, patient E between stages III and IV, and patient C at stage IV.

---

[1] A number of neologisms were produced by patients C and E in both monolingual and bilingual interactions. Note that patients C and E were the more severely demented of the four patients. Two English-Yiddish bilinguals reviewed the data and determined these were not Yiddish words. Often, however, they contained Yiddish phonological segments. Patient C produced twenty-nine neologisms, of which fifteen (52 percent) included Yiddish phonological sequences; patient E produced seven, of which six (88 percent) included Yiddish phonological sequences.

TABLE 10.3. General language behavior.

Language behavior	Patient B		Patient C		Patient D		Patient E	
	E[a]	Y[b]	E	Y	E	Y	E	Y
Naming problems	+[c]	N/A	+	+	+	−[d]	+	+
Paraphasic errors	+	−	+	+	+	−	+	+
Neologisms	−	−	+	+	+	−	+	+
Circumlocutions	−	−	+	+	+	−	+	+
Perseveration	+	−	+	+	+	+	+	+
Illogical responses	−	−	+	+	+	+	+	+
Topic loss	−	−	+	+	+	−	+	−

[a] E = English.
[b] Y = Yiddish.
[c] + = The problem listed was evidenced in our sessions.
[d] − = The problem listed was not evidenced in our sessions.

Results

General Language Abilities

The general language abilities of each patient are summarized in Table 10.3. In three out of the four cases, one language seemed more problematic than the other for each of the patients. In patient B's case this may be the result of the differential amount of testing performed in English and Yiddish, where there was greater testing in English. With patients D and E the differences between the two languages reflect our clinical sense that they were, indeed, differentially affected. It is important to keep in mind that subtle differences between languages may be present, even though on this chart language performance seems the same in each of the languages. For example, Patient E commonly used formulaic utterances (spontaneous singing, "familiar" phrases) in English and rarely used this type of utterance in Yiddish.

Language Choice

Two subjects, Patients B and D, always chose the appropriate language when speaking to the monolingual examiner. Patients D and E always chose the appropriate language when speaking to the bilingual examiner. Table 10.4 shows these results.

TABLE 10.4. Language choice.

Interaction	English		Yiddish	
Appropriate	Patient B,	Patient D	Patient D,	Patient E
Inappropriate	Patient C,	Patient E	Patient B,	Patient C

TABLE 10.5. Code-switches with bilingual interlocutor.

Patient	Number of code-switches	Number of utterances	+EQ[a]	−EQ[b]	−FM[c]
B	4	84	4 (100%)	0	0
C	87	338	72 (83%)	15 (17%)	3 (03%)
D	24	334	23 (96%)	1 (04%)	
E	57	349	50 (88%)	6 (11%)	1 (02%)

[a] + EQ = number of code-switches that follow the equivalence constraint.
[b] − EQ = number of code-switches that do not follow the equivalence constraint.
[c] − FM = number of code-switches that do not follow the free morpheme constraint.

Thus, only one subject, Patient D, consistently chose the appropriate language whether speaking to the monolingual or the bilingual examiner. Interestingly, she was the only subject who was born in the United States and may have learned English virtually simultaneously with her Yiddish, certainly at a younger age than the other subjects. One subject, Patient C, chose the wrong language in both interactions and was the most severely demented of all the patients. This suggests that ability correctly to make language choice reflects the overall stage of demented language decline.

Appropriate Code-Switching

All subjects were able to code-switch appropriately. Table 10.5 delineates the total number of code switches per subject when speaking in the presence of a bilingual person. (This included the bilingual examiner and the children of the subjects, who were sometimes present at the examination.) Each code-switch was evaluated to determine if it followed the equivalence and free morpheme constraints.

Example 1 is an example of a code-switch that follows Poplack's equivalence constraint.

EXAMPLE 1

The daughter, M., was asking her mother if her grandfather (Patient C's father) spoke Hebrew.
M.   And Hebrew Mom?
Patient C   Hebrew / noch an alterer noch*/ a Hebrew man.
            [Hebrew/still an old person; still/ a Hebrew man.]**
    Key: * Code-switched elements are between slashes.
          **Translated text is in brackets, under the actual text.

Example 1 follows the equivalence constraint rule because word order before and after the switch is the same in both languages: adverb/determiner, adjective, noun.

Example 2 is an example of a code-switch that does not follow Poplack's equivalency constraint.

EXAMPLE 2

> Patient E (referring to a passerby)
> oh, <u>dort se kimt de</u> /guests/.<u>Daner</u>/neighbors/ <u>zan</u>.
> [Here they come the/ guests. /Your/ neighbors/ (they) will be/.]

This does not follow Poplack's equivalency constraint because Yiddish allows verb final construction and English does not. This construction is not equivalent in English; however, according to Nishimura, it is a possible and an appropriate switch. Of interest is the fact that only the two most severely impaired patients, C and E, make these types of nonequivalent switches.

Example 3 is an example of a code-switch that does not follow the free morpheme constraint.

EXAMPLE 3

B.E.	[tell me the days of the week]
Patient D	muntik, dinstik, mittvoch, donnershtik, fraytik, shabbos.
	[Monday, Tuesday, Wednesday, Thursday, Friday, Saturday.]
B.E.	[After Saturday?]
Patient D	zintik, muntik, dinstik, mittvoch,/ THURshtik,/ ant shabbos.
	[Sunday, Monday, Tuesday, Wednesday, /THURSday,/ and Saturday.]
Key:	B.E. = bilingual examiner

Example 3 does not follow the free morpheme rule because THURS is not a free morpheme.

Inappropriate Code-Switching

Two subjects, Patients C and E, inappropriately code-switched with the monolingual examiner. Table 10.6 reports the number of inappropriate code-switches per subject. Each switch was analyzed to determine if it followed the linguistic constraints governing code-switching.

Notice that Patient C makes more inappropriate code-switches than Patient E, but all are grammatically correct according to the stricter Poplack constraint. This indicates a dissociation between linguistic and pragmatic appropriateness of code-switching.

TABLE 10.6. Code-switches with the monolingual examiner.

Patient	Number of code-switches	Number of utterances	+EQ[a]	−EQ[b]	−FM[c]
B	0	350	0	0	0
C	68	888	68 (100%)	0	0
D	0	944	0	0	0
E	23	1664	21 (91%)	2 (09%)	0

[a] + EQ = number of code-switches that follow the equivalence constraint.
[b] − EQ = number of code-switches that do not follow the equivalence constraint.
[c] − FM = number of code-switches that do not follow the free morpheme constraint.

TABLE 10.7. Grammatical category of code-switched elements.

Patient	Content words	Functors	Phrases
B	0	0	0
C	14	23	31
D	0	0	0
E	4	19	0

Next consider the number of code-switches as they relate to the grammatical category seen in Table 10.7.

According to Grosjean (1982), single-word code-switches usually occur on content words and not functors. The fact that the two of our subjects who did extensive code-switching had a large number of switches on functor words may be language specific. That is, we have observed that code-switching on functor words may be a general practice for Yiddish-English bilinguals and not a result of the dementia; one would need to test normal controls to determine if this is the case.

Translation

As to translation, one subject, Patient C, translated Yiddish into English either spontaneously or when asked for clarification when speaking to the monolingual examiner (Example 4). This subject, appropriately, did not translate when speaking to the bilingual examiner.

EXAMPLE 4

Patient C was talking about her life in Russia and about fighting in the war.
Patient C   "No, because I want to fight /ALEIN/."
M.E.   "You want to what?"
Patient C   "and I . . . I want to fight alone."
Key: M.E. = monolingual examiner.

Patient E engaged in spontaneous as well as requested translation when speaking to the bilingual examiner (Example 5).

EXAMPLE 5

B.E.   "Vus is 'holtz' auf English?
              [What is wood in English?]
Patient E   "Wood."
Key: B.E. = bilingual examiner.

Language Correction

An example of language correction is shown in Example 6. Patient E corrected the bilingual examiner's use of an incorrect word by supplying the correct word.

EXAMPLE 6

B.E.   Hant, aieh hob a pur bilders tse kiken.
              [Today, I have a few pictures to see.]
E.   "Tse zein."
              [To look at.]
Key: B.E. = bilingual examiner.

We grant that neither translation nor correction occurred particularly frequently with our subjects. Of course, we have no way of estimating how frequently they would have occurred had our subjects been normal controls. Note
that when correction of translation occurred in our subjects, they were appropriate, suggesting sparing of both the linguistic and pragmatic skills necessary to
perform them.

Discussion

Let us return to the research questions posed in the beginning of the chapter. The
first question, as to whether the language problems present in monolingual
demented subjects are also present in each of the languages of the bilingual
demented patients, is best answered by reference to Table 10.3. It is clear from
Table 10.3 that many of the language phenomena of monolingual SDAT can be
seen in bilingual demented patients, but dementia may affect each of the languages of the bilingual or multilingual differently.

The second question addressed the issue of problems of language choice and
code-switching in all bilingual demented patients. The data we collected in Table
10.4 indicate that not all bilingual demented patients have problems with language choice. When speaking to the bilingual examiner, two patients (D and E)
chose the appropriate language and two patients (C and B) did not follow the
interlocutor's lead. When speaking to the monolingual examiner, in the stronger
test of language choice, two patients (B and D) always chose the appropriate language. Two patients (C and E) did not.

Inappropriate code-switching, with the monolingual examiner, occurred
with two patients, C and E. Thus, problems with language choice and code-

TABLE 10.8. Severity of dementia and code-switching, language-choice problems.

Patient	Dementia stage	Code-switching problems		Language-choice problems	
		E[a]	Y[b]	E	Y
B	II	−	−	−	+
C	IV	+	+	+	+
D	III	−	+	−	−
E	III–IV	+	+	+	−

[a] E = English.
[b] Y = Yiddish.

switching did not necessarily occur in both languages for all patients. Only one patient, C, exhibited problems with language choice and code-switching with both examiners.

To determine if language choice and code-switching problems are related to the severity of dementia, consider the results in Table 10.8.

Clearly, the correlation between severity and code-switching problems is strong. Patient C was the most impaired patient, in stage IV, and also made the most frequent language-choice and code-switching errors. Patient E was the next most impaired, between stages III and IV, and made the next most errors. However, Patient D, the next most demented patient, showed less language-choice error than Patient B, the least demented patient. Therefore, there is a substantial correlation between severity of dementia and language-choice and code-switching problems. One possible explanation for Patient D's performance is that she learned both languages at the same time, from birth and at an earlier age, and therefore had more practice in bilingual language choice.

Finally, we consider the quality of the code-switching and language-choice errors of our bilingual demented patients. As Hyltenstam and Stroud (in press) report for their two subjects, our subjects' code-switching is virtually always linguistically correct, especially if we allow for Nishimura's extension of Poplack's rule on equivalence constraints between structurally distant languages. The pragmatic aspects of code-switching and of language choice, however, do seem to break down in most but not all of our subjects. It is generally understood that pragmatic abilities in demented patients remain intact longer than linguistic abilities (Causino et al., submitted). In fact, certain pragmatic abilities such as inference break down early. Other pragmatic skills, such as using social formulae, remain intact until late stages of dementia (Causino et al., submitted). Thus it seems that language choice and appropriate code-switching are intermediate between inference and formulae.

Our discourse analysis leads us to conclude, first, that bilingual demented patients exhibit many of the language problems reported for monolingual patients but, as with the aphasic bilingual, these may be differently exhibited in each of the languages.

Second, we saw that certain phenomena specific to bilingualism break down in dementia. In particular, normal bilingual subjects always select the appropriate language during interaction with a monolingual interlocutor. Furthermore, the healthy bilingual does not code-switch at all with a monolingual interlocutor. However, half of our demented bilingual patients no longer maintained the distinction between conversing with a bilingual and a monolingual, that is, they both chose the inappropriate base language and code-switched with either examiner.

Other sophisticated language behaviors were spared in certain patients, however, to our surprise. In two patients appropriate code-switching, translation abilities, and correction of the examiner's speech occurred. Moreover, these were the most impaired patients overall. Therefore, some aspects of bilingual discourse skills are maintained into late stages of dementia; these are skills that require both linguistic and pragmatic abilities.

Acknowledgments. We thank Angela Genovese for her assistance in data preparation and The Parker Jewish Geriatric Institute, New Hyde Park, New York, research staff, patients and families for their enthusiastic participation. This study was funded through a grant from the Research Foundation of the City University of New York #6-67453 and #6-66214.

References

Causino, M., Obler, L.K., Knoefel, J., & Albert, M. (submitted). Pragmatic abilities in late-stage SDAT. Boston VA Medical Center.

Dronkers, N., Koss, E., Friedland, R., & Wertz, R. (1986). "Differential" language impairment and language mixing in a polyglot with probable Alzheimer's disease. Presented at Interactional Neuropsychological Society Meeting.

Goodglass, H., & Kaplan, E. (1972). *The assessment of aphasia and related disorders.* Philadelphia: Lea and Febiger.

Grosjean, F. (1982). *Life with two languages: An introduction to bilingualism.* Cambridge, Mass.: Harvard University Press.

Hyltenstam, K., & Stroud, C. (in press). Bilingualism in Alzheimer's Disease: Two case studies. In K. Hyltenstam and L.K. Obler (Eds.), *Bilingualism across the lifespan: Aspects of acquisition, maturity and loss.* Cambridge: Cambridge University Press.

Hyltenstam, K., & Stroud, C. (1985). The psycholinguistics of language choice and code-switching in Alzheimer's dementia: Some hypotheses. *Scandinavian Working Papers on Bilingualism, 4,* 26–44.

Kaplan, E., Goodglass, H., & Weintraub, S. (1983). *Boston Naming Test.* Philadelphia: Lea and Febiger.

Lipski, J. (1978). Code-switching and the problems of bilingual competence. In M. Paradis (Ed.), *Aspects of bilingualism.* Columbia, S.C.: Hornbeim Press.

Nishimura, M. (1986). Intrasentential code-switching: The case of language assignment. In J. Vaid (Ed.), *Language processing in bilinguals: Psycholinguistics and neuropsychological perspectives.* Hillsdale, N.J.: Erlbaum.

Obler, L.K., & Albert, M. (1984). Language in aging. In M. Albert (Ed.), *Clinical neurology of aging.* New York: Oxford University Press.

Obler, L.K., & Albert, M. (1986). *Action naming test.* Experimental version. Boston VA Medical Center.

Poplack, S. (1978). Syntactic structure and social function in code-switching. *Centro de Estudios Puertorriqueños Working Papers, 2,* 1–32.

Poplack, S. (1979). "Sometimes I'll start a sentence in English Y TERMINO EN ESPANOL": Toward a typology of code-switching. *Centro de Estudios Puertorriquesños Working Papers, 4,* 1–79.

11
Gender-Specific Discourse Differences in Aphasia

Wolfgang U. Dressler, Ruth Wodak, and Csaba Pléh

Introduction

In an earlier study of text productions by nonaphasic Austrian speakers, Dressler and Pléh (1984) observed marked gender differences in story recall and in the retelling of pictorially represented (depicted) stories. In trying to interpret these differences in light of the available literature on gender differences, we found that these differences were perfectly consistent with previous findings by Wodak on gender-specific strategies used by nonaphasic speakers and, also, were compatible with the following general framework of language impairments proposed by Dressler (1982).

In a classification of phonological paraphasias, Dressler (1982) claimed that aphasia can impair all five aspects of language and language use as differentiated by Coseriu (1986): (1) Saussure's "parole," which is roughly equivalent to Chomsky's "performance" of a specific language; (2) sociolinguistic norms of a language as a social institution; (3) Saussure's *langue*, which is equivalent to Chomsky's "competence" as a (potential) system of regularities of an individual language; (4) language type (constituent typological elements of inflecting, agglutinating, isolating, etc., languages); and (5) linguistic universals, i.e., characteristics that hold for all natural languages and that, as such, constitute the basic human language faculty. Thus, in aphasia there are: (1) disturbances of performance, qualitatively similar to nonpathological slips of the tongue; (2) disturbances in application of sociolinguistic norms; (3) disturbances in linguistic competence that may be present in all aphasias (except amnestic aphasia/anomia and mild forms of other aphasias, e.g., at the end of the recovery) (Benson, 1979; Dressler and Pléh, 1984; Huber, 1981; Keller, 1980; Kertesz, 1979; Marshall, 1982; Poeck, 1983; Poeck et al. 1974); (4) in very severe cases, disturbances in constituent elements of the language type to which the patient's language belongs resulting in, for example, significant loss of inflection in an inflecting language or loss of intonation in a tonal language; and (5) disturbances in the human language faculty itself, as when no human language is possible and an artificial sign system must be used in therapy.

Gender-specific differences in German-speaking aphasics, the topic of our chapter, refer to sociolinguistic norms (the preceding point 2). In our view, it is unlikely that these observed effects reflect gender-specific changes in patients' basic language faculty or in their facility with a particular language type. With respect to linguistic competence, no gender-specific differences have been observed in speakers' knowledge of the grammatical system of German. And with respect to conceivable gender-specific differences in performance alone, we are unaware of any account phrased in these terms. Therefore, the most plausible locus of such differences is in sociolinguistic norms, where considerable differences in nonaphasic speakers have been documented in the form of divergent preferences for discourse strategies (Wodak, 1981a, 1981b, 1982, 1983a, 1983b).

There have been scarcely any studies on aphasic disturbances of sociolinguistic norms. Insofar as pragmatics is concerned, most aphasiologists seem to agree explicitly or implicitly that the pragmatic aspects of language behavior are not affected by aphasia (Cohen et al., 1979; de Bleser, 1987; Engel, 1977). However, de Bleser (1987, p. 281) has noted that "The non-fluent Broca's aphasic patient deviates not only in his linguistic performance but also in his dialogue behaviour," a matter of discourse pragmatics. Similarly, Dressler, Moosmüller, and Stark (1985) deal with aphasic disturbances in sociopragmatics, that is, how speech situations are defined differently by aphasic and normal speakers as reflected in the pragmatic aspects of their discourse.[1]

To date, the possible relevance of gender differences to sociolinguistics and to "sociopsycholinguistics" has not been considered in aphasiology. Work on prognosis in aphasia (Gloning et al., 1969) has not shown any significant gender-related differentiation in recovery. McGlone (1977, 1980; Kimura and Harshman, 1984; Pizzamiglio, Mammacari, and Razzano, 1985) has reported gender-related distinctions in cerebral lateralization, but these findings have not been related to gender-specific patterns of speech behavior. Moreover, in their critical review, Segalowitz and Bryden (1983, p. 363) conclude: "If men and women adopt different ways of approaching a particular task, we cannot be sure whether to attribute gender differences in laterality to differences in the cerebral representation processes or to differences in the strategy employed." The first alternative would seem to point to biologically determined intervening variables affecting language performance; however, no such gender-related differences were found by Benke, Gerstenbrand, and Kertesz (1987, 1988) using the Western Aphasia Battery. The second alternative (supported by Benke et al.) is consistent with our approach of looking for gender-related differences in adherence to sociolinguistic norms (see references and discussion in Wodak and Schulz, 1986). Thus, by looking for gender-related differences in the discourse of otherwise similarly impaired aphasic patients, we can gain some insight into which aspects of aphasic language are interpretable by reference to the language faculty proper and which are not. We can ask the question, for example, whether or not differences between a woman's and a man's speech, which might be characterized along the dimension of socio- (or partner) -centrism, disappear when language abilities are seriously impaired. If they do not disappear, one can argue that aphasia has not impaired previously acquired gender-specific discourse strategies, and that these characteristics of speech do not belong to the realm of language abilities in any narrow sense (either tied to language-specific, Chomskyan competence, or to a universal human language faculty). We suggest instead that these robust gender differences are regulated by acquired rules of social and cultural (and thus socialized) behavior. Thus, organic lesions resulting in aphasia would be expected to affect discourse in different ways than psychiatric diseases or acute psychological distress that may directly affect social behaviour (i.e., behavior acquired through socialization; Dressler and Wodak, 1986).

Recent research has illustrated significant behavioral differences attributable to socialization processes, such as identification with gender role models, usually the father, mother, or other primary caretaker (Wodak and Schulz, 1986). These differences occur at all levels of language—lexical, syntactic, semantic, and pragmatic—and in discourse—in monologues, dialogues, and other interactions and in oral as well as in written output. Moreover, such differences and indicators connect and correlate in specific ways with other sociolinguistic and psycholinguistic variables. Some of the results of this research, insofar as they relate to the language behavior of aphasics, are listed here.

In interaction processes, there is an asymmetry concerning the customary prerogatives of participants in conversations (Trömel-Plötz, 1984; Wodak, Feistritzer, Moosmüller, and Doleschal, 1988). These studies have established that a marked asymmetry exists between male and female speakers of equivalent status, class, and education. Women, on average, speak less and, at times, do not speak at all. Often they are interrupted, not taken seriously, or not supported. Topics initiated by women are often neglected, cut off, or cursorily dismissed.

Wodak (1986) has further demonstrated that significant gender-specific variations also exist, in both oral and written speech, in the way people express and deal with personal problems in a therapeutic setting. In addition to strong differences related to the social class of speakers, the topic of the discourse, and the degree of involvement with the problem under discussion, (middle-class) women on average tended to relate a story, while men tended to report a state of mind. Analogous differences were found in a large sample of written essays (on the topic "My Mother and I") by boys and girls in Austrian and American schools (Wodak and Schultz, 1986). Again, the girls tended to express their feelings, whereas the boys provided descriptions of their daily life, their sense of well-being, or of familiar people, but hid their feelings and personal involvement. It is interesting to note that these gender differences were much less prevalent in neurotic children: both male and female children suffering an acute psychological crisis showed their feelings openly. More specifically, neurotic boys tended to be expressive and to relate tales, while the girls told little stories and made evaluations. The number of personal reflections was low in both groups, probably because the involvement was so intense. Our inference is that psychological distress affects pragmatic aspects of language more than the underlying linguistic competence. We claim that exactly the opposite is true in aphasia: while language competence is disturbed, the pragmatic features remain intact—specifically, women relate, while men report and simply describe. In this Chapter, we direct our attention to the question of whether aphasic syndromes and aphasic speech therapy affect these gender-specific discourse strategies.

Speech Samples (Dressler and Pléh, 1984)

In this study (from our Viennese aphasia project[2]), we analyzed text productions of a sample of sixteen moderately impaired organic patients representing the following aphasic syndromes: Wernicke's (three male, two female), anomic (two male, two female), Broca's (two male, two female), and Global (two male, one female). All patients came from Vienna and the surrounding area. The ages and education levels of the male and female patients were comparable. All patients performed on two administrations using equivalent test batteries. The two testing sessions were separated by a month's interval during which patients received speech therapy.

Each test administration included four text productions. Thus, four texts were recorded before intensive speech therapy was administered to the patient and four after therapy. The four texts included in each test administration included two types. Each patient had to retell two pictorially presented (depicted) stories and had to recall two short stories that were read to them. The two depicted story stimuli consisted of four and six pictures, respectively, and the two (orally presented) short stories of eighteen and nineteen propositions, respectively (according to the analytic scheme provided by Labov and Waletzky, 1967). In total, our corpus consists of 128 relatively long texts (thirty-two for each of the four tasks; i.e., four texts recorded in each of two testing sessions for each of sixteen patients).

Analytic Scheme

The eight texts from each patient were tape recorded and then transcribed (using "narrow transcription," as defined by the International Phonetic Association) by a native speaker of German (H.K. Stark). Then, each transcript was translated (by E. Lindner) into standard orthography, along with indication of the standard meaning of dialect expressions and (in case of incomplete constructions and nonexisting word forms) with notation of the intended sentence or word. Neologisms and pauses were marked as well. These transcribed, normalized versions were compared again with the original tapes. The normalized texts were then segmented and coded by a fluent (though nonnative) Hungarian speaker of German. Next, the codings were checked by Austrian students who were unaware of the exact purpose of the research. Suggested corrections were evaluated by Pléh and Dressler and only then the coding was accepted as "final."

Each text produced by a patient was analyzed for a variety of different features, only some of which will be discussed. These features include: the number of sentences or sentence fragments; the functions of units (e.g., the number of descriptive sentences); various lexical statistics (e.g., noun types and tokens, verb types, and tokens); various forms of deixis: exophoric pronouns referring to the nonlinguistic content (e.g., to somebody represented in a picture) and place deixis; and intersentential relations denoted by various conjunctions (e.g., "and," "causal" conjunctions). In addition, the number of wrong (i.e., nonexistent or neologistic) words was tallied.

Statistical Analysis

Several dependent measures were defined in terms of the categories just listed, and a series of univariate analyses of variance were performed. Initially, each analysis of variance (ANOVA) included gender (male, female), therapy (before, after), and text (four levels consisting of two depicted and two orally presented texts) as factors. All the results presented next should be interpreted with extreme caution due to the small size of our sample and, since patient type was not included as a factor, in light of possible differences across different aphasic syndromes.

The corpus of narratives from the sixteen aphasic patients provided a good opportunity to look for gender-related differences, as has been done with texts produced by normal speakers (Klann-Delius, 1979; Wodak, 1983b; Wodak and Schulz, 1986). In particular, the relatively long speech samples obtained allowed examination of possible gender-related differences in aphasic speakers' use of cohesion and coherence indicators. The use of a task based on interpretation of pictures in addition to the purely verbal task of story recall provided an opportunity to study patients' tendencies toward descriptive versus narrative interpretations of stimuli.

The Descriptive Style of Male Patients

There was an overall higher number of sentences produced by male than female patients in the case of depicted stories, especially before therapy (before therapy means: 13.6 versus 8.1; after therapy means: 11.9 versus 7.5). The main effect of gender was marginally reliable, $F(1,14) = 3.74, p < 0.10$. More specifically, the male patients produced on the average almost twice as many "descriptive sentences" than did the female patients. Although there was a strong main effect of gender for this measure, $F(1,14) = 9.90, p < 0.01$, the similarly strong therapy times gender interaction $F(1,14) = 7.20, p < 0.02$) suggests that the relatively greater descriptivity of male patients' speech was much more pronounced before therapy (particularly in depicted stories). An influence of therapy is not surprising; the attention of patients is directed toward newly learned patterns, a factor that in turn reduces spontaneity. Also, and perhaps more important, is the fact that the same texts were presented before and after therapy; responding to the same stimuli a second time would further decrease patients' spontaneity. Moreover, gender-specific patterns and stereotypes may well be affected by long-term therapy, as they can be in psychotherapy (Wodak, 1981). All this suggests that in the depicted story task, a descriptive (and thus nonnarrative), approach was more available to men. The task of retelling depicted stories seems to have been interpreted—at least partially—by the male patients as one of picture description. This reinterpretation occurs with many aphasics but, in our study, it occurred significantly more often with men. This fits with the general male tendency toward analytic linguistic behaviour (Wodak, 1982).

Corresponding effects were noted in patients' use of diectic expressions. First, the male patients tended to use more exophoric pronouns in depicted stories than female patients (means: 4.3 versus 0.8), $F(1,14) = 3.00, p < 0.10$). Before therapy, the male patients also used more "place deixis," a category that is evidently related to descriptive interpretations of the task (means: 5.1 versus 2.5); but, after therapy, the use of place deixis (in line with a general decrease of descriptive expressions) decreased in men to 2.4 on the average, while the use of place deixis actually increased in women to 4.1. These divergent patterns were mirrored in a gender times therapy interaction, $F(1,14) = 4.79, p < 0.05$). This pattern, however, as would be expected on the basis of the preceding results, was really characteristic only of depicted stories. When just data from depicted texts were analyzed, the means for use of place deixis for male and female patients before therapy were 7.5 and 2.5, respectively, while after therapy the means were 2.4 and 4.6. [The gender times therapy interaction for just the depicted story data was marginally reliable; $F(1,14) = 3.69, p < 0.08$.]

In sum, these discourse measures indicate that for the male patients it was easier to consider the task connected with pictures as one of mere description, and that, under the influence of therapy or perhaps stimulus repetition, this tendency diminished. For female patients, perhaps as a consequence of recognizing the possibility of this compensatory strategy, the tendency to treat the depicted story task as one of picture description actually increased somewhat during therapy, as was reflected in their increased use of place deixis.

There were other distinguishing characteristics of male and female aphasics' discourse. For example, female patients used fewer neologistic (nonexistent) words than the male patients, $F(1,14) = 6.46, p < 0.02$. This tendency did not disappear when the length of patients' productions was taken into account by dividing the number of neologistic words by the sum of noun and verb tokens in the given text. For men, neologistic words amounted to as much as thirty-six percent of the word tokens, while for women the value was only fourteen percent, $F(1,14) = 4.63, p < 0.05$. This effect was, again, much clearer in depicted stories (36 percent versus 8 percent) than in recall of orally presented stories (36 percent versus 20 percent). This result comes as no surprise. The pattern of female aphasic speech behavior corresponds to what has previously been documented in the speech of (normal, adult) Austrian women (Lutz and Wodak, 1987; Moosmüller, 1988a, 1988b). Note in this regard that patients' spontaneous, subjective reactions during testing and their comments after tests clearly indicate that aphasia tests are interpreted as examinations. In general, in test situations and in interviews, (normal) female speakers tend to be more hesitant in answering questions; they rather prefer not to answer than to answer incorrectly. In addition to more hesitation, they produce more tag questions and other indicators associated with insecurity. By comparison, men hesitate less, are more self-assured, and are ready to give wrong answers (Wodak, 1983a; Lutz, 1984).[3]

Aphasic women strive for more explicit coherence. The gender of patients had a very clear influence on the use of conjunctions. Women used about twice as many conjunctions as men (means: 11.4 versus 4.6 per story), $F(1,14) = 5.39$, $p < 0.05$. Although the higher rate of use by women was evident in all types of conjunctions, only in the cases of "and" and "causal" did it reach statistical significance. This difference in the use of conjunctions can be interpreted in the following way. Women tend to be more sociocentric (e.g., partner oriented) and evaluative (Wodak, 1983a), even when they are producing rather mutilated texts. They make more efforts to mark relations between propositions and to differentiate them, even when the propositions are unclear and incomplete.

Discussion

The sociopsychological theory of text planning (as developed by Wodak, 1983a, 1983b; Wodak and Schulz, 1986) posits that the perception and structuring of reality is patterned according to culture-, class-, gender-, and disease-specific socialization. Consequences of these interspeaker differences are manifest in organization at the macro-level of discourse (its macrostructure), in discourse type, and in speaker strategies. Research with children and adults of Western Europe and North America has shown that women are socialized toward holistic, gestaltlike thinking and speech behavior. These tendencies seem not to be inborn, but due to gender-specific socialization (Wodak, 1981a, 1981b, 1983a; Wodak and Schulz, 1986). Related work has elaborated quantitative differences across speakers of varying social class, gender, age, and disease category, both at the discourse level (e.g., use of conjunctions and particles) and in sociolinguistics (Dressler, 1982; Dressler and Wodak, 1982; Wodak, 1982). Our results, based on an analysis of aphasic discourse, fit well in both models. Men prefer descriptive sentences and score better on the task of retelling depicted stories, which they often transform into a picture description task. Women, on the other hand, prefer narrations and evaluations, i.e., reflective speech patterns (Wodak, 1981b). This explains their increased use of conjunctions and their sociocentric behavior, which stand in contrast to male descriptive strategies. Also, men seem to use more "wrong words" than women, because they are often more self-assured, have less of a minority complex, and are more daring in asserting wrong things than are women, who prefer to remain silent in the same circumstances (similar results in Lutz, 1984).

Several of the observed effects of socialization, while not impaired by aphasia, may be sensitive to the effects of therapeutic intervention or, perhaps more likely, the fact that the patients responded to the same texts on two occasions. Indeed, we expect that only long-term psychotherapy (Wodak, 1981a) may effect an irreversible change on the gender-specific socialization taking place over the life span in the home, at school, and in the work place. Still, the possibility remains that some – although not all – of these gender-specific differences between male and female aphasics are greatly diminished as a result of therapy. In other words, it is unwise to rule out homogeneous, nongender-specific therapy as a potential mechanism for socialization unhindered by patients' aphasic symptoms.

Finally, our analysis supports differentiation of the discourse effects of aphasia from those of psychological distress (Dressler and Wodak, 1986). The pragmatic phenomena considered here were not impaired by aphasia. In contrast, in neurotic syndromes that are linked to disruptions in socialization in the face of intact language competence, it is precisely pragmatic speech strategies that are affected. Such distinctions have to be taken into account both in theoretical evaluations and in designing therapy programs. In this way our results shed light both on the nature of aphasic impairment and on the proper psycho- and sociological evaluation of aphasic therapy.

Notes

1. For comparable results, refer to research on bilingualism and bilingual aphasia; e.g., Paradis (1978, Chapter IV) and Paradis and Lebrun (1983).
2. Project 3632 of the Fonds zur Förderung der Wissenschaftlichen Forschung. In the interim, eighty aphasics have been given two administrations of a test battery (conceived by the late Karl Gloning⁺, Wolfgang U. Dressler, and Jacqueline Ann Stark) consisting of thirty-two subtests, four of which were used for this study. For this chapter, we originally wanted to have analyses for four groups of equal size, with the groups defined on the basis of standard neurological and neuropsychological criteria. However, a careful neurolinguistic analysis revealed that one of the four originally tested Global aphasics had to be reclassified as a Wernicke's aphasic. Fortunately, the resulting unequal distribution of cell frequencies did not prevent us from use analysis of variance.
3. For comparison, refer to Quinting (1981) and Dressler and Pléh (1984).

References

Beaugrande, R. de, & Dressler, W.U. (1981). *Einführung in die Textlinguistik.* Tübingen: Niemayer. *Introduction to text linguistics.* London: Longman.

Benke, Th., Gerstenbrand, F., & Kertesz, A. (1988). Sex differences in interhemispheric language organization. In E. Scherzer, R. Simon, & J. Stark (Eds.), *Proceedings First European Conference on Aphasiology* (pp. 232–236). Vienna: Allgemeine Unfallversicherungsanstalt.

Benke, Th., Wagner, M., & Gerstenbrand, F. (1988). *Acht Hypothesen zur zerebralen Asymmetrie bei Männern und Frauen.* Innsbruck: Mitteilungen aus dem Institut für Sprachwissenschaft der Universität Innsbruck, Report 5.

Benson, D.F. (1979). *Aphasia, alexia and agraphia.* New York: Churchill Livingstone.

Cohen, R., Kelter, S., & Woll, G. (1979). Conceptual impairment in aphasia. In *Semantics from different points of view.* Berlin.

Coseriu, E. (1968). Sincronía, diacronía y tipología. Actas del XI. Congresso Intern. de linguística y filogía románicas, Madrid, C.S.I.C., 269–283.

De Bleser, R. (1987). The communicative impact of non-fluent aphasia on the dialog behaviour of linguistical unimpaired partners. In F. Lowenthal & F. Vandamme (Eds.) *Pragmatics and education* (pp. 273–285). New York: Plenum.

Dressler, W.U. (1982). A classification of phonological paraphasias. *Wiener Linguistische Gazette, 29,* 3-16.

Dressler, W.U., & Wodak, R. (1982). Sociophonological methods in the study of sociolinguistic variation in Viennese German. *Language and Society, 11,* 339-370.

Dressler, W.U., & Pléh, C. (1984). Zur narrativen Textkompetenz von Aphatikern. In W.U. Dressler & R. Wodak (Eds.), *Normale und abweichende Texte* (pp. 1-45). Hamburg: Buske.

Dressler, W.U., Moosmüller, S., & Stark, H.K. (1985). Sociophonology and aphasia. In W.U. Dressler & L. Tonelli (Eds.), *Natural phonology from Eisenstadt* (pp. 45-52). Padova: CLESP.

Dressler, W.U., & Wodak, R. (1986). Disturbed texts. In J. Petöfi (Ed.), Text connectedness from psychological point of view (pp. 141-149). Hamburg: Buske.

Engel, D. (1977). Textexperimente mit Aphatikern. Tübingen: Narr.

Gloning, K., Heiss, W.D., Trappl, R., & Quatember, R. (1969). Eine experimentell-statistische Untersuchung zur Prognose der Aphasie. *Nervenarzt, 40,* 491-494.

Huber, W. (1981). Aphasien. *Studium Linguistik, 11,* 1-21.

Keller, E. (1980). Competence and performance in aphasia within a performance model of language. *Montreal Working Papers in Linguistics, 14,* 213-219.

Kertesz, A. (1979). Aphasia and associated disorders: Taxonomy, localization and recovery. New York: Grune and Stratton.

Kimura, D., & Harshman, R.A. (1984). Sex differences in brain organization for verbal and non-verbal functions. In De Vries et al. (Eds.), *Progress in Brain Research, 61,* 423-439.

Klann-Delius, G. (1981). Sex and language acquisition—Is there any difference? *Journal of Pragmatics, 5,* 1-15.

Labov, W., & Waletzky, J. (1967). Narrative analysis; oral versions of personal experience. In J. Helm (Ed.), *Essays on the verbal and visual arts* (pp. 12-44). Seattle: University of Washington.

Lutz, B. (1984). Verständlickeit und Verstehen non Nachrichten mit einer empirischen Analyse der Rezeption von Rundfunknachrichten. Master's thesis, University of Vienna.

Lutz, B., & Wodak, R. (1987). *Information für Informierte.* Vienna: Verlag der Österreichischen Akademie der Wissenschaften.

Marshall, J.C. (1982). What is a symptom complex. In M. Arbib et al. (Eds.), *Neural models of language processes* (pp. 389-410). New York: Academic.

McGlone, J. (1977). Sex differences in the cerebral organization of verbal functions in patients with unilateral lesions. *Brain, 100,* 775-793.

McGlone, J. (1980). Sex differences in human brain organization: A critical survey. *The Behavioral and Brain Sciences, 3,* 215-227.

Moosmüller, S. (1988). Phonological variation in parliamentary discussions. In R. Wodak (Ed.), *Language, power and ideology.* Amsterdam: Benjamins.

Paradis, M. (Ed.) (1978). *Aspects of bilingualism.* Columbia S.C.: Hornbeam Press.

Paradis, M., & Lebrun, Y. (Eds.). (1983). La neurolinguistique du bilingualisme. *Langages, 18,* 72.

Pizzamiglio, L., Mammucari, A., & Razzano, C. (1985). Evidence for sex differences in brain organization in recovery of aphasia. *Brain and Language, 25,* 213-223.

Poeck, K., et al. (1975). Die Aphasien. In A. Bischoff et al. (Eds.), *Aktuelle Neurologie* (pp. 159-169). 2, 3. Stuttgart: Thieme.

Quinting, G. (1971). *Hesitation phenomena in adult aphasic and normal speech.* The Hague: Mouton.

Segalowitz, S.J., & Bryden, M.P. (1983). Individual differences in hemispheric representation of language. In S. Segalowitz (Ed.), *Language functions and brain organization* (pp. 341–372). New York: Academic.

Trömel-Plötz, S. (Ed.). (1984). *Gewalt durch Sprache.* Frankfurt/Main: Fischer.

Wodak, R. (1981a). *Das Wort in der Gruppe.* Vienna: Verlag der Österreichischen Akademie der Wissenschaften.

Wodak, R. (1981b). Women relate, men report. *Journal of Pragmatics*, *5*, 261–285.

Wodak, R. (1982). Die Sprache von Müttern und Töchtern. Ein soziophonologischer Vergleich. *Wiener Linguistische Gazette*, Beiheft 1.

Wodak, R. (1983a). *Hilflose Nähe?—Mütter und Töchter erzählen.* Vienna: Österreichischer Bundesverlag.

Wodak, R. (1983b). Arguments in favour of a sociopsycholinguistic theory of textplanning. Sex specific behavior revisited. *Klagenfurther Beiträge zur Sprachwissenschaft*, *9*, 313–350.

Wodak, R. (1986). *Language behavior in therapy groups.* Los Angeles: University of California Press.

Wodak, R., & Schulz, M. (1986). *The language of love and guilt.* Los Angeles: University of California Press.

Wodak, R., Feistritzer, G., Moosmüller, S., & Doleschal, U. (1987). *Sprachliche Behandlung von Frau und Mann.* Vienna: Schriftenreihe zur sozialen und beruflichen Stellung der Frau 16.

Author Index

Many thanks to Marianne Corre and Lucien for their help in preparing this index.

Subject Index